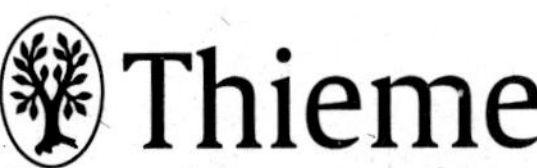
Thieme

Dx-Direct!

Direct Diagnosis in Radiology

Pediatric Imaging

Gundula Staatz, MD
Head of Pediatric Radiology Section
Department of Diagnostic Radiology
Friedrich Alexander University
Erlangen-Nuremberg, Germany

Dagmar Honnef, MD
Department of Radiology
University Hospital RWTH Aachen
Aachen, Germany

Werner Piroth, MD
Center for Diagnostic and Interventional Radiology
HELIOS Medical Center Wuppertal
University Medical Center
Witten/Herdecke, Germany

Tanja Radkow, MD
Department of Radiology
Friedrich Alexander University
Erlangen-Nuremberg, Germany

264 Illustrations

Indian Edition
Thieme Medical and Scientific Publishers Private Ltd
N-26, Sector 18, Noida, U.P - 201301 (India)
Email : customerservice@thieme.in
www.thieme.com

Thieme
Stuttgart · New York · New Delhi

Library of Congress Cataloging-in-Publication Data is available from the publisher.

This book is an authorized and revised translation of the German edition published and copyrighted 2007 by Georg Thieme Verlag, Stuttgart, Germany. Title of the German edition: Pareto-Reihe Radiologie: Kinderradiologie.

Translator: John Grossman, Schrepkow, Germany

Illustrator: Emil Wolfgang Hanns, Schriesheim, Germany

Rüdigerstrasse 14, 70469 Stuttgart, Germany
http://www.thieme.de
Thieme New York, 333 Seventh Avenue, New York, NY 10001, USA
http://www.thieme.com

Cover design: Thieme Publishing Group
Typesetting by Ziegler + Müller, Kirchentellinsfurt, Germany

ISBN 978-3-13-145171-2
(TPS, Rest of World)
ISBN 978-81-907698-8-4
(India)

1 2 3 4 5 6

Reprint 209 : Pediatric Imaging
Published by Thieme Medical and Scientific Publishers Private Ltd
N-26, Sector 18, Noida, U.P - 201301 (India)
Email : customerservice@thieme.in
www.thieme.com
Printed by Saurabh Printers Pvt. Ltd., New Delhi

1 Lung and Mediastinum

Normal Thymus · *D. Honnef, W. Piroth* 1
Respiratory Distress Syndrome (RDS) · *D. Honnef, W. Piroth* 6
Pulmonary Interstitial Emphysema (PIE) · *D. Honnef, W. Piroth* 9
Bronchopulmonary Dysplasia (BPD) · *D. Honnef, W. Piroth* 12
Meconium Aspiration Syndrome · *D. Honnef, W. Piroth* 15
Congenital Lobar Emphysema · *D. Honnef, W. Piroth* 17
Congenital Cystic Adenomatoid Malformation (CCAM) · *D. Honnef, W. Piroth* 19
Pulmonary Sequestration · *D. Honnef, W. Piroth* 22
Bronchogenic Cyst · *D. Honnef, W. Piroth* 25
Congenital Diaphragmatic Hernia · *D. Honnef, W. Piroth* 28
RSV Bronchiolitis · *D. Honnef, W. Piroth* 31
Lobar and Segmental Pneumonia · *D. Honnef, W. Piroth* 33
Tuberculosis · *T. Radkow, G. Staatz* 36
Cystic Fibrosis · *D. Honnef, W. Piroth* 41
Foreign Body Aspiration · *D. Honnef, W. Piroth* 44
Mediastinal Teratoma · *D. Honnef, W. Piroth* 47
Thoracic Neuroblastoma · *T. Radkow, G. Staatz* 51
Thoracic Hodgkin Lymphoma · *D. Honnef, W. Piroth* 54

2 Cardiovascular System

Arteria Lusoria · *D. Honnef, W. Piroth* 57
Double Aortic Arch · *D. Honnef, W. Piroth* 59
Coarctation of the Aorta · *D. Honnef, W. Piroth* 62
Pulmonary Artery Sling · *D. Honnef, W. Piroth* 66
Ebstein Anomaly · *D. Honnef, W. Piroth* 69
Tetralogy of Fallot · *D. Honnef, W. Piroth* 71
Transposition of the Great Arteries (TGA) · *D. Honnef, W. Piroth* 74
Ventricular Septal Defect (VSD) · *D. Honnef, W. Piroth* 77
Atrial Septal Defect (ASD) · *D. Honnef, W. Piroth* 80
Patent Ductus Arteriosus (PDA) · *D. Honnef, W. Piroth* 83
Anomalous Pulmonary Venous Connection · *D. Honnef, W. Piroth* 86

3 Neck

Fibromatosis Colli · *G. Staatz* 90
Cervical Cysts · *D. Honnef, W. Piroth* 92
Cervical Lymphadenitis · *G. Staatz* 95
Retropharyngeal Abscess · *D. Honnef, W. Piroth* 98
Hashimoto Thyroiditis · *G. Staatz* 101

4 Gastrointestinal Tract

Meconium Plug Syndrome · *D. Honnef, W. Piroth* 103
Necrotizing Enterocolitis (NEC) · *D. Honnef, W. Piroth* 105
Intestinal Nonrotation and Malrotation · *D. Honnef, W. Piroth* 108
Volvulus (Small Bowel and Large Bowel Volvulus) · *D. Honnef, W. Piroth* 112
Esophageal Atresia · *D. Honnef, W. Piroth* 115
Small Bowel Atresia · *D. Honnef, W. Piroth* 119
Anal Atresia · *D. Honnef, W. Piroth* 122
Hypertrophic Pyloric Stenosis (HPS) · *D. Honnef, W. Piroth* 126
Hirschsprung Disease (Congenital Megacolon) · *D. Honnef, W. Piroth* 128
Intussusception · *D. Honnef, W. Piroth* 131
Appendicitis · *D. Honnef, W. Piroth* 135
Crohn Diseas · *D. Honnef, W. Pirothe* 138
Meckel Diverticulum · *D. Honnef, W. Piroth* 143
Inguinal Hernia · *D. Honnef, W. Piroth* 145
Biliary Atresia · *D. Honnef, W. Piroth* 148
Choledochal Cyst · *D. Honnef, W. Piroth* 151
Cholecystolithiasis · *D. Honnef, W. Piroth* 156
Hepatoblastoma · *D. Honnef, W. Piroth* 159
Abdominal Trauma · *D. Honnef, W. Piroth* 162

5 Urogenital Tract

Vesicoureteral Reflux · *D. Honnef, W. Piroth* 166
Ureteropelvic Junction Obstruction · *D. Honnef, W. Piroth* 170
Multicystic Dysplastic Kidney · *G. Staatz* 174
Duplex Kidney · *D. Honnef, W. Piroth* 177
Urethral Valve · *D. Honnef, W. Piroth* 181
Acute Pyelonephritis · *D. Honnef, W. Piroth* 184
Nephrocalcinosis · *D. Honnef, W. Piroth* 188
Wilms Tumor (Nephroblastoma) · *D. Honnef, W. Piroth* 190
Adrenal Hemorrhage · *D. Honnef, W. Piroth* 195
Neuroblastoma · *D. Honnef, W. Piroth* 198
Pelvic Rhabdomyosarcoma · *D. Honnef, W. Piroth* 201
Sacrococcygeal Teratoma · *D. Honnef, W. Piroth* 205
Ovarian Teratoma · *G. Staatz* 209
Epididymitis · *G. Staatz* 213
Testicular Torsion · *G. Staatz* 215

6 Musculoskeletal System

Rickets · *D. Honnef, W. Piroth* 218
Transient Synovitis of the Hip (Irritable Hip) · *T. Radkow, G. Staatz* 222
Osteomyelitis and Septic Arthritis · *D. Honnef, W. Piroth* 225
Fibrous Cortical Defect and Nonossifying Fibroma · *D. Honnef, W. Piroth* 230
Aneurysmal Bone Cyst · *D. Honnef, W. Piroth* 233
Enchondromatosis · *D. Honnef, W. Piroth* 237
Osteochondroma (Osteocartilaginous Exostosis) · *G. Staatz* 241
Osteoid Osteoma · *D. Honnef, W. Piroth* 245
Ewing Sarcoma · *T. Radkow, G. Staatz* 249
Osteogenic Sarcoma · *D. Honnef, W. Piroth* 253
Langerhans Cell Histiocytosis · *D. Honnef, W. Piroth* 257
Acute Lymphatic Leukemia (ALL) · *T. Radkow, G. Staatz* 263
Developmental Dysplasia of the Hip (DDH) · *T. Radkow, G. Staatz* 266
Slipped Capital Femoral Epiphysis · *T. Radkow, G. Staatz* 271
Legg–Calvé–Perthes Disease · *T. Radkow, G. Staatz* 275
Hemangioma and Arteriovenous Malformation (AVM) · *T. Radkow, G. Staatz* 280
Lymphangioma · *D. Honnef, W. Piroth* 284
Pediatric Fractures · *T. Radkow, G. Staatz* 288
Battered Child Syndrome (Child Abuse) · *D. Honnef, W. Piroth* 292

7 Central Nervous System

Craniosynostosis · *D. Honnef, W. Piroth* 296
Midline Anomalies · *T. Radkow, G. Staatz* 301
Dandy–Walker Malformation · *T. Radkow, G. Staatz* 305
Intraventricular Hemorrhage · *T. Radkow, G. Staatz* 308
Periventricular Leukomalacia (PVL) · *T. Radkow, G. Staatz* 311
Hypoxic-Ischemic Brain Damage · *T. Radkow, G. Staatz* 315
Orbital Cellulitis · *T. Radkow, G. Staatz* 319
Neurocutaneous Syndromes (Phakomatoses) · *T. Radkow, G. Staatz* 322
Tumors of the Posterior Cranial Fossa · *T. Radkow, G. Staatz* 329
Brainstem Gliomas · *T. Radkow, G. Staatz* 334
Tethered Cord · *T. Radkow, G. Staatz* 337
Craniocerebral Trauma · *T. Radkow, G. Staatz* 340

Index 345

3D	Three-dimensional
ACTH	Adrenocorticotropic hormone
AFP	α-fetoprotein
A-P	Anteroposterior
BPD	Bronchopulmonary dysplasia
CCAM	Congenital cystic adenomatoid malformation
CMV	Cytomegalovirus
CNS	Central nervous system
CSF	Cerebrospinal fluid
CT	Computed tomography, computed tomogram
DMSA	Dimercaptosuccinic acid
DSA	Digital subtraction angiography
DTPA	Diethylene-triaminepenta-acetic acid
DWI	Diffusion-weighted imaging
ECMO	Extracorporeal membrane oxygenation
ERCP	Endoscopic retrograde cholangiopancreatography
FFE	Fast field echo
FISP	Fast imaging with steady precession
FLAIR	Fluid attenuated inversion recovery
GCS	Glasgow Coma Scale
GE	Gradient echo
HASTE	Half Fourier single shot turbo spin echo
hCG	Human chorionic gonadotrophin
HU	Hounsfield unit
MALT	Mucosal associated lymphoid tissue
MAPCA	Major aortopulmonary collateral arteries
MIBG	Meta-iodobenzyl-guanidine
MIP	Maximum intensity projection
MPR	Multiplanar reconstruction
MRCP	MR cholangio-pancreatography
MRI	Magnetic resonance imaging
NCPAP	Nasal continuous positive airway pressure
Nd:YAG	Neodymium:yttrium aluminum garnet
PCO2	Carbon dioxide partial pressure
PDA	Patent ductus arteriosus
PEEP	Positive end-expiratory pressure
PET	Positron emission tomography
PNET	Primitive neuroectodermal tumors
PO2	Oxygen partial pressure
PPV	Positive pressure ventilation
PVL	Periventricular leukomalacia
RARE	Rapid acquisition with relaxation enhancement
RDS	Respiratory distress syndrome
RSV	Respiratory syncytial virus
SE	Spin echo
SPIR	Spectral presaturation inversion recovery
SSFP	Steady state free precession
SSFSE	Single shot fast spin echo
STIR	Short tau inversion recovery
TSE	Turbo spin echo
VACTERL	Vertebral, anal, cardiac, tracheoesophageal, renal, limp defects
VCUG	Voiding cystourethrog-raphy
WHO	World Health Organization

Definition

Lies in the superior anterior mediastinum • Two lobes, fused in the center • The left lobe is usually larger than the right • Size, shape, and extent are highly variable • Usually disappears by age 6 years, except for a small remnant.

Imaging Signs

- **Chest radiograph findings**
  Broad upper mediastinum • Sail sign: triangular lateral expansion.
- **Ultrasound findings**
  Appears horseshoe-shaped on cross-sectional images in infants • Appears triangular or oval on longitudinal sections • Homogeneous echo pattern • Finely granular echo texture (more echogenic than the liver, less echogenic than the thyroid).
- **CT findings**
  Convex margin • Rectangular or triangular shape depending on age • No compression of adjacent structures (trachea and vascular structures) • Isodense to muscle prior to puberty • Enhances homogeneously.
- **MRI findings**
  Configuration as on CT images • Hyperintense on T2-weighted images • Nearly isointense to muscle on T1-weighted images.

Clinical Aspects

- **Typical presentation**
  Common in infants • Diminishes in size during early childhood.
- **Therapeutic options**
  None.
- **Course and prognosis**
  Disappears in stress situations such as acute illness or steroid therapy • Reappears after recovery or termination of steroid therapy ("rebound phenomenon").
- **Complications**
  Primary disorders of the thymus are rare.

Differential Diagnosis

Hyperplasia of the thymus	– Occurs in disorders such as thyroid hyperfunction or myasthenia gravis – Occurs in response to stress situations such as burns
Thymoma	– Thymoma is present in 15–25% of patients with myasthenia gravis – Peak age: 20 years – Fifty percent are malignant

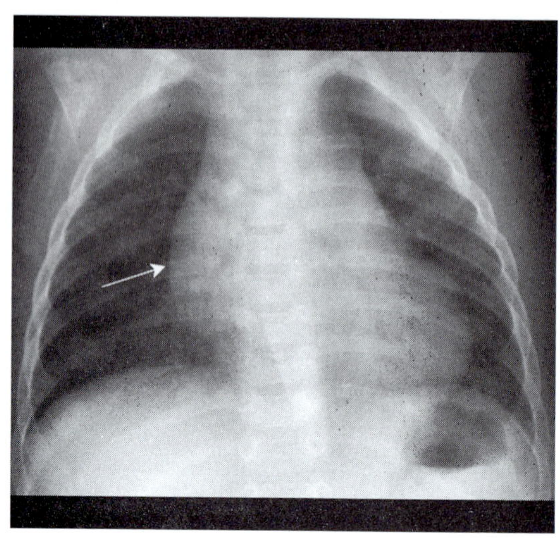

Fig. 1.1 Chest radiograph (A-P). Wide superior mediastinum with a thymus of physiologic size in a newborn. The right mediastinal contour is defined by the thymus (arrow).

Thymus cyst
- Rudiment of the third pharyngeal pouch
- More common on the left than right
- Occasional wall calcifications
- Cystic structure with slight density and echogenicity; differential diagnosis includes teratoma

Histiocytosis of the thymus
- Incidence: 0.2–1.0/100 000 children
- 60–70% of all cases occur before the age of 2 years
- Histiocytosis X shows a predilection for the male sex (2:1 ratio)
- Up to 10% of all cases are congenital

Lymphoma
- Most common cause of a mass in the anterior mediastinum in children

Benign teratoid tumor
- Epidermoid, dermoid, teratoma
- Calcifications, fatty tissue
- Well demarcated

Malignant teratoid tumor
- Choriocarcinoma, seminoma, embryonal carcinoma, yolk sac tumor, gemistocytic germinal cell tumor, teratocarcinoma
- Calcification is less common than in teratoma
- Infiltration of adjacent structures
- Lobulation can be a sign of malignancy

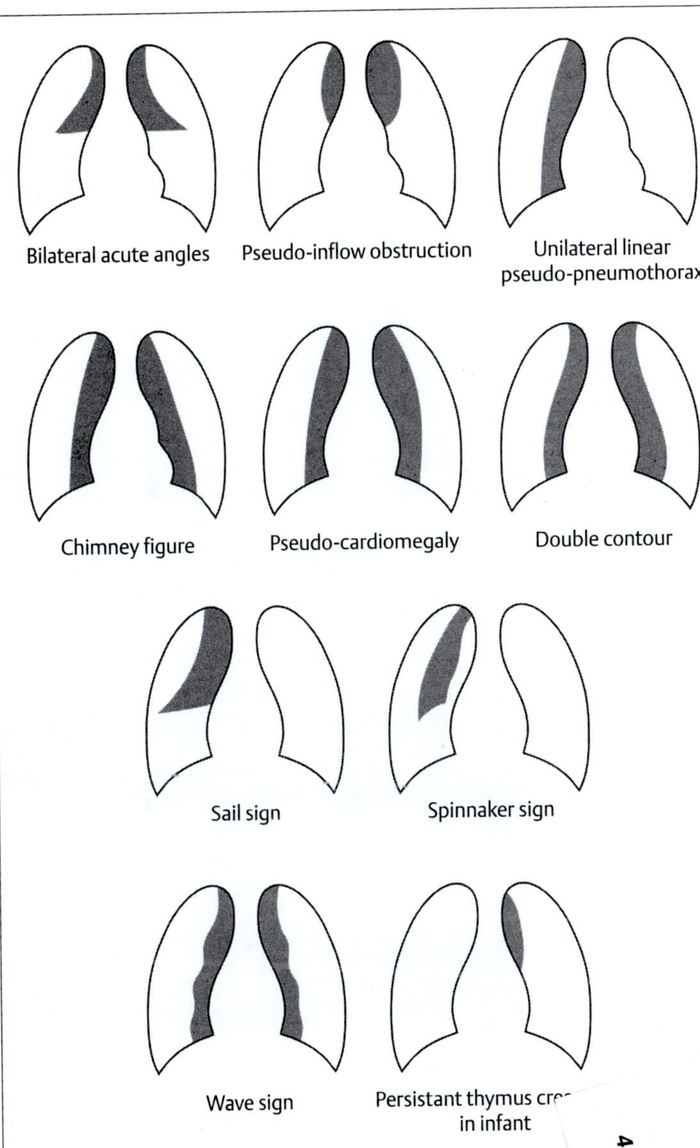

Fig. 1.2 Forms of the thymus (from Ebel KD, Willich E, Richter E. Diffe in der Pädiatrischen Radiologie. Stuttgart: Thieme; 1995).

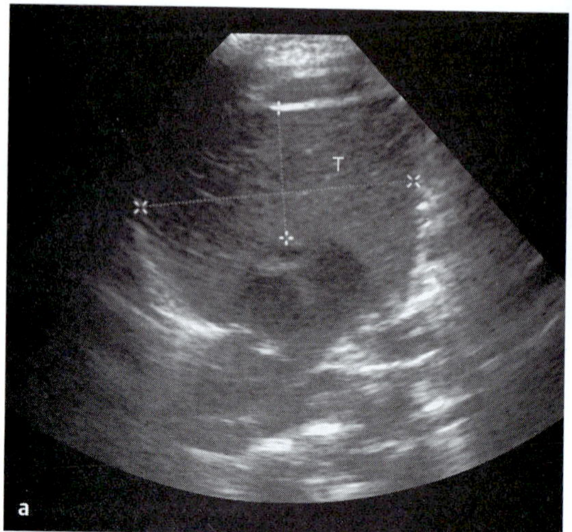

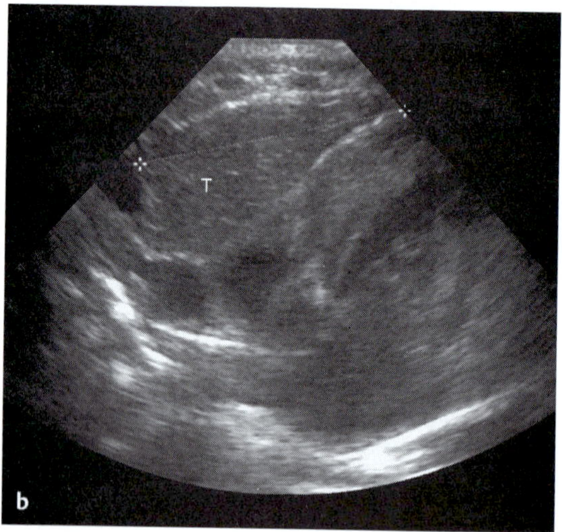

Fig. 1.3 a, b Superior mediastinum above the throat. Ultrasound. Thymus (T) in the axial (**a**) and sagittal (**b**) planes. Typical homogeneous, finely granular echo texture.

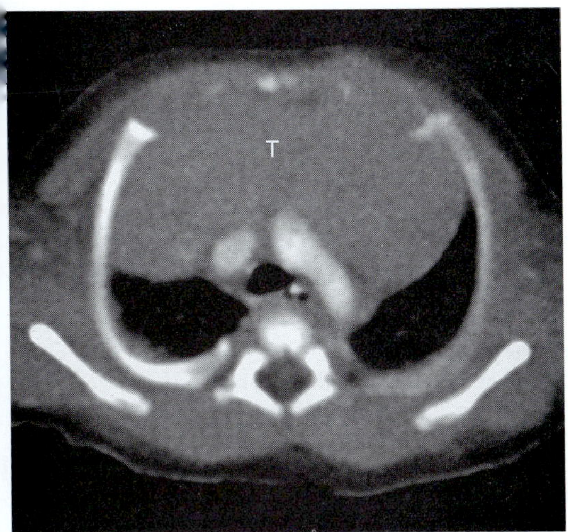

Fig. 1.4 Axial chest CT after intravenous contrast administration. The large mass (isodense to soft tissue) in the anterior superior mediastinum is consistent with a hypertrophic thymus (T).

Tips and Pitfalls

- Misinterpreting a normal thymus as an abnormal mediastinal mass.
- Ultrasound examination to visualize the normal echo texture will suffice to clarify equivocal findings.
- When in doubt, additional radiographs may be obtained in 6 weeks to check whether findings remain unchanged.

Selected References

Adam EJ et al. Sonography of the thymus in healthy children: frequency of visualization, size, and appearance. Am J Roentgenol 1993; 161: 153–155

Ebel KD et al. Differential Diagnosis in Pediatric Radiology. Stuttgart, Thieme, 1999

Frush DP et al. Imaging evaluation of the thymus and thymic disorders in children. In: Pediatric Chest Imaging. Berlin: Springer; 2001

Mendelson DS et al. Imaging of the thymus. Chest Surg Clin North Am 2001; 11: 269–293

Definition

- **Epidemiology**
  Occurs in 50–80% of premature infants < 28 weeks' gestation or with birth weight < 1000 g.
- **Etiology, pathophysiology, pathogenesis**
  Primary surfactant deficiency due to immaturity of the lungs • Microatelectasis • Reduced functional residual capacity • Intrapulmonary shunts • Reduced pulmonary compliance.

Imaging Signs

- **Chest radiograph findings**
  - *Grade I:* Alveolar collapse produces a fine reticulogranular appearance.
  - *Grade II:* Also includes positive findings on air bronchogram extending into the periphery of the lung.
  - *Grade III:* Findings also include ill-defined contours of the heart and diaphragm • Thickening of the interstitium and interstitial edema produce veil-like shadowing.
  - *Grade IV:* "White lung": Homogeneous shadowing of the entire lung.

  A normal chest radiograph obtained 6 hours after birth excludes RDS • Pleural effusion rarely occurs.

Clinical Aspects

- **Typical presentation**
  Postpartum respiratory insufficiency • Expiratory stridor • Cyanosis • Tachypnea • Nasal flaring • Intercostal retractions.
- **Therapeutic options**
  Early intubation and respiration with PEEP • Administration of artificial surfactant through endotracheal tube.
- **Course and prognosis**
  Reasons for failure to improve following surfactant administration include: very immature lung, sepsis, persistent patent ductus arteriosus, and heart defect.
- **Complications**
  Pulmonary interstitial emphysema • Pneumothorax • Pneumomediastinum • Pneumopericardium • Superinfection • Bronchopulmonary dysplasia • Pulmonary hemorrhage.

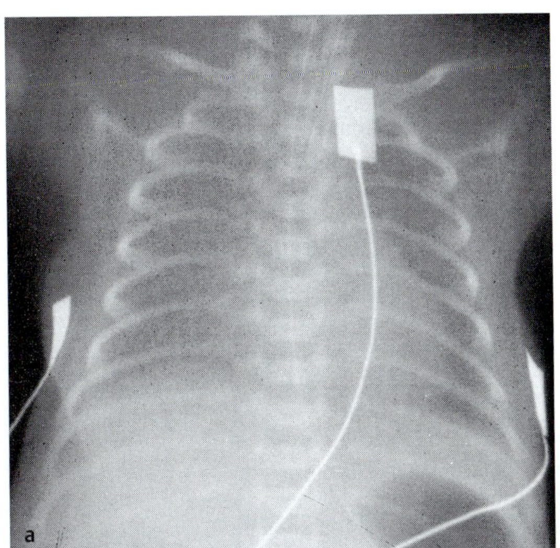

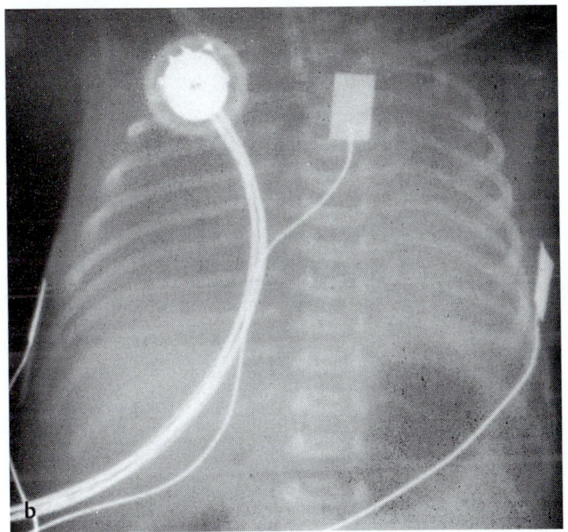

Fig. 1.5 a, b Respiratory distress syndrome. A-P chest radiograph. Typical radiographic appearance of grade III (**a**) and IV (**b**) respiratory distress syndrome.

Differential Diagnosis

Transient tachypnea (wet lung disease)	– Due to aspiration of amniotic fluid and/or insufficient drainage of prenatal alveolar fluid – Normalizes within the first 24–48 hours
Group B streptococcal pneumonia	– Most common type of pneumonia in newborns – Often associated with pleural effusion – Bilateral granular opacification with some patchy, confluent shadowing
Bilateral pulmonary hemorrhage	– No characteristic changes – Difficult to identify (bloody tracheal secretion)
Hypoplastic left heart syndrome	– Cardiomegaly, round heart – Apex of the heart elevated due to right heart atrophy

Tips and Pitfalls

- Misinterpreting an image obtained in maximal expiration.
- Chest findings in neonatal intensive care must always be evaluated in conjunction with clinical data (i.e., course of pregnancy and birth, amniotic fluid findings).

Selected References

Ainsworth SB. Pathophysiology of neonatal respiratory distress syndrome: implications for early treatment strategies. Treat Respir Med 2005; 4: 423–437

De Mello DE. Pulmonary pathology. Semin Neonatol 2004; 9: 311–329

Swischuk LE et al. Immature lung problems: can our nomenclature be more specific? Am J Roentgenol 1996; 917–918

Definition

- **Epidemiology**
  Occurs in 30–40% of premature infants (< 32 weeks' gestation, birth weight < 1200 g) receiving positive pressure ventilation.
- **Etiology, pathophysiology, pathogenesis**
  Barotrauma due to high-pressure ventilation with PEEP • Rupture of overextended alveoli and terminal bronchioles • Air leaks into the pulmonary interstitium and lymph vessels • Reduced pulmonary compliance.

Imaging Signs

- **Chest radiograph findings**
  Distended alveoli appear as round radiolucencies (bubbles) measuring 1–1.5 mm • Diffusely distributed (visualized only on inspiration) • After rupture, multiform, primarily cystoid and linear radiolucencies measuring approximately 2 mm are visualized • Findings may be asymmetric (visible on inspiration and expiration) • Linear radiolucencies show changes in diameter which become narrower toward the periphery, in contrast with air bronchogram findings • Larger pseudocysts with mass effect may be present • Pneumothorax and/or pneumomediastinum may occur • The lung itself is usually rigid and collapses only slightly.

Clinical Aspects

- **Typical presentation**
  Occurs within the first few days of life (acute condition) • Usually there is preexisting RDS with respiratory insufficiency • Radiographic changes usually precede clinical symptoms.
- **Therapeutic options**
  Reduce peak ventilation pressure • Accept higher PCO_2 values • High-frequency ventilation • Consider other methods of respiratory support • Position the infant on the affected side • Regular radiologic follow-up is indicated.
- **Course and prognosis**
  Usually temporarily detectable where respiration parameters have not been properly adjusted • Typical complications occur.
- **Complications**
  Pseudocysts • Pneumothorax • Pneumomediastinum • Pneumopericardium (intervention is indicated in the event of imminent cardiac tamponade) • Air embolism.

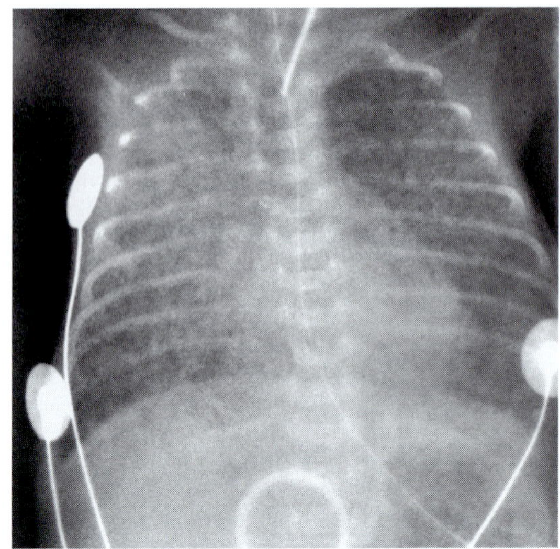

Fig. 1.6 Pulmonary interstitial emphysema. Chest radiograph (A-P). Bilateral pulmonary interstitial emphysema in hyaline membrane disease and high-pressure ventilation.

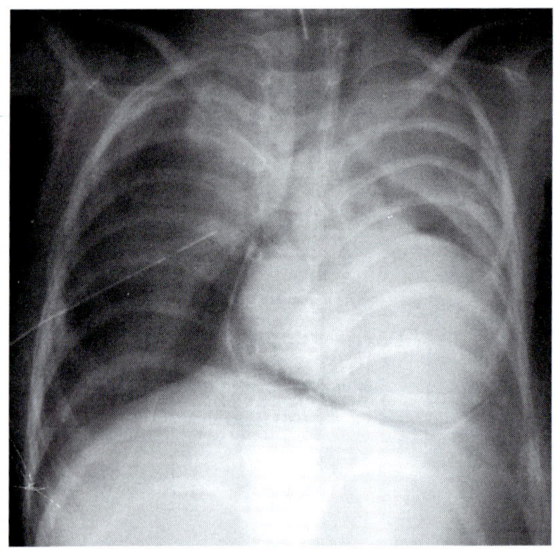

Fig. 1.7 Pulmonary interstitial emphysema (PIE). Chest radiograph (A-P). Right pneumothorax (with drain in situ), pneumomediastinum, and pneumopericardium. Normal position of central venous catheter and endotracheal tube.

Differential Diagnosis

BPD	- Round areas of reduced transparency (pseudocysts) - Typically occur only after the first week of life - Varying degrees of severity
CCAM	- Typically present at birth - Cystic radiolucencies are usually larger and do not change over time

Tips and Pitfalls

- Increased transparency of the lung mimics an improvement in findings (note that interstitial air does not participate in gas exchange).
- Can be confused with air bronchogram.
- Can be misinterpreted as a pneumatocele or circumscribed pneumothorax (for example, air trapped in the inferior pulmonary ligament).

Selected References

Donnelly LF et al. Localized lucent chest lesions in neonates. Am J Roentgenol 1999; 212: 837–840

Pursnani SK et al. Localized persistent interstitial pulmonary emphysema presenting as a spontaneous tension pneumothorax in a full term baby. Pediatr Surg Int 2006; 22: 613–616

Definition

- **Epidemiology**
  Occurs in 15–30% of premature infants < 28 weeks' gestation or with birth weight < 1000 g • Rare in preterm infants > 32 weeks' gestation.
- **Etiology, pathophysiology, pathogenesis**
  Lung is immature • After oxygen administration (80–100%), intubation, and ventilation • Infection • Injury to the alveoli, bronchial mucosa, and pulmonary vascular structures leads to necrosis, edema, epithelial metaplasia, and structural changes in the intima and media.

Imaging Signs

- **Chest radiograph findings**
  Stages according to Weinstein:
  - *Grade 1:* Dull, weak densities that give the lung a veil-like appearance.
  - *Grade 2:* Linear reticular densities located primarily in the central region.
  - *Grade 3:* More pronounced linear reticular densities extending into the periphery of the lung.
  - *Grade 4:* Grade 3 findings along with small, well demarcated cystic changes primarily in the basal region.
  - *Grade 5:* Pronounced areas of density and cystic areas of the same size (cysts are larger than in grade 4 and primarily in the basal region).
  - *Grade 6:* Cystic areas are larger than the areas of density, giving the lung a bubbly appearance.

  BPD can be asymmetric when it occurs secondary to chronic atelectasis or pneumothorax.

Clinical Aspects

- **Typical presentation**
  Tachypnea • Intercostal retractions • Nasal flaring • Increased heart rate • Cyanosis • Prolonged expiration • Stridor • Signs of right heart strain • Failure to thrive.
- **Therapeutic options**
  Prevention: Prenatal administration of corticosteroids • Early administration of surfactant • Early detection and treatment of a persistent patent ductus arteriosus • Vitamin A supplementation • Restriction of artificial ventilation.
  Treatment: Oxygen • Postnatal administration of corticosteroids • Inhalational anti-inflammatory treatment • Diuretics • Bronchodilators.
- **Course and prognosis**
  Recurrent respiratory infections in the first 2 years of life.
- **Complications**
  Bacterial superinfection.

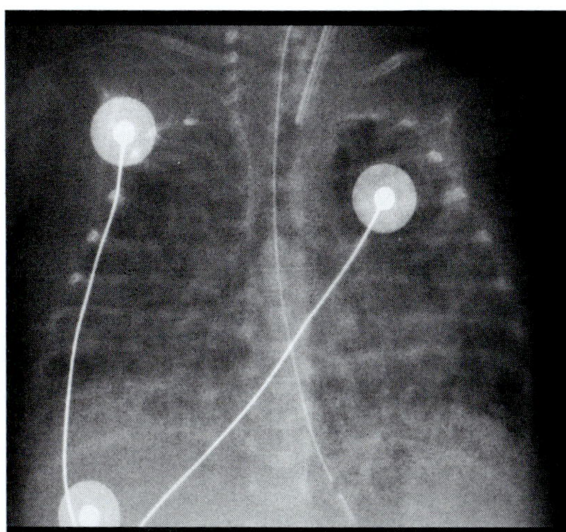

Fig. 1.8 Premature infant with grade 5 bronchopulmonary dysplasia (BPD). Chest radiograph (A-P). The pronounced bilateral pulmonary opacities and cystic areas are immediately obvious.

Table 1.1 Clinical stages according to Jobe and Bancalari

Gestational age	< 32 weeks	≥ 32 weeks
	Oxygen over 21 % for at least 28 days plus	
	At 36 weeks' gestation*	On postpartum day 56*
Mild BPD	No need for O_2	No need for O_2
Moderate BPD	< 30 % O_2 required	< 30 % O_2 required
Severe BPD	≥ 30 % O_2 required and/or positive pressure (PPV or NCPAP)	≥ 30 % O_2 required and/or positive pressure (PPV or NCPAP)

* Or on discharge if sooner.

Differential Diagnosis

Grade 1
- RDS

Grades 2–4
- Overhydration or infusion
- Pulmonary edema in patent ductus arteriosus

Grades 5, 6
- Interstitial emphysema
- Total anomalous pulmonary venous connection with pulmonary obstruction
- Congenital pulmonary lymphangiectasia
- Viral pneumonia
- Congenital tuberculosis

Tips and Pitfalls

- Additional infections such as RSV bronchiolitis can be detected only by comparing findings with previous imaging studies.
- Knowledge of the patient's history and respiratory status is essential to the diagnosis in a newborn.
- BPD should be considered whenever uncharacteristic lung changes are detected.

Selected References

Bland RD. Neonatal chronic lung disease in the post-surfactant era. Biol Neonate 2005; 88: 181–191

Jobe AH et al. Bronchopulmonary dysplasia. Am J Respir Crit Care Med 2001; 163: 1723–1729

Weinstein MR et al. A new radiographic scoring system for bronchopulmonary dysplasia. Newborn Lung Project. Pediatr Pulmonol 1994; 18: 284–289

Definition

- **Epidemiology**
  Usually occurs in term or postmature infants • Amniotic fluid contains meconium in 10–15% of births • Symptomatic meconium aspiration occurs in about 10% of cases.
- **Etiology, pathophysiology, pathogenesis**
  Stress such as fetal hypoxia • This results in reflexive discharge of meconium • Intrauterine aspiration of amniotic fluid containing meconium • Aspirated meconium initially obstructs the bronchioles • Later, there is chemical pneumonitis with localized overinflation and consolidation.

Imaging Signs

- **Chest radiograph findings**
  Radiologic changes depend on the severity of aspiration • Severe cases have almost radiopaque, coarse, patchy, partially confluent alveolar opacities, some of which are surrounded by cystoid radiolucencies (combinations of focal areas of insufficient ventilation and overinflated lung tissue) • Findings are usually distributed asymmetrically • Pulmonary interstitial edema, pneumothorax, and pneumomediastinum may occur (in 20–40% of cases) • Associated pleural effusion may occur.

Clinical Aspects

- **Typical presentation**
  Severe perinatal asphyxia • "Pea soup" amniotic fluid • *Umbilical cord blood gas analysis:* Severe metabolic acidosis • Often there is no spontaneous respiration • Flaccid muscle tone • Bradycardia • Baby is pale/cyanotic • Dyspnea • Expiratory stridor • Auscultatory findings include rattling • Newborn is covered in meconium.
- **Therapeutic options**
  Thorough cleaning of nose and mouth • Airway suction • Intubation and high-frequency ventilation • Bronchial lavage (can remove surfactant) • Administration of sodium bicarbonate for acidosis • ECMO is indicated when all else fails.
- **Course and prognosis**
  The risk of persistent fetal circulation is high (persistent pulmonary hypertension with right–left shunt via patent fetal vessels such as a ductus arteriosus or foramen ovale).
- **Complications**
  Bacterial superinfection.

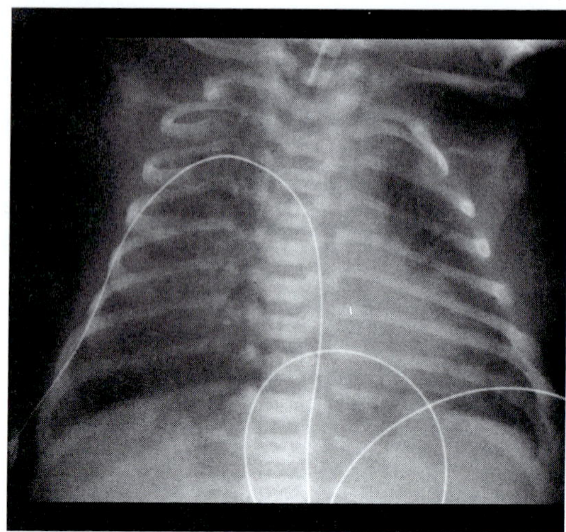

Fig. 1.9 Meconium aspiration syndrome. Chest radiograph (A-P). Newborn with coarse, patchy, partially confluent opacities following meconium aspiration.

Differential Diagnosis

Neonatal pneumonia	– Indistinguishable
Transient neonatal tachypnea	– Usually secondary to caesarean section – Resolves within 24–48 hours

Tips and Pitfalls

- In the first few days, the clinical picture is essential to distinguish this disorder from transient tachypnea in the newborn.
- Imaging studies cannot distinguish this disorder from neonatal pneumonia.

Selected References

Dargaville PA et al. Surfactant therapy for meconium aspiration syndrome: current status. Drugs 2005; 65: 2569–2591

Gooding CA et al. Roentgenographic analysis of meconium aspiration of the newborn. Radiology 1971; 100: 131–140

Velaphi S et al. Intrapartum and postdelivery management of infants born to mothers with meconium-stained amniotic fluid: evidence-based recommendations. Clin Perinatol 2006; 33: 29–42

Definition

- **Epidemiology**
  Predilection for male sex (3:1 ratio) • Associated with patent ductus arteriosus and ventricular septal defect in 15% of cases.
- **Etiology, pathophysiology, pathogenesis**
  Bronchial cartilage anomaly • Endobronchial obstruction such as mucosal fold or mucus plug • Bronchial compression e.g., caused by patent ductus arteriosus or aberrant left pulmonary artery • Congenital bronchial stenosis or alveolar malformations • Valve mechanism and partial collapse of distal lung segments.

Imaging Signs

- **Chest radiograph and CT findings**
  Hyperinflated lung segment or lobe (left upper lobe: 43% of cases; right middle lobe: 32%; right upper lobe: 20%) • Partial collapse of adjacent lung segments due to compression • Mediastinum is shifted to the contralateral side • Flattening of the ipsilateral hemidiaphragm • Pulmonary vascular structures are spread apart.
- **Ultrasound findings**
  Prenatal visualization of echogenic or cystic areas of the lung.

Clinical Aspects

- **Typical presentation**
  Tachypnea • Dyspnea • Coughing • Progressive cyanosis • Muffled sound of respiration over the affected side • Hoarseness • Bulging of the chest on the affected side.
- **Therapeutic options**
  Resection of the affected lung segment.
- **Course and prognosis**
  Nonprogressive cases are potentially reversible • Resection is curative.
- **Complications**
  Mortality is about 10% • Superinfection.

Differential Diagnosis

Bronchial atresia	– Usually in the apical posterior left upper lobe – Fingerlike perihilar opacity (mucus plug distal to the atresia)
Pulmonary cysts	– Congenital: no history – Acquired: usually secondary to trauma – Primarily subpleural

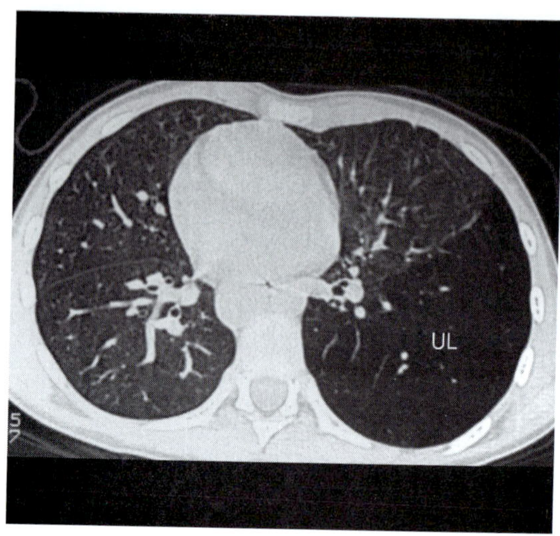

Fig. 1.10 Congenital lobar emphysema. Chest CT (mid-lung window). Marked overinflation of the left lower lobe. Slight changes in the left upper lobe from compressive atelectasis. Mediastinum is displaced to the right.

Pneumatocele	– Large air-filled cyst created by a valve mechanism, often larger than 10 cm – Predilection for: middle and lower lobes – Primarily secondary to pneumonia in infants and young children
CCAM	– Multiple air-filled cystic structures of varying size
Congenital diaphragmatic hernia	– Primarily in the left hemithorax – Left hemidiaphragm cannot be identified – Air-filled bowel loops in the thorax

Tips and Pitfalls

Immediately after delivery the affected lung lobe may still be filled with amniotic fluid and can appear very dense due to lack of ventilation.

Selected References

Donnelly LF et al. Localized lucent chest lesions in neonates. Am J Roentgenol 1999; 212: 834–840

Olutoye O et al. Prenatal diagnosis and management of congenital lobar emphysema. J Pediatr Surg 2000; 35: 792–795

Ozcelik U et al. Congenital lobar emphysema: evaluation and long-term follow-up of thirty cases at a single center. Pediatr Pulmonol 2003; 35: 384–391

Definition

- **Epidemiology**
  Rare congenital lung disorder • No sex predilection.
- **Etiology, pathophysiology, pathogenesis**
  Adenomatoid proliferation of terminal bronchioles during fetal development • Proliferation of smooth muscle cells in the cyst wall • Absence of cartilage in the bronchial wall • Cysts are lined with cuboidal and columnar epithelium.

Imaging Signs

- **Chest radiograph and CT findings**
  Lobulated, well demarcated cystic mass lacking pulmonary structure • Occasionally air and fluid signs are present • Usually unilateral (80% of cases) • No lobe predilection • Mediastinum is shifted toward the contralateral side (87% of cases) • Partial collapse of adjacent lung segments due to compression • Ipsilateral lung is hypoplastic.
- **CT classification and histopathologic findings (Stocker et al.)**

Table 1.2 Stocker classification

Type	Frequency	Characteristics
I	50%	• Isolated or multiple large cysts (2–10 cm) • Grouping around a dominant large cyst • No alveolar pulmonary tissue
II	40%	• Multiple small cysts (< 10–20 mm) • Epithelial lining
III	10%	• Isolated solid masses with bronchus-like structures • Ciliated cuboidal epithelium with microscopic cysts

- **Prenatal ultrasound findings**
  Solid or cystic mass • Mediastinal displacement • Polyhydramnios (66% of cases) due to esophageal compression • Fetal ascites (71% of cases) • Fetal hydrops (8–47% of cases).

Clinical Aspects

- **Typical presentation**
  A third of affected infants do not have symptoms (incidental finding) • Two-thirds have immediate postnatal respiratory distress (cyanosis) • Recurrent bronchitis or pneumonia.
- **Therapeutic options**
  The treatment of choice is surgical resection.

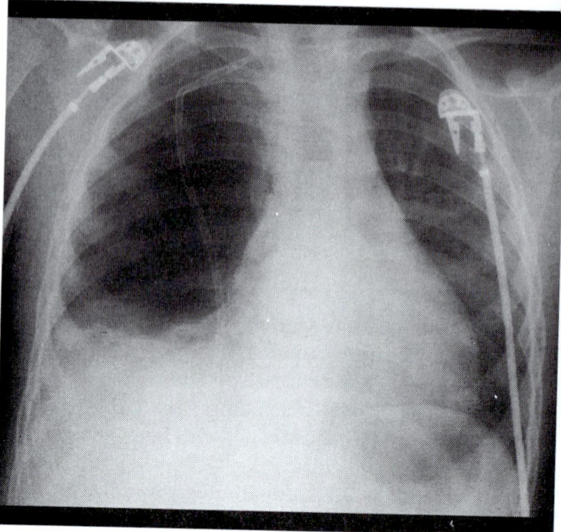

Fig. 1.11 Congenital cystic adenomatoid malformation (CCAM). Chest radiograph (A-P). Pronounced transparency of the right hemithorax, mediastinal displacement to the left, moderately impaired ventilation in the right basal lung segments. Drain in the right upper lobe.

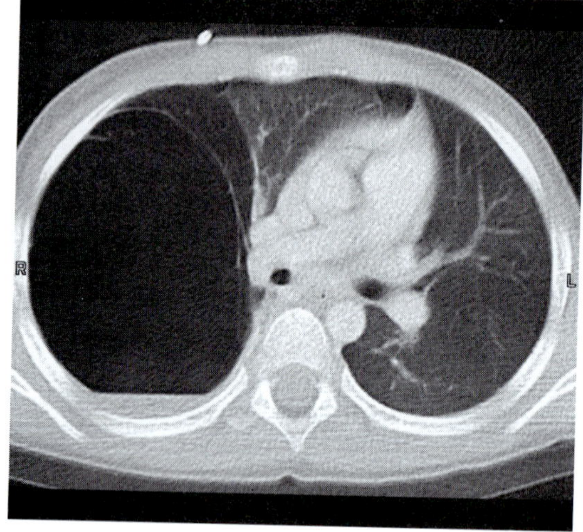

Fig. 1.12 CT (mid-lung window). Large intrapulmonary lesion on the right with air and fluid sign. Type I CCAM according to Stocker (with the kind permission of Prof. R. Buchmann, Dept of Pediatric Radiology, Arkansas Children's Hospital Little Rock, USA).

- **Course and prognosis**
  - *Type I:* Excellent prognosis after resection.
  - *Type II:* Poor prognosis as it is often associated with other severe abnormalities.
  - *Type III:* Poor prognosis due to pulmonary hypoplasia and hydrops.
- **Complications**
  Transformation into rhabdomyosarcoma is rare but can occur.

Differential Diagnosis

Pneumatocele	– Large air-filled cyst (bulla) – Created by valve mechanism – Larger than 10 cm
Bronchogenic cyst	– Small isolated cyst close to the midline
Cystic bronchiectasis	– Continuous with the bronchial system – Known pulmonary disorder such as cystic fibrosis
Pulmonary sequestration	– Usually contains no air in the prenatal phase – Typically located in the left lower lobe – Air inclusions in superinfection
Congenital diaphragmatic hernia	– Primarily in the left hemithorax – Left hemidiaphragm cannot be identified – Air-filled bowel loops in the thorax – Air and fluid signs less common than in CCAM – Appearance varies with patient positioning and respiratory phase
Congenital lobar emphysema	– Overinflated lung segment, no cysts
Cavitary necrosis complicating pneumonia or pulmonary abscess	– Clinical findings are crucial – History (i.e., previous imaging studies) and dynamics are important – Cavitary necrosis from ischemia and necrosis of inflamed consolidated lung parenchyma – Pulmonary abscess is demarcated by a thick marginal wall
Pulmonary cysts	– Usually posttraumatic – Primarily subpleural

Tips and Pitfalls

Without a patient history and clinical correlation, this disorder is easily confused with other disorders considered in the differential diagnosis above.

Selected References

Kim WS et al. Congenital cystic adenomatoid malformation of the lung: CT-pathologic correlation. Am J Roentgenol 1997; 168: 47–53

Leeuwen KV et al. Prenatal diagnosis of congenital cystic adenomatoid malformation and its postnatal presentation, surgical indication and natural history. J Pediatr Surg 1999; 34: 794–799

Stocker JT et al. Congenital cystic adenomatoid malformation of the lung: classification and morphological spectrum. Hum Pathol 1977; 8: 155–171

Definition

- **Epidemiology**
  Prevalence 0.1–1.7% • Usually diagnosed before age 10 years.
- **Etiology, pathophysiology, pathogenesis**
  Congenital anomaly of a pulmonary lobe • Lobe has its own systemic arterial supply (usually from the aorta) • Nonfunctional degenerative lung tissue • *Synonym:* Bronchopulmonary foregut malformation (occasionally associated with gastrointestinal anomalies).
  Intralobar form: Covered by visceral pleura of the normal lung • Frequency 75–86% of all cases • Often only diagnosed in adulthood • No sex predilection • Rarely occurs with other congenital malformations • *Location:* Posterobasal lower lobe (ratio of left to right = 3:2) • Rarely, there is communication with the bronchial tree • Systemic arterial supply is usually from the distal thoracic aorta, less often from the abdominal aorta or one of its branches • Venous drainage is via the pulmonary veins.
  Extralobar form: Separate pleural covering • Frequency 14–25% of all cases • Usually diagnosed in the neonatal period • Occurs eight times as often in males than females • Often associated with other congenital malformations such as diaphragmatic defect, CCAM, cardiac malformations • Usually on the left side between lower lobe and diaphragm • Supplied by systemic arteries • Drainage is via larger systemic veins (inferior vena cava, azygos vein, hemiazygos vein) • No communication with the bronchial tree.

Imaging Signs

- **Chest radiograph findings**
  Homogeneous density close to the diaphragm • Isodense to soft tissue • Well demarcated • Round, oval, or triangular • Air and fluid signs may be present with infection • Recurrent pneumonia or signs of chronic bronchitis may be present in adjacent tissue • Pleural effusion may be present.
- **CT and MRI findings**
  Fluid and air-filled cysts may be present • Mass with inhomogeneous density pattern • Inhomogeneous enhancement (rare) • CT or MR angiography can visualize vascular anatomy.
- **Prenatal ultrasound**
  Hyperechoic homogeneous mass • Doppler ultrasound can often identify the vascular structures supplying and draining the sequestration.
- **Angiographic findings**
  Demonstrates the thoracic and abdominal aorta with aberrant systemic arteries and venous drainage.

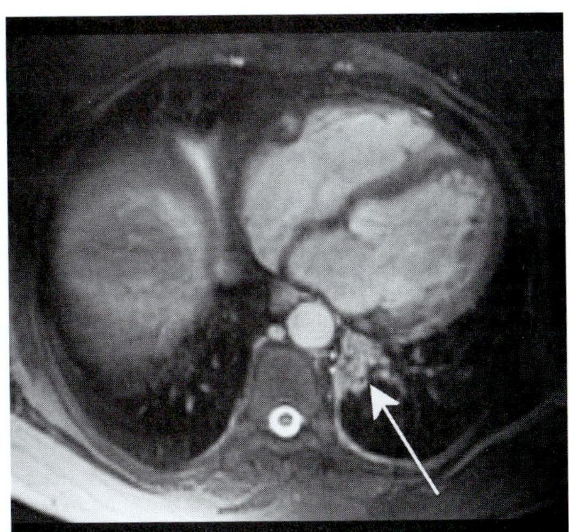

Fig. 1.13 Lung sequestration. MR image (axial GE sequence). The lung sequestration is visualized as a hyperintense mass (arrow) in a typical location in the left lower lobe.

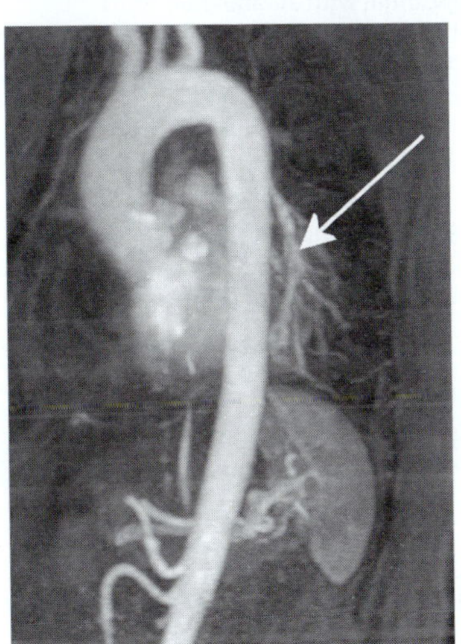

Fig. 1.14 MR image (maximum intensity projection, contrasted 3D MR angiography). Well established arterial supply to the sequestration (arrow), here via the left coronal artery (origin is not clearly visualized on the maximum intensity projection).

Clinical Aspects

- **Typical presentation**
  Can remain asymptomatic for a long time • Chronic recurrent pneumonia • Hemoptysis.
- **Therapeutic options**
  Symptomatic treatment with broad-spectrum antibiotics • Curative treatment by surgical resection • Curative or preoperative embolization of the systemic blood supply.
- **Course and prognosis**
  Disorder is cured by resection or embolization.
- **Complications**
  Superinfection of the pulmonary sequestration.

Differential Diagnosis

Chronic pneumonia	– Typical clinical findings with no detectable anomalies of pulmonary sequestration (in particular normal vascular anatomy)
Solitary abscess or pneumonia with abscess formation	– Round shadow, often with air and fluid signs – Primarily in the posterior upper and lower lobes – Usually a sequela of staphylococcal infection – Pneumatocele can occur where there is communication with the bronchial system
Pulmonary contusion	– History of trauma – Resolves within 3–10 days
Pulmonary arteriovenous fistula	– Predilection for the left lower lobe – Typical radiographic morphology – Arterial supply from the pulmonary arteries

Tips and Pitfalls

Pulmonary sequestration should be considered in cases of recurrent pneumonia.

Selected References

Berrocal T et al. Congenital anomalies of the tracheobronchial tree, lung, and mediastinum: embryology, radiology, and pathology. Radiographics 2004; 24: e17

Bratu I et al. The multiple facets of pulmonary sequestration. J Pediatr Surg 2001; 36: 784–790

Corbett HJ et al. Pulmonary sequestration. Paediatr Respir Rev 2004; 5: 59–68

Definition

▸ **Epidemiology**

Accounts for 5–11 % of mediastinal mass in children • Mediastinal lesions show no sex predilection • Intrapulmonary bronchogenic cysts affect boys more often than girls.

▸ **Etiology, pathophysiology, pathogenesis**

Derived from abnormal budding of the embryonal foregut • Spherical hollow space • Connection with the bronchial tree is usually obliterated • Lined with respiratory epithelium.

Intrapulmonary form (15%): Often communicates with the bronchial system • Can contain air and clear or mucoid secretion • Lined with respiratory epithelium • Does not have its own blood supply • Occurs twice as often in the lower lobe than in the upper lobe.

Mediastinal form (85%): Normally does not communicate with the bronchial system • Cysts are paratracheal (normally on the right side), carinal (most common form), or hilar • Usually fluid filled • Locations include the posterior mediastinum (50%), pericarinal region (35%), and superior mediastinum (14%), usually on the right side.

Imaging Signs

▸ **Chest radiograph findings**

Intrapulmonary: Round or oval mass • Usually air filled • Air and fluid signs may be present • Usually solitary • Two-thirds of all cysts occur in the lower lobe • Long-term follow-up demonstrates changes in size.

Mediastinal: Round or oval mass • Usually air filled • Air and fluid signs may be present • Usually unilocular • Extrapulmonary site in the middle mediastinum • Often on the right side • Bronchial compression leads to obstructive emphysema or atelectasis • Impression of the trachea and occasionally esophagus as well • Subcarinal cysts widen the angle of the bifurcation • Long-term follow-up demonstrates changes in size.

▸ **CT findings**

Density depends on the cyst contents • Well demarcated mass • Wall does not enhance • Marginal enhancement suggests superinfection • No central enhancement after contrast administration • Malignant degeneration can occur where a solid component is present.

▸ **MRI findings**

Signal intensity on T1-weighted images depends on cyst contents • High signal intensity on T2-weighted images • Contrast behavior is identical to CT • Malignant degeneration can occur where a solid component is present.

▸ **Ultrasound findings**

Examination can demonstrate cyst depending on its location.

▸ **Barium swallow**

A mediastinal cyst will cause impression or displacement of the esophagus.

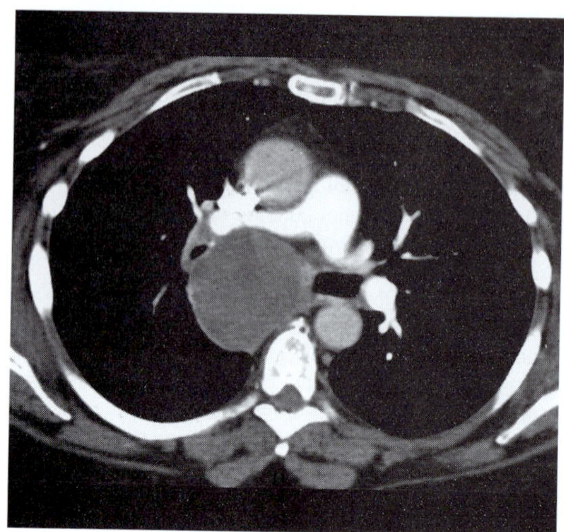

Fig. 1.15 Bronchogenic cyst. Contrast CT of the chest. Oval cystic infracarinal mass with central density values around 10 HU. Location and morphology are typical of a bronchogenic cyst.

Clinical Aspects

- **Typical presentation**
  Cysts are asymptomatic in 50% of cases • Often an incidental finding on routine radiographs • RDS in newborns and infants • Older children exhibit signs of respiratory tract obstruction • Whistling • Stridor • Cyanosis • Respiratory distress • Chronic coughing • Substernal symptoms • Recurrent pneumonia • Upper respiratory tract infections • Intrapulmonary lesions can lead to hemoptysis.
- **Therapeutic options**
  Treatment of choice is surgical resection • Antibiotic treatment is indicated for repeated lung infections.
- **Course and prognosis**
  Excellent prognosis after resection.
- **Complications**
  Superinfection.

Differential Diagnosis

▸ **Intrapulmonary bronchogenic cyst**

Round pneumonia	– No signs of a mass – Follow-up demonstrates dynamic changes
Primary pulmonary tumor	– Extremely rare pulmonary blastoma, plasma cell granuloma, or infantile myofibromatosis
Congenital cystic adenomatoid malformation	– Multiple air-filled cystic structures of varying size
Cavitary necrosis complicating pneumonia or pulmonary abscess	– Clinical findings are crucial – History (i.e., previous imaging studies) is important – Dynamics in short-term follow-up

▸ **Mediastinal bronchogenic cyst**

Enteric cyst	– Often associated with vertebral malformations (usually cranial to the cyst) – Usually bilateral – Genuine enteric duplications lined with gastric or intestinal mucosa
Cystic teratoma	– Not purely cystic; calcification densities and/or structures with fat density are also demonstrated
Thymus cyst	– Can exhibit calcifications in its wall – Multilocular
Cyst arising from ectopic thyroid tissue	– Ectopic thyroid tissue with typical signal characteristics and contrast uptake dynamics
Neuroenteric cyst	– Posterior mediastinum – Associated with neurofibromatosis and meningocele

Tips and Pitfalls

- Lesions in atypical locations are difficult to distinguish from other disorders considered in the differential diagnosis.
- Fluid with a high protein content can mimic a solid process on CT.
- Cysts can recur following interventional cyst aspiration (follow-up is indicated).

Selected References

Ashizawa K et al. Anterior mediastinal bronchogenic cysts: demonstration of complicating malignancy by CT and MRI. Br J Radiol 2001; 74: 959–961

Berrocal T et al. Congenital anomalies of the tracheobronchial tree, lung, and mediastinum: embryology, radiology, and pathology. Radiographics 2004; 24: e17

McAdams et al. Bronchogenic cyst: imaging features with clinical and histopathologic correlation. Radiology 2000; 56: 441–446

Nobuhara KK et al. Bronchogenic cysts and esophageal duplications: common origins and treatment. J Pediatr Surg 1997; 32: 1408–1413

Definition

- **Epidemiology**
  Incidence: 1:2500 live births • Twice as common in boys than girls.
- **Etiology, pathophysiology, pathogenesis**
  Defective closure of the pleuroperitoneal foramina or insufficient development of the muscular components of the diaphragm • Herniation of abdominal organs. The earlier the diaphragmatic hernia occurs, the more pronounced the ipsilateral or contralateral pulmonary hypoplasia will be.
  Bochdalek hernia: 85–90% of cases • Herniation through the vertebrocostal trigone (posterolaterally) • 80% of hernias occur on the left side.
  Anterior hernias: Morgagni hernia: right retrosternal hernia • Larrey hernia: left retrosternal defect with herniation through the sternocostal triangle.
  Late-onset hernia: Presumably the liver or spleen initially prevents herniation • Intraabdominal pressure increases after birth • Can also occur in Group B streptococcal pneumonia.

Imaging Signs

- **Chest radiograph findings**
  Immediately after birth a soft tissue density is seen in the affected hemithorax • Later after birth, air-filled bowel loops may be seen in the hemithorax • The ipsilateral hemidiaphragm cannot be identified • There is conspicuously little gas in the abdomen • Hypoplasia of the ipsilateral lung • Mediastinum is displaced toward the contralateral side • Cardiopulmonary findings are initially normal in the late-onset form • Gastric tube lies in the hemithorax (contrast administration is not usually necessary) • In a right diaphragmatic hernia, the liver herniates, rarely the bowel.
- **CT findings**
  Not usually required to confirm the diagnosis • Helpful in excluding other apparently cystic thoracic disorders • Intrathoracic bowel loops are readily demonstrated.
- **Fetal MRI findings**
  Demonstrates intrathoracic bowel structures (hyperintense on T2-weighted images) or parenchymal organs • Fetal lung volume can be determined by fetal MRI of the lung to estimate the severity of pulmonary hypoplasia.
- **Prenatal ultrasound findings**
  Intrathoracic mass • Inhomogeneous echo pattern • Peristaltic deformations may be present • Heart is displaced • Fluid-filled stomach cannot be identified within the abdomen.

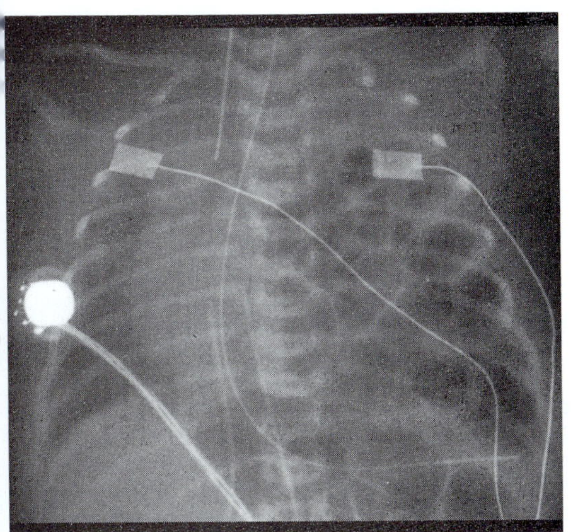

Fig. 1.16 Newborn with a large congenital left diaphragmatic hernia. Chest radiograph (A-P). The herniated bowel loops have caused pulmonary hypoplasia on the left side and mediastinal displacement to the right.

Clinical Aspects

- **Typical presentation**
  RDS may be present.
- **Therapeutic options**
  Surgical hernia repair • In the case of prenatal diagnosis, in utero surgical treatment is an option • Management of pulmonary hypoplasia and RDS • ECMO may be required in severe cases.
- **Course and prognosis**
  Stillborn infant (35% of cases) • Death in the neonatal period (35% of cases) • Surgical mortality is 40–50%.
- **Complications**
  Bilateral pulmonary hypoplasia • Postoperative pulmonary hypertension • Pneumothorax may occur from ventilation of the hypoplastic lung • Associated with anomalies of the central nervous system (28% of cases), gastrointestinal tract (20%), cardiovascular system (13–23%), and urogenital tract (15%).

Differential Diagnosis

CCAM	– Multiple air-filled cystic structures of varying size – No sunken abdomen – Normal distribution of abdominal intestinal gas
Fluid-filled congenital lobar emphysema	– Normal distribution of abdominal intestinal gas – Diaphragm is well demarcated

Tips and Pitfalls

Bowel loops may be misinterpreted as a mass or pleural effusion in an immediate postpartum examination when the gastrointestinal tract has not yet filled with gas.

Selected Reference

Donnelly LF et al. Correlation between findings on chest radiography and survival in neonates with congenital diaphragmatic hernia. Am J Roentgenol 1999; 173: 1589–1593

Barnewolt CE et al. Percent predicted lung volumes as measured on fetal magnetic resonance imaging: a useful biometric parameter for risk stratification in congenital diaphragmatic hernia. J Pediatr Surg 2007; 42: 193–197

McCarten K et al. Delayed appearance of right diaphragmatic hernia associated with group B streptococcal infection in newborns. Radiology 1981; 139: 385–389

Definition

- **Epidemiology**
  Most common viral infection in infants and young children • Primarily occurs before the age of 2 years.
- **Etiology, pathophysiology, pathogenesis**
  Pathogen: Respiratory syncytial virus (RSV) • Accounts for over 50% of cases of acute bronchiolitis • Bronchiolar edema affects infants much more severely than older children, who develop the full clinical picture of bronchiolitis less often • Risk factors include chronic pulmonary disease and chronic cardiac disease • Incubation period is 5 days • Ciliary and goblet cell necrosis, and necrosis of the bronchial glands • Swelling of the respiratory mucosa with increased mucus production • Stenosis and obstruction of the respiratory tract.

Imaging Signs

- **Chest radiograph findings**
  Usually there is bilateral overinflation • Subsegmental atelectasis • Peribronchial cuffing (thickening of the bronchial wall) • Bilateral perihilar streaky densities • Nodular infiltrates may also be present • Hilar lymphadenopathy • Rarely pleural effusion.

Clinical Aspects

- **Typical presentation**
  Dyspnea • Cyanosis • Wheezing • Asthmalike symptoms • Abnormal auscultatory findings.
- **Therapeutic options**
  Oxygen • Bronchospasmolytic agents.
- **Course and prognosis**
  Usually resolves within 2 weeks • Mortality is less than 1%.
- **Complications**
  RSV bronchiolitis can be life-threatening in children with other disorders such as BPD or congenital heart defects • Dehydration • Secondary bacterial superinfection.

Differential Diagnosis

Neonatal period	– Group B streptococcal infection – Staphylococcal infecton (*Staphylococcus aureus* is found in about 90% of pleural effusions and empyemas and in 40–60% of cases of pneumatocele or pneumothorax) – CMV infection (no hilar lymphadenopathy or perihilar interstitial opacities) – *Candida albicans* infections

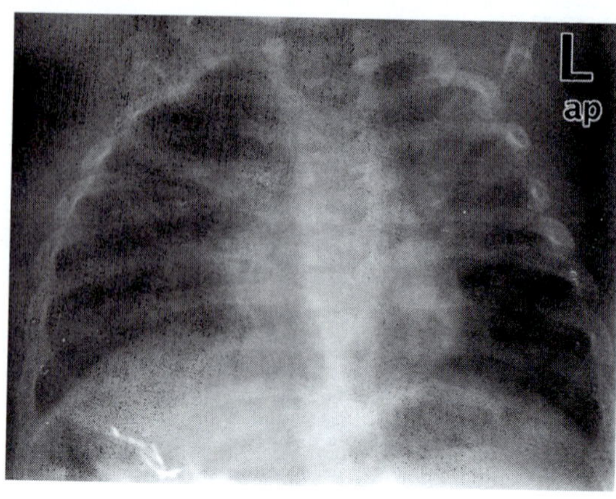

Fig. 1.17 RSV bronchiolitis. Chest radiograph of sitting patient (A-P). Overinflation of the left lung in particular, bilateral nodular infiltrates and atelectasis in both upper segments.

Infants	– Chlamydial infection (bilateral interstitial opacities, discrepancy between slight clinical symptoms and severe radiographic findings) – *Mycoplasma pneumoniae* infection
School-age children	– *Mycoplasma pneumoniae* infection (most common pathogen, rise in complement fixation titer is diagnostic, usually with bilateral hilar lymphadenopathy; interstitial pattern in the early stage, later alveolar pattern) – Influenza A viral infection – *Haemophilus influenzae* infection – Streptococcal infection – Staphylococcal infection (see above) – *Klebsiella* infection

Tips and Pitfalls

Without a patient history and clinical correlation, this disorder is easily confused with other infections considered in the differential diagnosis.

Selected References

Barr FE et al. The pharmacological mechanism by which inhaled epinephrine reduces airway obstruction in RSV associated bronchiolitis. J Pediatr 2000; 136: 699–700

Brooks AM et al. Predicting deterioration in previously healthy infants hospitalized with respiratory syncytial virus infection. Pediatrics 1999; 104: 463–467

Kirks DR. Practical Pediatric Imaging: Diagnostic Radiology of Infants and Children. Philadelphia: Lippincott-Raven, 1998

Swischuk LE. Imaging of the Newborn, Infant, and Young Child. Philadelphia: Williams & Wilkins; 1997; 111–116

Swischuk LE. Emergency Imaging of the Acutely Ill or Injured Children. Philadelphia: Williams & Wilkins; 2000: 1–15

Definition

- **Epidemiology**
  Rare in children younger than 2 years.
- **Etiology, pathophysiology, pathogenesis**
  Complication of lower respiratory tract infection • Hematogenous spread • Aspiration • Usually involves a circumscribed alveolar space • *Most common pathogen: Streptococcus pneumoniae* (70% of cases) • *Less common pathogens: Haemophilus influenzae, Mycoplasma pneumoniae, Moraxella catarrhalis, Chlamydia pneumoniae, Staphylococcus aureus.*

Imaging Signs

- **Chest radiograph findings**
  A single imaging plane is usually sufficient • Partially confluent alveolar opacities • Homogeneous segmental or lobar opacities • May also occur as a spherical lesion, mimicking a mass • Volume of the affected pulmonary lobe is increased • Adjacent fissure is displaced • Usually limited to a single pulmonary lobe • Associated pleural effusion may be present • Positive air bronchogram • Staphylococcal pneumonia may subsequently lead to formation of pneumatoceles.
- **CT findings**
  Usually not required in the absence of complications • *Empyema:* Thickening and enhancement of the parietal pleura, extrapleural soft tissue, and subcostal fatty tissue • *Pulmonary abscess:* Air and/or fluid-filled cavity with a thick, enhancing wall • *Cavitary necrosis:* Air and/or fluid-filled areas without enhancement of the walls in pneumonic areas of the lung with slight opacity • Used for guiding percutaneous drainage of empyema or pulmonary abscess.
- **Ultrasound findings**
  Peripheral pneumonia: Hypoechoic area in the air-filled lung • *Parapneumonic effusion:* Anechoic fluid in the pleural fissure • *Complicated effusion and/or empyema:* Pleural thickening, septation, fibrin strands, hyperechoic effusion components.

Clinical Aspects

- **Typical presentation**
  Dyspnea • Cyanosis • Wheezing • Fever • Coughing • Leukocytosis • Elevated C-reactive protein • Rattling respiration noise over the affected lung segment.
- **Therapeutic options**
  Antibiotics.
- **Course and prognosis**
  Usually resolves within 2 weeks • Radiographic follow-up is not necessarily indicated (may be advisable in a complication clinical course).
- **Complications**
  Parapneumonic effusion • Pleural empyema • Pneumatocele • Cavitary necrosis • Pulmonary abscess.

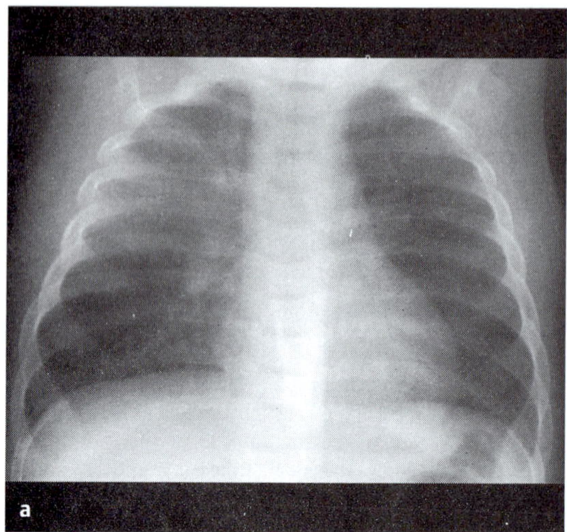

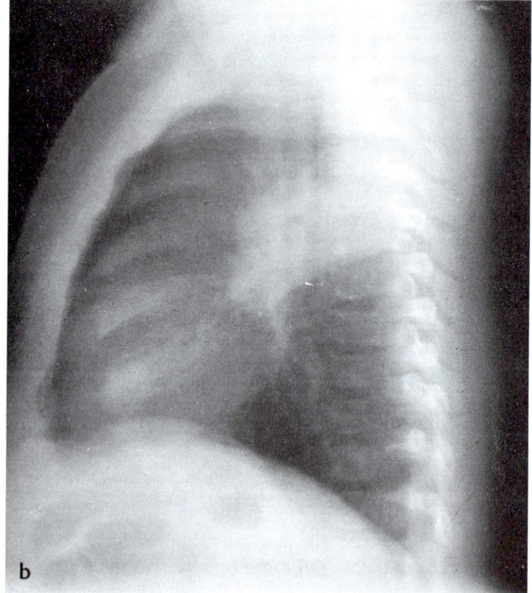

Fig. 1.18 a, b Segmental pneumonia in the upper lobe. Chest radiographs in two planes. Homogeneous shadowing of the right posterior upper lobe segment. No associated effusion, no marked ventilation disturbances or overinflation.

Differential Diagnosis

Masses from other causes	– Such as bronchogenic cysts or neuroblastoma – No air bronchogram – Second imaging plane may be helpful

Tips and Pitfalls

Inflammation can be misinterpreted as a mass.

Selected References

Coote N et al. Diagnosis and investigation of bacterial pneumonias. Paediatr Respir Rev 2000; 1: 8–13

Donnelly LF. Fundamentals of Pediatric Radiology. Philadelphia: Saunders; 2001

Virkki R et al. Differentiation of bacterial and viral pneumonia in children. Thorax 2002; 57: 438–441

Definition

- **Epidemiology**
  Incidence is 2.3:100 000 children • Children younger than 5 years are at greatest risk.
- **Etiology, pathophysiology, pathogenesis**
  Pathogen: Mycobacterium tuberculosis • The lung is the most common site of involvement (72% of cases) • Spread is via droplets • Incubation period is weeks to months • Stages include primary and postprimary tuberculosis.
  Primary tuberculosis: Children • Inhaled bacteria enter the bronchioles and alveoli • Focal inflammation • *Primary (Ranke's) complex:* Primary focal lesion in the pulmonary parenchyma (the Ghon focus), centripetal lymphangitis, and regional lymphadenitis in the hilum.
  - *Uncomplicated course:* Lesions in the pulmonary parenchyma and lymph nodes become fibrotic and calcify.
  - *Complicated course* (such as in newborns, infants, and immunosuppressed patients): Lymphatic, hematogenous, and canalicular seeding • Dissemination throughout the entire lung (miliary tuberculosis) and other organs.

  Postprimary tuberculosis: Adolescents and adults • Usually occurs years after the primary infection due to reinfection or renewed compromise to the immune system • Generalized disease and spread to organs.

Imaging Signs

- **Chest radiograph findings**
  Primary stage:
  Solitary small patch of infiltrate in the periphery of the lung (especially in the middle segments of the lung) with an acute primary focus • Ipsilateral polycyclic thickening of the hilum or widening of the mediastinum due to enlargement of the paratracheal lymph nodes • There may be streaky densities between the hilum and the primary focus • *Additional findings with enlarged hilar lymph nodes:* Local emphysema, partial or total collapse of the lung, secondary pneumonia • Pleural effusion (10% of cases) • With defective cell-mediated immunity, primary progressive pneumonia occurs with massive mediastinal lymphadenopathy and infiltration of the middle and lower lung segments • Miliary tuberculosis results from lymphatic and hematogenous spread following initial infection (especially in newborns)—finely nodular pattern in both lungs, enlarged hilar and mediastinal lymph nodes.
  Postprimary stage:
  - Solitary tuberculous foci in the apex of the lung: Simon apical focus • Assmann tuberculous infiltrate • Occasionally exudative pleuritis.
  - Miliary tuberculosis: Micronodular focal lesions especially in the upper lobes, more in the cranial areas than caudal areas • Unilateral or bilateral pleural effusion • Hilar or mediastinal lymph nodes are rarely involved.
  - Landouzy septicemia: Very rare • Occurs with immunodeficiency • Multiple extensive necroses without any tissue reaction.

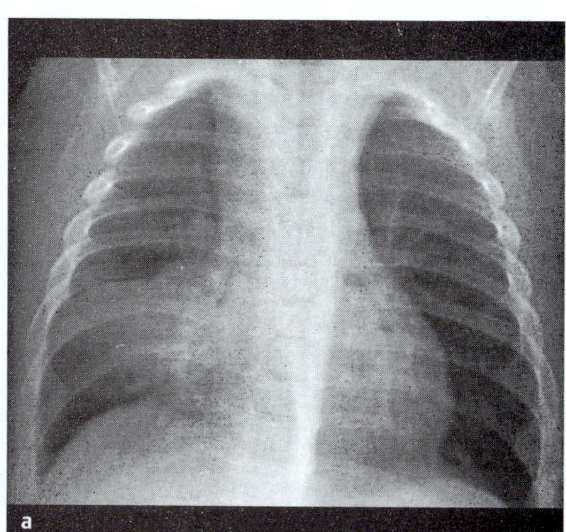

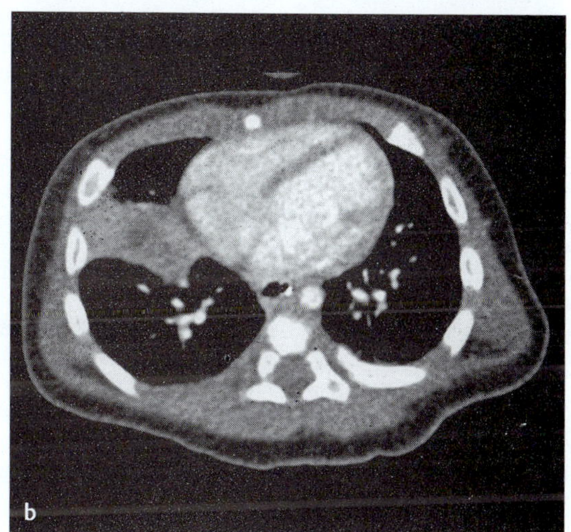

Fig. 1.19 a, b Tuberculosis. Chest radiograph (A-P) (**a**), axial contrast CT (**b**). Infant with primary tuberculosis and primary progressive pneumonia. Patchy infiltrate in the right middle lobe (**a, b**) with liquefaction (**b**).

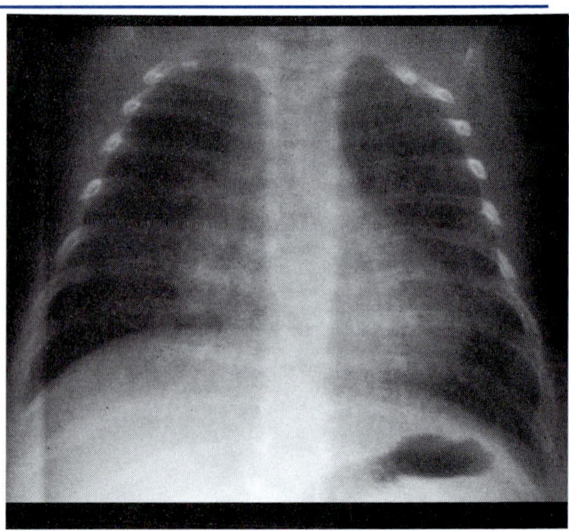

Fig. 1.20 Six-month-old infant with miliary tuberculosis. Chest radiograph (A-P). Disseminated finely nodular foci in both lungs. Enlarged hilar lymph nodes primarily on the right side.

Organ stage:

- Exudative tuberculosis: Nodular and/or patchy infiltrates • Predilection for the apical and posterior segment of the upper lobe and apical segment of the lower lobe.
- Cavernous tuberculosis: Thin-walled air-filled cavernous lesions.
- Fibrous cirrhotic tuberculosis: Pleural blistering • Apical streaky or bandlike parenchymal densities • Hilar displacement due to scarring • Calcifications • Bullous emphysema may be present • Bronchiectasis • Shrunken lung.

► **Contrast CT findings**

Method of choice in uncertain cases • Very sensitive in detecting enlarged hilar and mediastinal lymph nodes.

Primary stage: Enlarged lymph nodes may cause bronchial compression and tracheal displacement • Lymph node liquefaction (hypodense after contrast administration) • Lymph node calcifications • Infiltration with liquefaction in primary progressive tuberculous pneumonia • Multiple, sharply demarcated diffusely distributed intrapulmonary nodules in miliary tuberculosis.

Postprimary stage: Infiltration • Nodules • Cavernous lesions • Thickening of the bronchial wall.

► **MRI**

May be useful in excluding seeding to other organs.

► **Ultrasound**

Useful in detecting and quantifying pleural effusions.

Clinical Aspects

- **Typical presentation**
  Primary tuberculosis: Often subclinical • Signs of mild infection • Erythema nodosum occurs rarely • Rarely there are pulmonary symptoms such as coughing, sputum, or superinfection with fever due to compression from enlarged lymph nodes • Rarely there is progressive disease with lobar infiltration, development of cavernous lesions, and pleuritis.
  Postprimary tuberculosis: Anorexia • Fatigue • Weight loss • Chills • Night sweats • Coughing • Hemoptysis • Chest pain • *Lymph nodes:* Slightly painful swelling, occasionally with fistulas, usually in the neck and groin nodes.
  Miliary tuberculosis: Sudden onset with fever • Unspecific signs of sepsis • Pulmonary symptoms occur relatively late.
- **Therapeutic options**
  Isoniazid • Rifampicin • Pyrazinamide • Ethambutol • Streptomycin • Prothionamide.
- **Course and prognosis**
  The disorder usually subsides after the primary complex manifests itself • Clinical course is severe in newborns, infants, and immunosuppressed patients • Prognosis varies with the clinical manifestation • Prognosis is poor for patients with disseminated tuberculosis, miliary tuberculosis, and meningitis.
- **Complications**
  Pleural effusion • Pneumothorax • Atelectasis • Bronchiectasis • Bronchial stenosis • Endobronchial tuberculosis • Miliary tuberculosis • Pericardial effusion • Constrictive pericarditis • Cor pulmonale • Hematogenous seeding leading to involvement of bones, bowel, kidneys, central nervous system, and eye (rare).

Differential Diagnosis

Viral pneumonia	– Bilateral increase in perihilar signs, rarely unilateral – Thickening of the bronchial wall – Overinflation, atelectasis
Bacterial pneumonia	– Confluent alveolar densities – Homogeneous segmental or lobar opacities – Pleural effusion may be present
Fungal infections	– Lobar, interstitial, or bronchopneumonic infiltration – Pleural effusion is rare – Pleural effusion and involvement of the chest wall suggest actinomycosis or nocardiosis
Hodgkin disease	– Chimneylike widening of the mediastinum – Hilar lymphomas are not invariably present – Vascular compression is common – Bronchial obstruction is rare – Pleural effusion is rare

Non-Hodgkin lymphoma	– Usually unilateral mediastinal mass – Often not clearly demarcated from the lung
Sarcoidosis	– Bilateral hilar and/or mediastinal lymphadenopathy – Interstitial granulomatous changes

Tips and Pitfalls

- Tuberculosis should be considered in infants with unilateral enlarged hilar lymph nodes.
- An infiltrate initially suspected to be tuberculous that resolves within 3–6 weeks is inconsistent with tuberculosis.
- In cases of suspected tuberculosis, obtain an additional lateral chest radiograph for better visualization of the hilar lymph nodes. When in doubt, CT is helpful.

Selected References

Marais BJ et al. A proposed radiological classification of childhood intra-thoracic tuberculosis. Pediatr Radiol 2004; 34: 886–894

Powell DA et al. Tuberculosis in children: an update. Adv Pediatr 2006; 53: 279–322

Starke JR. Diagnosis of tuberculosis in children. Pediatr Infect Dis J 2000; 19: 1095–1096

Definition

- **Epidemiology**
  Most common congenital metabolic disorder in Europe (prevalence 1:2500) • No sex predilection • Rare in Africans and Asians • Risk of disease is 25% in patients with heterozygous parents and 1:50 where the mother has clinically important disease.
- **Etiology, pathophysiology, pathogenesis**
  Autosomal recessive genetic defect (CFTR, chromosome 7) • Defective chloride transport • Exocrine glands excrete increased quantities of highly viscous mucus • Alveolar and bronchial obstruction results • Trapped air leads to overinflated lung segments • Recurrent bacterial superinfection • Bronchiectasis.

Imaging Signs

- **Chest radiograph findings**
  Lung findings are normal in newborns • Earliest sign is focal and/or generalized overinflation • Thickening of the bronchial wall occurs later • Linear densities from peribronchial interstitial inflammation • *Bronchiectasis:* Round nodular shadows (mucopurulent plugging in bronchiectasis) or ring shadows (patent bronchiectasis) • Nodular infiltrates in bacterial superinfection • Atelectasis • Bullae • Enlarged hila (enlarged lymph nodes and/or pulmonary hypertension) • Interstitial emphysema • The upper lobe is affected more often than other segments of the lung • Cor pulmonale with signs of right heart strain occurs in the late stage.
- **CT (high-resolution CT) findings**
  Superior to plain radiography, especially in the early phase • Early characteristic findings include a mosaic perfusion pattern and air trapping on expiration • Thickening of the bronchial wall • Inflammatory interstitial streaky densities • Bronchiectasis (cylindrical, sacciform) • Mucus plugging • Acute infiltrates • Atelectasis • Bullae • Emphysema • Hilar lymphadenopathy • In the presence of complications, CT can detect or exclude aspergillosis or abscess • May be used prior to lung transplantation.

Clinical Aspects

- **Typical presentation**
  Initial manifestation involves gastrointestinal tract obstruction (meconium ileus or other pathology) in 10–15% of cases • Recurrent pulmonary infections • Obstruction • Chronic coughing • Failure to thrive • Sinusitis • Gallstones • Pancreatic insufficiency with diabetes mellitus and steatorrhea • Cirrhosis of the liver.
- **Therapeutic options**
  Mucolytic agents • Antibiotics • Physical therapy to help patient cough up viscous mucus • Increased caloric intake • Pancreatic enzymes • Insulin • Bronchial artery embolization in cases of hemoptysis • Lung transplant.

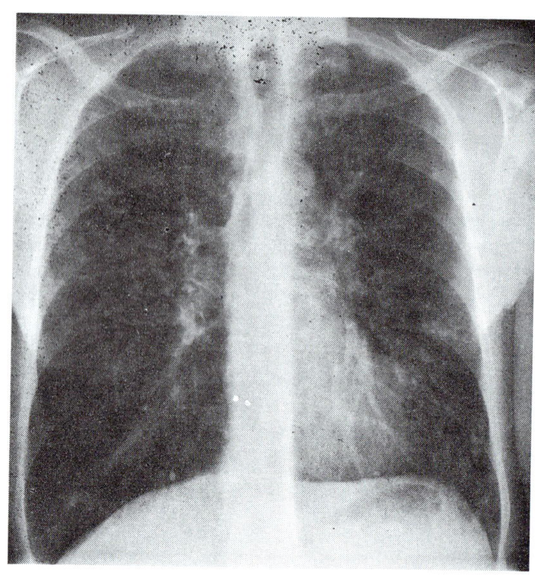

Fig. 1.21 Cystic fibrosis. Chest radiograph (A-P). Full picture of cystic fibrosis. Marked bilateral overinflation, bronchiectasis with severe mucopurulent plugging, bilateral fibrosis and scarring of the lung, bilateral hilar lymphadenopathy. No acute pneumonic infiltrates. No cor pulmonale.

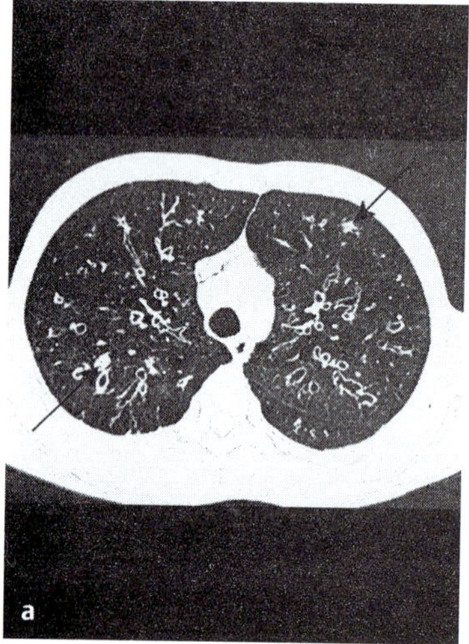

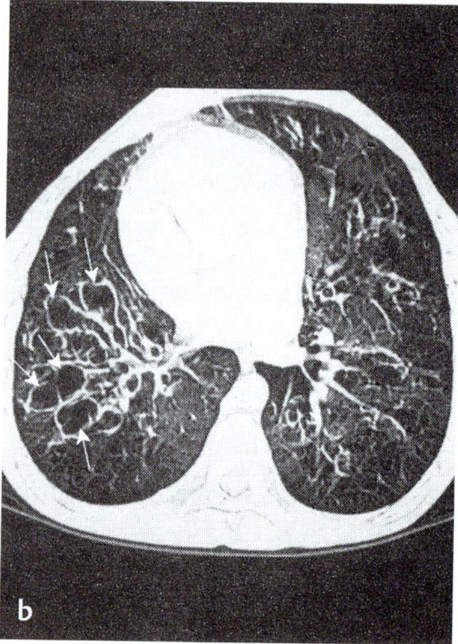

Fig. 1.22 a, b Cystic fibrosis. High-resolution CT. Thickening of the bronchial walls and increased interstitial densities. Cylindrical bronchiectasis, occasionally with mucopurulent plugging (**a**, arrows). Another patient with severe sacciform bronchiectasis, especially in the right lower lobe (**b**, arrows). Mosaic perfusion pattern indicative of regional hypoperfusion (**b**).

- **Course and prognosis**
  Prognosis depends on clinical course • Pulmonary findings are usually the decisive factor • Average life expectancy is over 40 years.
- **Complications**
  Pneumothorax • Pneumonia • Aspergillosis • Hemoptysis • Cor pulmonale • Pulmonary hypertension • Findings equivalent to meconium ileus (distal bowel obstruction syndrome) • Cirrhosis of the liver with portal hypertension • Pancreatic insufficiency.

Differential Diagnosis

Asthma	– History of allergy – Reversible pulmonary obstruction with thickening of the bronchial wall, overinflation, air trapping, and atelectasis – Bronchiectasis with mucoid impaction occurs less often in cases complicated by allergic bronchopulmonary aspergillosis
Primary ciliary dyskinesia syndrome	– Congenital dysfunction of the respiratory epithelium – Recurring sinus and bronchial infection – Situs inversus (Kartagener syndrome: complete situs inversus with bronchiectasis and sinusitis) – Less severe pulmonary pathology
Recurrent aspiration	– Common with neuromuscular disorders – Bronchiectasis often present in the lower lobe and posterior segments

Tips and Pitfalls

Misinterpreting the early signs of cystic fibrosis as an asthmatic disorder.

Selected References

Khoshoo V et al. Meconium ileus equivalent in children and adults. Am J Gastroenterol 1994; 89: 153–157

Moskowitz SM et al. Cystic fibrosis lung disease: genetic influences, microbial interactions, and radiological assessment. Pediatr Radiol 2005; 35: 739–757

Rossi UG et al. Radiology of chronic lung disease in children. Arch Dis Child 2005; 90: 601–607

Definition

- **Epidemiology**
  Age predilection: 5 months to 4 years.
- **Etiology, pathophysiology, pathogenesis**
  Aspiration of a foreign body (approximately 10% are radiopaque) into the tracheobronchial system • The commonly aspirated foreign bodies are peanuts, pieces of carrot, and plastic parts of toys • This may create a valve mechanism leading to overinflation of the affected lung segment • Complete bronchial obstruction causes atelectasis of the affected lung segment • Primarily involves the main bronchus • No clear predilection for either side • Aspirated food can absorb water and swell up • Oil, salt, and protein components in peanuts can irritate the mucosa and lead to edema and granulation tissue.

Imaging Signs

- **Chest radiograph findings**
  Films obtained on inspiration can be perfectly normal • A film should also be obtained on expiration • Obstructive emphysema is usually present • Volume of the affected lung can be normal or reduced • Asymmetric lung transparency • Atelectasis • Infiltrates • Pneumothorax and/or pneumomediastinum.
- **Fluoroscopic findings**
  Fluoroscopy and spot views show mediastinal deviation toward the normal side on expiration • Paradoxical movement of the diaphragm • Overinflation of the affected side is more pronounced on expiration.
- **Decubitus views**
  Indicated only where expiration films cannot be obtained • Horizontal projection with patient in right or left lateral position • The "lower" lung is normally less well ventilated • The lower lung does not collapse where the aspirated foreign body creates a valve mechanism.
- **CT findings**
  Uncertain cases require CT with thin slices (multidetector CT) • Highly sensitive in visualizing foreign bodies • Visualizes late sequelae of foreign body aspiration (chronic bronchitis, bronchiolitis obliterans, and bronchiectasis) • May detect other disorders considered in differential diagnosis.
- **MRI findings**
  Indicated in exceptional cases such as an aspirated peanut not detected on bronchoscopy • With their high fat content, peanuts appear hyperintense on T1-weighted images and contrast sharply against the hypointense lung tissue.

Clinical Aspects

- **Typical presentation**
  Coughing • Dyspnea • Cyanosis • Fever • Therapy-resistant stridor • May be asymptomatic.

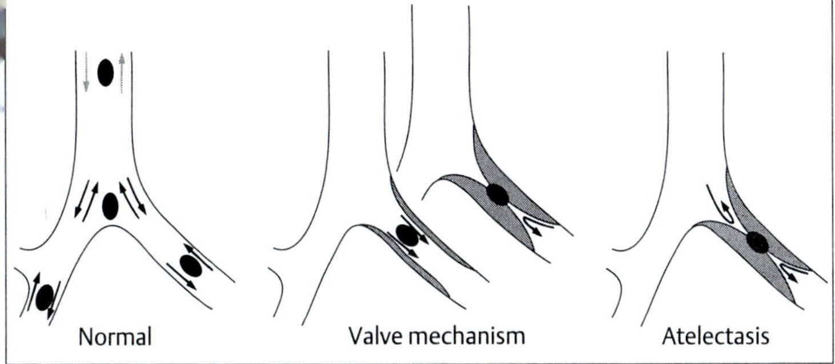

Fig. 1.23 Sequelae of foreign body inspiration according to the location and size of the foreign body (from Benz-Bohm G. Kinderradiologie. Stuttgart: Thieme; 2005).

- **Therapeutic options**
  Bronchoscopic extraction.
- **Complications**
  Therapy-resistant or recurrent pneumonia • Atelectasis • Pneumothorax and/or pneumomediastinum with bronchial wall rupture.

Differential Diagnosis

Bronchial asthma	– History – Symmetric overinflation of both sides of the lung – Thickening of the bronchial wall – Atelectasis
Bronchiolitis obliterans	– Overinflation with flattening of the diaphragm – Peribronchial infiltrates – Atelectasis – Mosaic perfusion pattern on high-resolution CT, bronchiectasis
Swyer-James syndrome	– Special form of bronchiolitis obliterans – Unilaterally increased transparency of the lung – Volume of the affected side is normal or reduced
Extrinsic tracheobronchial compression	– Pulmonary sling – Duplication of the aortic arch – Descending aorta on the right side
Endobronchial tumor	– Carcinoid

Tips and Pitfalls

- A very small foreign body may not cause any bronchial obstruction.
- Consider bilateral aspiration with symmetric ventilation.
- Migrating foreign bodies are associated with changing findings.

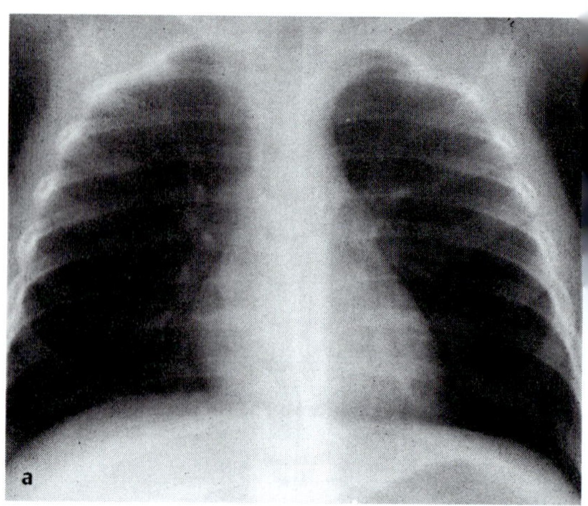

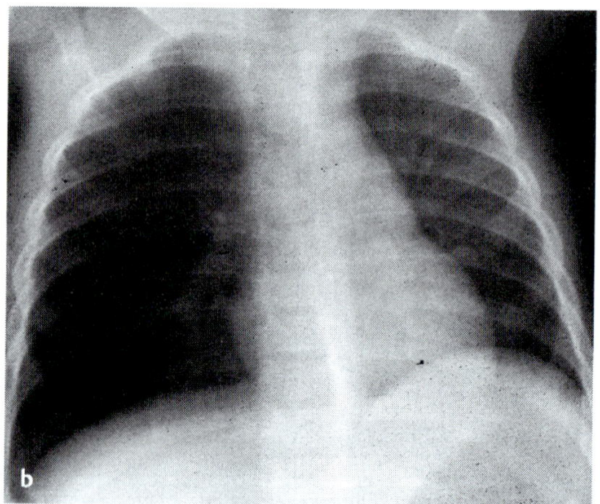

Fig. 1.24 a, b Foreign body aspiration. A-P spot views of the chest under fluoroscopy on inspiration (**a**) and expiration (**b**). Marked overinflation of the right lung with transient mediastinal shift to the contralateral side and paradoxical diaphragm movement on expiration. Aspiration of a peanut into the right main bronchus with resulting valve mechanism.

Selected References

Donnelly LF et al. The multiple presentations of foreign bodies in children. Am J Roentgenol 1998; 170: 471–477

Imaizumi H et al. Definitive diagnosis and location of peanuts in the airways using magnetic resonance imaging techniques. Ann Emerg Med 1994; 23: 1379–1382

Kosucu P et al. Low-dose MDCT and virtual bronchoscopy in pediatric patients with foreign body aspiration. Am J Roentgenol 2004; 183: 1771–1777

Definition

- **Epidemiology**
  Accounts for a quarter of the tumors of the anterior mediastinum in children • The anterior mediastinum is the second most common site of extragonadal teratomas • Frequently occur in Klinefelter syndrome • Usually detected only in early childhood and at school age.
- **Etiology, pathophysiology, pathogenesis**
  Disseminated pluripotential primordial germ cells • Consists of all three germ layers • Can contain tissue such as hair, bone, and fat.
  - Mature teratoma (solid).
  - Cystic teratoma (dermoid cyst).
  - Immature teratoma.
  - Malignant teratoma (teratocarcinoma, rare in children).
  - Mixed teratoma.

Imaging Signs

- **Chest radiograph findings**
  Well demarcated • In the anterosuperior mediastinum • Can exhibit variable density • Calcifications occur in 20–43% of all lesions (more common in benign forms) • Lobulation suggests malignancy • Presence of a tooth is pathognomonic • Pleural effusion suggests malignancy.
- **CT findings**
  Tumor of mixed density • Very sensitive in detecting fat, calcification, and cystic components • Septal or peripheral enhancement • Often indistinguishable from thymus • Lobulation suggests malignancy • Malignant form may be associated with infiltration of adjacent structures and metastases.
- **MRI findings**
  Particularly well suited for demonstrating the cystic character of the lesion (hyperintense on T2-weighted images) • Minute quantities of fat can be detected using the chemical shift (phase-contrast) technique • Patient is not subjected to ionizing radiation.

Clinical Aspects

- **Typical presentation**
  Often an asymptomatic incidental finding • Symptoms occur in large tumors with mass effect • Coughing • Dyspnea • Chest pain • Pulmonary infection • Rare in newborns; occurrence is associated with severe respiratory distress.
- **Therapeutic options**
  Surgical resection • Combined radiation and chemotherapy for malignant variant.
- **Course and prognosis**
  Treatment is curative (5-year survival rate is 100%).

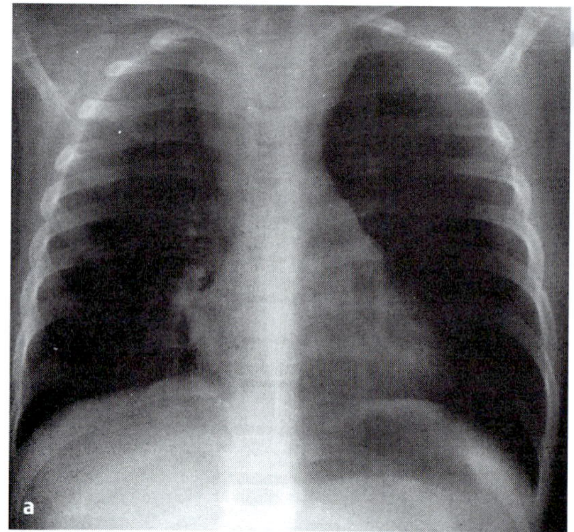

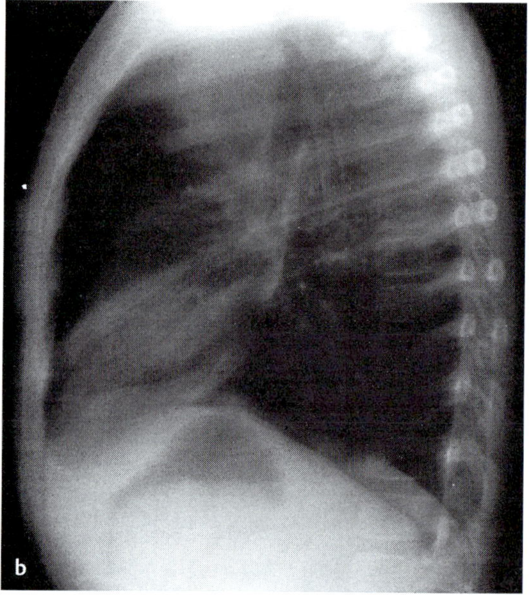

Fig. 1.25 a, b Mediastinal teratoma. A-P (**a**) and lateral (**b**) chest radiographs. Pronounced mass in the anterosuperior mediastinum with marked bilateral widening of the mediastinal shadow.

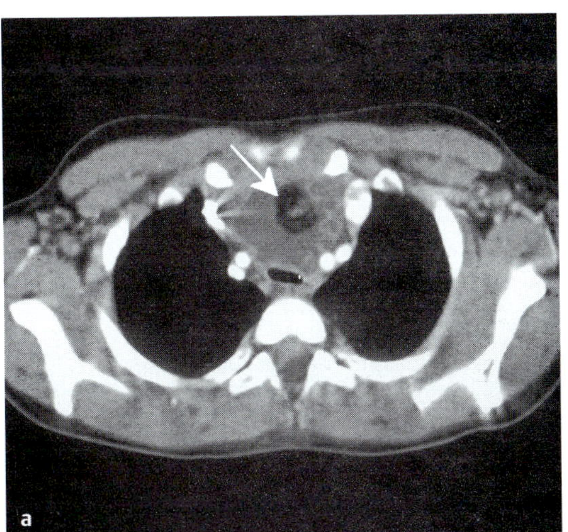

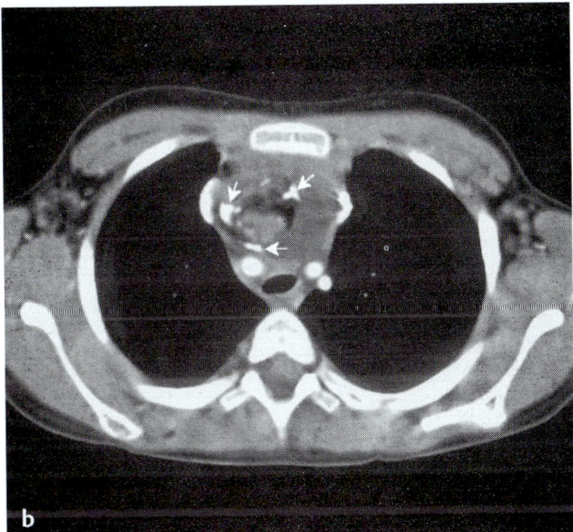

Fig. 1.26 a, b Contrast CT of the chest. The large mediastinal mass is clearly visualized. Pronounced displacement of the mediastinal vascular structures. The tumor contains fat, a pathognomonic finding (**a**, large arrow), and calcifications (**b**, small arrows).

▸ **Complications**

Compression and displacement of adjacent structures • Hemorrhaging from the tumor or vascular erosion • Shortness of breath due to rapid increase in size • Fistulas • Degeneration: in older children up to 10% of lesions become malignant.

Differential Diagnosis

Thymus	– Homogeneous density – Typical configuration – Typical ultrasound morphology – Size correlates with age
Thymoma	– Rare in children (age range 40–60 years) – Clinical symptoms with myasthenia gravis
Retrosternal goiter	– Rare in children – Pathology is regressive – Continuous with the thyroid
Mediastinal lymphoma	– Extrathoracic involvement is possible – "Chimney" configuration of the mediastinum – Usually homogeneous density on CT, occasionally with enhancement – No calcifications

Tips and Pitfalls

Can be misinterpreted as thymus or thymoma.

Selected References

Drevelegas A et al. Mediastinal germ cell tumors: a radiologic-pathologic review. Eur Radiol 2001; 11: 1925–1932

Erasmus JJ, McAdams HP, Donnelly LF, Spritzer CE. MR imaging of mediastinal masses. Magn Reson Imaging Clin N Am 2000; 8: 59–89

Jeung MY et al. Imaging of cystic masses of the mediastinum. Radiographics 2002; 22: 79–93

Definition

- **Epidemiology**
  Accounts for 8% of all pediatric cancer cases • The second most common solid tumors after brain tumors • Primarily occur in infants and young children (88% of patients are younger than 4 years old) • Boys are affected more often than girls (1.3:1).
- **Etiology, pathophysiology, pathogenesis**
  Sporadically occurring embryonal tumor of the sympathetic nervous system • Genetic factors are involved • Can mature into ganglioneuroblastoma or ganglioneuroma • 15% of lesions occur in the chest • 20% occur in the posterior mediastinum • In 50% of cases, the lesion has already metastasized at the time of diagnosis (lymph nodes, bone marrow, bone, liver, and skin) • Catecholamine metabolites are present in urine in 90% of cases • See neuroblastoma of the urogenital tract for staging.

Imaging Signs

- **Chest radiograph findings**
  Paravertebral • Round • Sharply demarcated • Erosion of the ribs or vertebral body • Pedicle erosion • Widening of the intercostal space • Calcifications.
- **MRI findings**
  Primary method of local staging • Usually homogeneously hyperintense on T2-weighted images • Hypointense on T1-weighted images • Marked enhancement • May exhibit intraspinal growth (hourglass tumors) • Spinal cord compression • Intracranial metastases may occur.
- **CT findings**
  Staging • Images usually show a large inhomogeneous mass that enhances with contrast • Hemorrhaging and necrosis are present in 50% of cases • Fine nodular calcifications are present in up to 85% of cases • Organ displacement • Tumorous sheath around vascular structures • No invasion of vascular structures • Lymphadenopathy • Metastases • Penetration into the spinal canal.
- **Nuclear imaging findings**
  MIBG (metaiodobenzylguanidine) imaging • Visualizes primary lesion and remote metastases • Tc (technetium) imaging may be indicated with bone involvement.
- **Ultrasound**
  Mass with inhomogeneous echogenicity • Better suited for abdominal diagnostics.

Clinical Aspects

- **Typical presentation**
  Usually asymptomatic • Mild respiratory tract obstruction • Stridor • Chronic coughing • Dysphagia • Bone pain • Headache • Fever • Weight loss • Swollen lymph nodes • Neurologic symptoms with intraspinal growth • Horner syndrome with cervical growth.

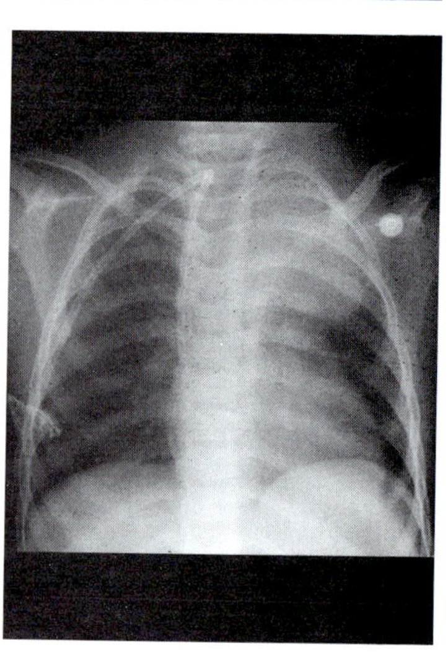

Fig. 1.27 Thoracic neuroblastoma in a 4-year-old girl. Chest radiograph (A-P). Large, sharply demarcated mass in the apex of the left lung. Hickman catheter in situ.

- **Therapeutic options**
  Surgical treatment • Chemotherapy • Radiation therapy • Bone marrow or stem cell transplantation in disseminated disease.
- **Course and prognosis**
  Depends on patient's age (infants younger than 12 months have a better prognosis), stage of the disease, location of the tumor and its genetic factors (poor prognosis with amplification of the N-myc oncogene) • Thoracic neuroblastoma has a better prognosis than abdominal neuroblastoma.
- **Complications**
  Neurologic complications (including paraplegia) with intraspinal tumor growth • Infections during treatment • Iatrogenic late sequelae • Recurrence.

Differential Diagnosis

Posterior pneumonia	– No rib erosion – No intraspinal mass – Positive air bronchogram
Bronchogenic cyst	– Can occur in paraspinal location – Cyst density values
Lymphoma	– Usually in anterior mediastinum (Hodgkin disease) – Usually homogeneous density, no calcifications
Pulmonary sequestration	– Typically in the lower lobe – Air inclusions in superinfection
Thoracic spondylodiskitis	– Widening of the paravertebral soft tissue – Height reduction in the disk interspace – Margins of the endplates are ill-defined

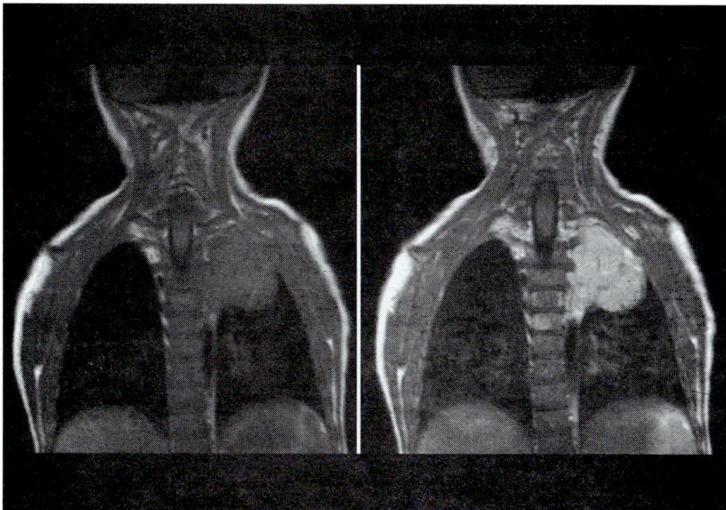

Fig. 1.28 Coronal T1-weighted MR images before and after contrast administration. Hypointense mass in the posterior mediastinum showing marked contrast enhancement (same patient as in Fig. 1.27).

Tips and Pitfalls

- Be alert to widening of the paravertebral shadow, enlargement of the neural foramina, and pedicle erosion.
- Can be mistaken for pneumonia.
- Fine nodular calcifications within the tumor are suggestive of the diagnosis.

Selected References

Kushner BH. Neuroblastoma: A disease requiring a multitude of imaging studies. J Nucl Med 2004; 45: 1172–1288

Mehta K et al. Imaging neuroblastoma in children. Crit Rev Comput Tomogr 2003; 44: 47–61

Pfluger T et al. Integrated imaging using MRI and 123 I metaiodobenzylguanidine scintigraphy to improve sensitivity and specificity in the diagnosis of pediatric neuroblastoma. Am J Roentgenol 2003; 181: 1115–1124

Strollo DC et al. Primary mediastinal tumors: part II. Tumors of the middle and posterior mediastinum. Chest 1997; 112: 1344–1357

Definition

▸ **Epidemiology**

Occurs rarely before age 3 years • Peak occurrence is at 15–35 years and after 65 years • Accounts for 5% of all malignant pediatric neoplasms • Boys are affected more often than girls (1.4:1).

▸ **Etiology, pathophysiology, pathogenesis**

Etiology remains unclear • Viruses have been postulated as causes • No hereditary risk factors.

- Nodular lymphocyte-predominant Hodgkin lymphoma.
- Classic Hodgkin lymphoma with four subtypes (lymphocyte predominance, nodular sclerosis [75% of tumors in the anterior mediastinum], mixed cellularity, lymphocyte depletion).

Stages (modified Ann Arbor classification):

- *Stage I:* Involvement limited to one lymph node region.
- *Stage II:* Involvement of two or more lymph node regions on the same side of the diaphragm.
- *Stage III:* Involvement of one or more lymph node regions on both sides of the diaphragm.
- *Stage IV:* Diffuse involvement of organs such as bone marrow and liver.
- *A:* No defined generalized symptoms.
- *B:* With fever, night sweats, weight loss.

Imaging Signs

▸ **Chest radiograph findings**

Enlarged hilar lymph nodes, occasionally with polycyclic margins • "Chimney" mediastinum (bilaterally widened superior mediastinum) • Tracheal displacement or stenosis • Occasionally, associated pleural effusion • Rarely pulmonary involvement with round focal lesions.

▸ **CT findings**

Demonstrates extent of lymph node involvement • Tumorous sheath around vascular structures without early compression • Sensitive in detecting pulmonary involvement • Primary method of thoracic staging • CT-guided aspiration can provide histologic information (needle core biopsy, Reed–Sternberg cells).

▸ **Ultrasound findings**

Useful in examining peripheral lymph node sites (such as neck ultrasound) • Initial abdominal staging.

▸ **MRI findings**

Not a routine study for thoracic staging • Mediastinal involvement • Recommended for cervical and abdominal staging • Bony structures.

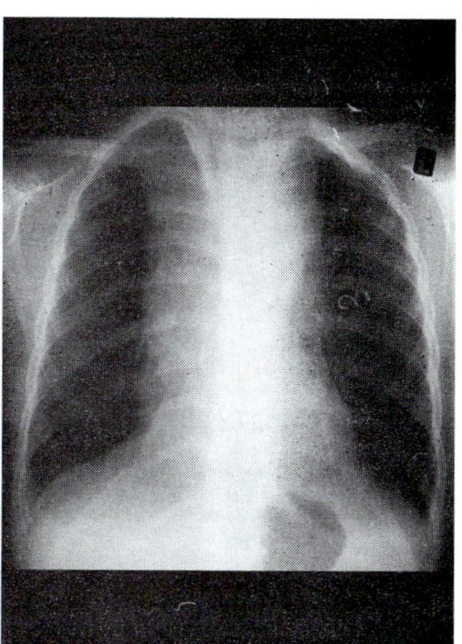

Fig. 1.29 Thoracic Hodgkin lymphoma. Chest radiograph (A-P). Pronounced mediastinal tumor masses with typical “chimney” configuration.

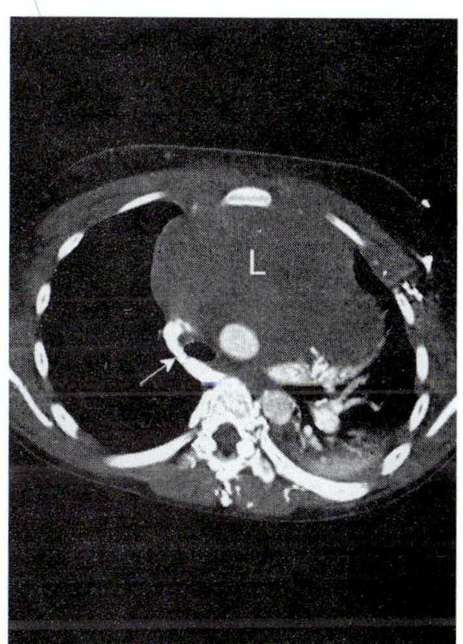

Fig. 1.30 Contrast CT of the chest. Massive mediastinal lymphoma (L) enveloping the central mediastinal vascular structures. The superior vena cava is completely compressed with collateral venous flow through the azygos vein (arrow) and veins of the chest wall.

Clinical Aspects

- **Typical presentation**
  Swollen lymph nodes • Type B symptoms (fever, weight loss, night sweats) • Superior inflow tract congestion • Hemoptysis • Splenomegaly.
- **Therapeutic options**
  Chemotherapy • Radiation therapy.
- **Course and prognosis**
  Cure rate of 90% with proper treatment.
- **Complications**
  Infections during treatment • Bone marrow transplants may be required • Pericardial infiltration (occasionally with pericardial effusion) • Thymus infiltration • Recurrence.

Differential Diagnosis

Non-Hodgkin lymphomas	– Mediastinal involvement is less common (50% of cases) – Often in middle or posterior mediastinum – There may be pulmonary involvement with cavitary necrosis of round focal lesions – Pleural effusion
Thymoma	– Rare in children (age range 40–60 years) – Myasthenia gravis
Teratoma	– Typically contains calcification and fat
T-cell leukemia, T-cell lymphoma of the thymus	– Not clearly distinguishable on imaging studies – More often associated with pleural effusion

Tips and Pitfalls

Can be misinterpreted as isolated enlarged paratracheal, paraaortic, or hilar lymph nodes (usually unspecific).

Selected References

Luker GD, Siegel MJ. Mediastinal Hodgkin disease in children: response to therapy. Radiology 1993; 189: 737–740

Schwartz CL. Special issues in pediatric Hodgkin's disease. Eur J Haematol Suppl 2005; 66: 55–62

White KS. Thoracic imaging of pediatric lymphomas. J Thorac Imaging 2001; 16: 224–237

Definition

- **Epidemiology**
  Most common vascular malformation of the aortic arch • Prevalence is 0.5% of the normal population, 30% of individuals with Down syndrome.
- **Etiology, pathophysiology, pathogenesis**
  An aberrant right subclavian artery arising distal to the left subclavian artery • Usually courses posterior to the esophagus to the right side • Rarely courses between the trachea and esophagus • Rarely, with a right aortic arch, the left subclavian artery will cross to the contralateral side posterior to the esophagus • Dysphagia because of esophageal compression • Stridor from tracheal compression.

Imaging Signs

- **Chest radiograph findings**
  Usually normal.
- **Barium swallow findings**
  Lateral view shows typical posterior impression of the esophagus • A-P view shows slight left caudal impression of the esophagus in a right cranial direction.
- **CT and MRI findings**
  Images precisely visualize the vascular anatomy and surrounding mediastinal structures • Delineation of associated malformations • Conventional angiography is not required.

Clinical Aspects

- **Typical presentation**
  Usually asymptomatic (incidental finding) • Rarely dysphagia • Extremely rarely patients present with coughing and stridor from tracheal impression.
- **Therapeutic options**
  Surgical transsection and mobilization of the aberrant right subclavian artery • Reimplantation of the artery into the ascending aorta may be indicated in symptomatic cases.
- **Complications**
  Infants with dysphagia who refuse food can develop dystrophy • Tracheal compression can lead to pulmonary complications.

Differential Diagnosis

Aberrant left subclavian artery	– Posterior impression – A-P film shows right caudal impression of the esophagus in a left cranial direction
Duplication of the aortic arch	– Bilateral impression of the esophagus – The right arch is usually more developed than the left arch

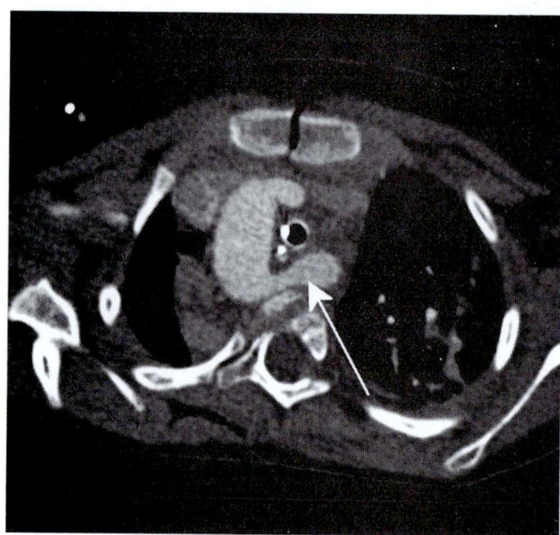

Fig. 2.1 Arteria lusoria. Contrast-enhanced CT. Right aortic arch, right descending aorta. The left subclavian artery courses posterior to the trachea and esophagus (gastric tube) to the left (arrow). Postoperative air inclusions secondary to sternotomy. Endotracheal tube.

Tips and Pitfalls

Do not neglect to visualize the esophagus in dystrophy of uncertain etiology and in recurrent bronchopulmonary infection.

Selected References

Bove T et al. Tracheobronchial compression of vascular origin. Review of experience in infants and children. J Cardiovasc Surg 2001; 42: 663–666

Donnelly LF et al. Aberrant subclavian arteries: cross-sectional imaging findings in infants and children referred for evaluation of extrinsic airway compression. AJR Am J Roentgenol 2002; 178: 1269–1274

Ulger Z et al. Arteria lusoria as a cause of dysphagia. Acta Cardiol 2004; 59: 445–447

Definition

- **Epidemiology**
  Accounts for 55% of vascular rings. Usually, there are no additional malformations.
- **Etiology, pathophysiology, pathogenesis**
  Persistent fourth branchial arterial arch • Two aortic arches arise from a single aorta • The arches join to form a single descending aorta • In 75% of cases, a left descending aorta is present • Each arch gives rise to a common carotid and a subclavian artery • In 80% of cases, the left arch is smaller, is further caudal, and courses anterior to the esophagus and trachea • The right arch usually courses posterior to the esophagus.

Imaging Signs

- **Chest radiograph findings**
  Tracheal compression (usually more severe on the right than left) • Tracheal stenosis and displacement • Paratracheal soft tissue may appear prominent.
- **Barium swallow findings**
  Broad horizontal impression at the level of T3 and T4 vertebrae • The A-P view shows bilateral esophageal compression • No longer indicated as a standard diagnostic study.
- **CT and MRI findings**
  CT angiography or MR angiography is indicated for preoperative planning • Visualization of double aortic arch and compression of esophagus and/or trachea • Multiplanar and 3D reconstructions have replaced conventional angiography.

Clinical Aspects

- **Typical presentation**
  Stridor • Dyspnea • Recurrent pneumonia in early childhood, occasionally immediately after birth • rarely dysphagia • Occasionally asymptomatic.
- **Therapeutic options**
  Thoracotomy with surgical transsection of the smaller arch.
- **Course and prognosis**
  Persistent respiratory problems due to tracheomalacia (aortopexy may be indicated).
- **Complications**
  Severe, life-threatening tracheal compression.

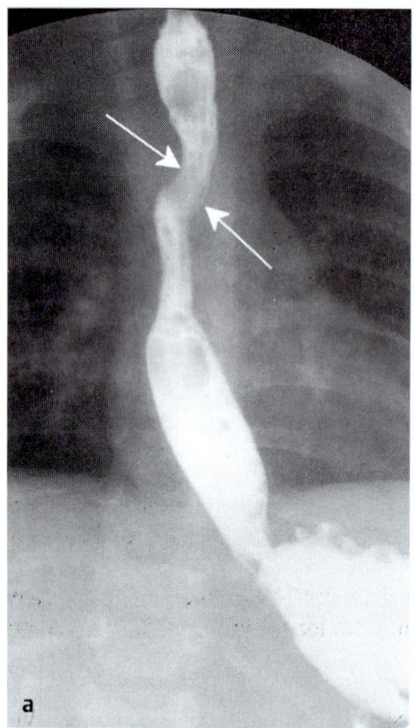

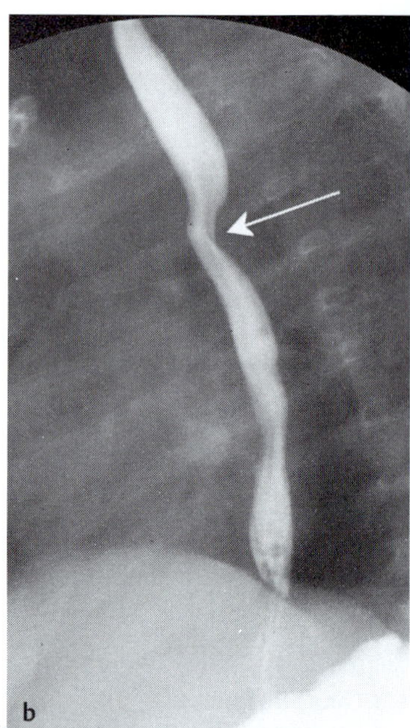

Fig. 2.2 a, b Double aortic arch. A-P (**a**) and lateral (**b**) views of barium swallow. Typical narrowing of the esophagus at the level of the aortic arch (arrows).

Differential Diagnosis

Right aortic arch with aberrant left subclavian artery	– Usually distinguishable only on cross-sectional images – Right retroesophageal aortic arch from which the left subclavian artery arises as the last branch of the abnormal arch – Ligamentum arteriosum extending from the descending aorta to the left pulmonary artery, compressing the trachea and esophagus
Aberrant origin of the left pulmonary artery	– Posterior tracheal compression on chest radiograph
Mediastinal tumor	– Further diagnostic workup with CT and/or MRI

Tips and Pitfalls

- Missing an arteria lusoria on an equivocal chest radiograph.
- Additional diagnostic studies are indicated wherever typical symptoms are present.

Selected References

Cerillo AG et al. Sixteen-row multislice computed tomography in infants with double aortic arch. Int J Cardiol 2005; 99: 191–194

Funabashi N et al. Images in cardiovascular medicine. Double aortic arch with a compressed trachea demonstrated by multislice computed tomography. Circulation 2004; 110: 68–69

Yilmaz M et al. Vascular anomalies causing tracheoesophageal compression: a 20-year experience in diagnosis and management. Heart Surg Forum 2003; 6: 149–152

Definition

- **Epidemiology**
  Accounts for 5–8% of all congenital heart defects • Sex predilection: Four times more common in boys than in girls.
- **Etiology, pathophysiology, pathogenesis**
  Stenosis at the junction of the aortic arch and descending aorta • Concentric hypertrophy of the left ventricle due to increase in systemic vascular resistance.
  - *Preductal:* Infantile type • Long hypoplastic aortic segment distal to the origin of the brachiocephalic trunk • Often combined with cardiac anomalies • Usually associated with patent ductus arteriosus
  - *Postductal:* Adult type • Short stenosis distal to the origin of the ductus arteriosus • Usually no cardiac anomalies • Often an incidental finding • Ductus arteriosus is usually obliterated.

  Arterial hypertension in the upper half of the body • Hypotension distal to the stenosis.
  Collaterals: From the subclavian artery to the intercostal arteries, anterior spinal artery, internal thoracic artery, lateral thoracic arteries, cervical arteries.
  Associated malformations: Bicuspid aortic valve (25–50% of cases), intracardiac anomalies (up to 30% of cases, e.g., ventricular septal defect), Turner syndrome (up to 36%), cerebral aneurysms, mycotic aneurysm distal to the coarctation, Shone complex (supravalvular mitral stenosis, “parachute” mitral valve, subaortic stenosis and coarctation of the aorta), additional anomalies of the supraaortic vessels.

Imaging Signs

- **Chest radiograph findings**
  Rib notching (>age 10) • Widening of the upper mediastinum to the right (dilation of the ascending aorta proximal to the stenosis) • “Triple” sign (notching of the left superior margin of the mediastinum at the junction of the aortic arch and descending aorta).
  Symptomatic aortic coarctation: Signs of cardiac insufficiency • Generalized cardiomegaly • Pulmonary hyperemia • Pulmonary venous congestion.
  Asymptomatic aortic coarctation: Apex of the heart is normal or elevated • Supraaortic vessels are dilated (hypertension).
- **Barium swallow**
  No longer a standard study (“reverse triple” sign, epsilon sign).
- **Echocardiographic findings**
  Location and extent of the stenosis.

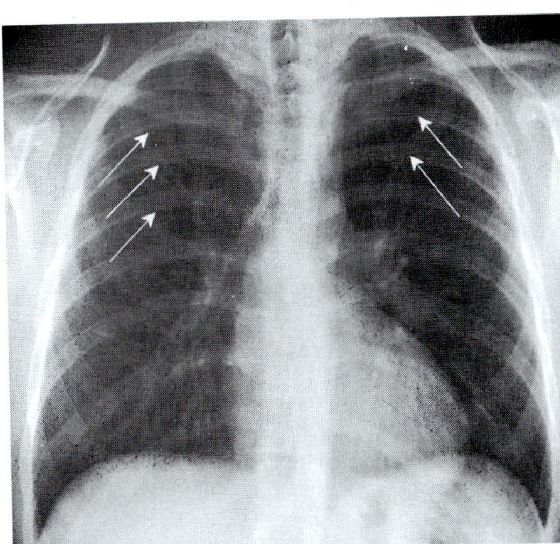

Fig. 2.3 Coarctation of the aorta. A-P chest radiograph. Moderate coarctation of the aorta with typical rib notching that develops with collateral circulation via the intercostal arteries.

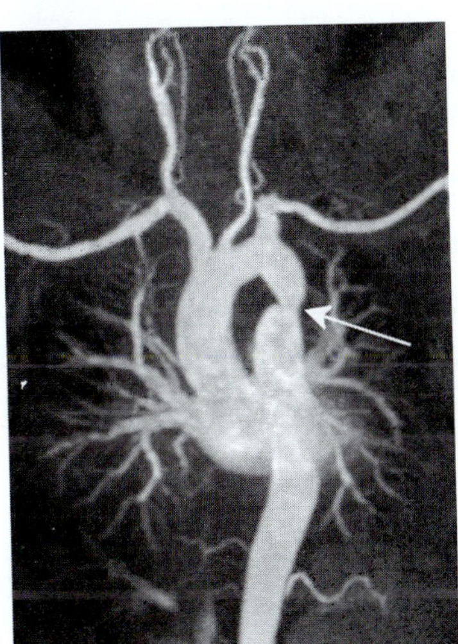

Fig. 2.4 MIP reconstruction of a contrast-enhanced 3D MR angiogram. Postductal coarctation of the aorta (arrow).

- **MRI findings**
  - *ECG-triggered T1-weighted SE images (black blood):* Location and extent of the stenosis (sagittal-oblique plane through the aortic arch) • Axial diameter of the stenosis (paraxial-oblique plane).
  - *Gradient echo cine sequences (white blood):* Anatomy (sagittal-oblique plane) • Systolic flow jet (black) • Aortic regurgitation (bicuspid aortic valve).
  - *Phase-contrast angiography:* Flow gradient • Collaterals.
  - *3D contrast-enhanced MR angiography:* Anomalous origins of the vessels arising from the aortic arch • Collaterals.
- **Angiography**
  Not necessarily indicated • Interventional procedure • Pressure gradient.

Clinical Aspects

- **Typical presentation**
  Severe stenosis and lack of collateral circulation leads to cardiac insufficiency in infants • Condition may long remain asymptomatic • Bruit also audible between the scapulae and over the abdominal aorta • Hypertension in the upper half of the body • There may be associated stroke • Headache • Epistaxis • Recurrent lower leg pain • Weakened femoral pulse • Pulsation or systolic murmur in the throat.
- **Therapeutic options**
  - *Medical:* Prostaglandin can be administered to newborns to delay closure of the ductus arteriosus to ensure perfusion of the lower body • Management of cardiac insufficiency.
  - *Surgical:* Resection of the aortic coarctation and ductus arteriosus tissue • End-to-end anastomosis • Prosthetic patch aortoplasty.
  - *Interventional:* Balloon angioplasty (palliative or in residual stenosis).
- **Course and prognosis**
  Mortality: 11 % prior to the age of 6 months • Surgical risk of isolated postductal aortic coarctation: 0–3.5 %.
- **Complications**
  Renal insufficiency due to decreased perfusion of the lower half of the body. *Postoperative:* Residual stenosis (32 % of cases) • Chronic persistent hypertension • Mesenteric arteritis • Recurrent stenosis following surgery in newborns is common (15–20 % of cases) • Postoperative aneurysm (24 % of patients receiving patch angioplasty).

Differential Diagnosis

Discontinuous aortic arch	– Complete discontinuity – Blood flows into the descending aorta via patent ductus arteriosus
Pseudo-coarctation	– Kinking of the aortic arch without stenosis
Takayasu arteritis	– Inflammatory process of the aortic wall – Contrast enhancement of the vascular wall – Involvement of the supraaortic vessels – Chronic course leads to stenosis or occlusion of the aorta and its branches

Tips and Pitfalls

Typical radiographic appearance is often absent in the early phase • Further imaging studies are indicated.

Selected References

Dähnert W. Radiology Review Manual. Coarctation of Aorta. Philadelphia: Lippincott Williams & Wilkins; 2002: 622–623

Didier D et al. Coarctation of the aorta: pre- and postoperative evaluation with MRI and MR angiography: correlation with echocardiography and surgery. Int J Cardiovasc Imaging 2005; 3: 1–19

Fiore AC et al. Comparison of angioplasty and surgery for neonatal aortic coarctation. Ann Thorac Surg 2005; 80: 1659–1665

Uddin MJ et al. Surgical management of coarctation of the aorta in infants younger than five months: a study of 51 Patients. Ann Thorac Cardiovasc Surg 2000; 6: 252–257

Definition

- **Epidemiology**
  Accounts for 3–6% of all malformations of the aortic arch.
- **Etiology, pathophysiology, pathogenesis**
  Etiology is not clear • Defective development of sixth branchial arterial arch • The left pulmonary artery arises from the right pulmonary artery • The left pulmonary artery courses between the trachea and esophagus, passing to the left above the right main bronchus.

Imaging Signs

- **Chest radiograph findings**
  Posterior tracheal compression in the distal segment or directly precarinal • Distal trachea or right main bronchus may be anteriorly displaced • Left hilum is displaced caudally • Lung volume may be asymmetric • Emphysema or atelectasis of the right and/or left half of the lung due to bronchial compression.
- **Barium swallow findings**
  Anterior compression of the esophagus • Not part of standard diagnostic procedure.
- **CT and MRI findings**
  CT angiography or MR angiography is indicated for preoperative planning • Visualization of pulmonary artery sling and tracheal compression • Multiplanar and 3D reconstructions have replaced conventional angiography.

Clinical Aspects

- **Typical presentation**
  Stridor • Dyspnea • Recurrent pneumonia in early childhood, occasionally immediately after birth • Rarely dysphagia • Can be asymptomatic.
- **Therapeutic options**
  Reimplantation of the aberrant vessel.
- **Course and prognosis**
  Symptoms often persist postoperatively (due to hypoplasia or dysplasia of the trachea and main bronchi).
- **Complications**
  Often associated with other congenital disorders such as heart defects (e.g., patent ductus arteriosus or atrial septal defect).

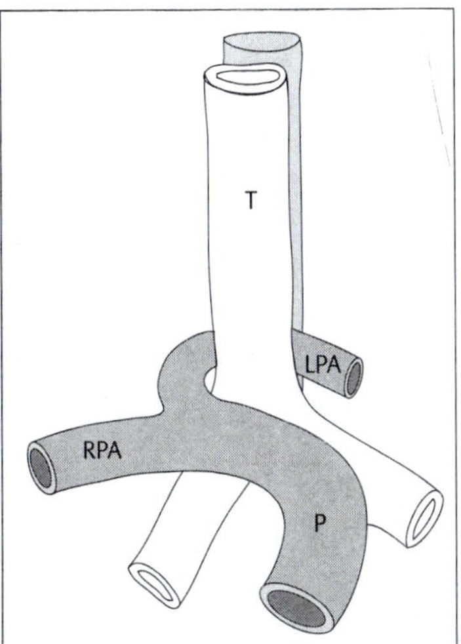

Fig. 2.5 Pulmonary artery sling. Schematic diagram of vascular anatomy (anterior aspect) (from Benz-Bohm G. Kinderradiologie. Stuttgart: Thieme; 2005).

LPA: Left pulmonary artery
P: Pulmonary artery
RPA: Right pulmonary artery
T: Trachea

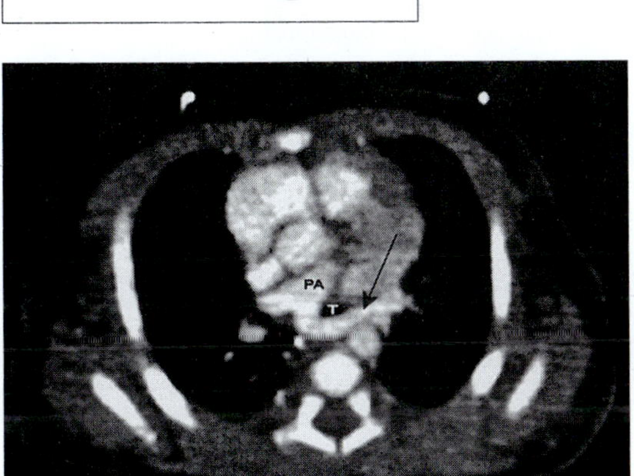

Fig. 2.6 CT after contrast administration. Left pulmonary artery sling (arrow) arising from the right pulmonary artery (PA) and coursing to the left between the trachea (T) and esophagus (marked by a gastric tube).

Differential Diagnosis

Right aortic arch with aberrant left subclavian artery	– Usually distinguishable only on cross-sectional images – Right retroesophageal aortic arch from which the left subclavian artery arises as the last branch of the abnormal arch – Ligamentum arteriosum extending from the descending aorta to the left pulmonary artery, compressing the trachea and esophagus
Duplication of the aortic arch	– Tracheal compression, usually more severe on the right than on the left – Tracheal compression at the right margin often more severe than at the left margin – Posterior tracheal compression and displacement
Mediastinal tumor	– Further diagnostic workup with CT and/or MRI

Tips and Pitfalls

Missing this pathology on an equivocal chest radiograph.

Selected References

Bove T et al. Tracheobronchial compression of vascular origin. Review of experience in infants and children. J Cardiovasc Surg 2001; 42: 663–666

Sebening C et al. Vascular tracheobronchial compression syndromes – experience in surgical treatment and literature review. Thorac Cardiovasc Surg 2000; 48: 164–174

Woods RK et al. Vascular anomalies and tracheoesophageal compression: a single institution's 25-year experience. Ann Thorac Surg 2001; 72: 434–439

Definition

- **Epidemiology**
  Accounts for less than 1% of all congenital heart defects • No sex predilection • Usually occurs spontaneously • Probably increasingly seen in children of mothers taking lithium (for depression) during the first trimester of pregnancy.
- **Etiology, pathophysiology, pathogenesis**
  The rudimentary septal and posterolateral tricuspid leaflets are displaced into the right ventricle • Usually there is tricuspid insufficiency • The right ventricle is small and atrialized • Occasionally only the outflow tract remains • Therefore only a small volume is ejected into the pulmonary vascular system (which is possibly, in addition, hypoplastic) • 50% of cases involve a patent foramen ovale or an atrial septal defect (septum secundum defect) • Degree of increased resistance of the pulmonary flow tract determines the extent of the right-to-left shunt through patent foramen ovale • Volume overload to the right heart • Eventually left ventricular dysfunction may be present because of massive right-sided cardiomegaly.

Imaging Signs

- **Chest radiograph findings**
  Massive right heart ("box-shaped" heart) • Small vascular pedicle due to hypoplastic segment of the pulmonary artery • Lung perfusion may be reduced depending on the severity of the right-to-left shunt.
- **Echocardiographic findings**
  Displaced tricuspid valve with atrialized portion of right ventricle • Patent foramen ovale or atrial septal defect (septum secundum defect) with shunt flow • Tricuspid regurgitation.
- **MRI findings**
  - *ECG-triggered T1-weighted SE images, long axis:* Visualization of the anatomy.
  - *GE cine-MRI and SSFP sequences:* Valve morphology and function • Volumetric measurements.
  - *Phase-contrast angiography:* Shunt flow.
- **Angiography**
  Seldom required for primary diagnosis.

Clinical Aspects

- **Typical presentation**
  Approximately in 50% of cases, patients are asymptomatic at the time of birth • Cyanosis • Right heart insufficiency • Cardiac arrhythmia (typically atrial fibrillation) • Systolic and diastolic murmurs in the parasternal left fourth intercostal space • Minimal exercise tolerance.
- **Therapeutic options**
  Medical management of cardiac arrhythmia • Reconstruction or replacement of the tricuspid valve • Correction of associated heart defects, such as repair of an atrial septal defect.

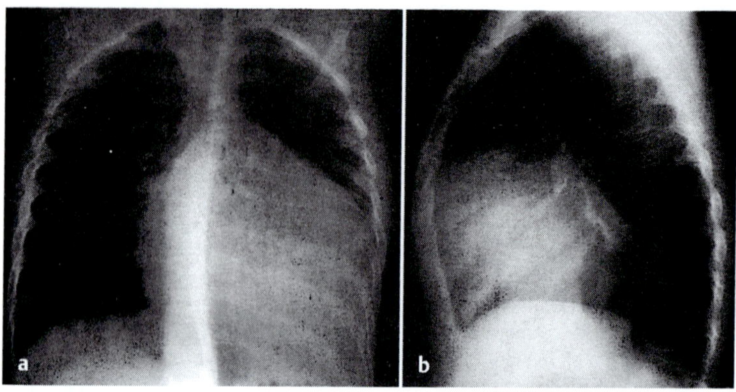

Fig. 2.7 a, b Uncorrected Ebstein anomaly. A-P (**a**) and lateral (**b**) chest radiographs. Massive enlargement of the right heart with box shape and moderately reduced delineation of pulmonary vascular structures.

- **Course and prognosis**
  Depends on the hemodynamic situation • Child may not have any symptoms.
- **Complications**
  Sudden cardiac death in atrial arrhythmia • Paradoxical embolism in atrial septal defect with stroke.

Differential Diagnosis

Large pericardial effusion	– Acyanotic – Distinguishable on ultrasound
Large atrial septal defect	– Acyanotic – Increased lung perfusion – Left-to-right shunt at the level of the atrium
Multivalvular defect or tricuspid insufficiency	– Echocardiography is diagnostic

Tips and Pitfalls

Can be mistaken for pericardial effusion or multivalvular defect.

Selected References

Ammash NM et al. Mimics of Ebstein's anomaly. Am Heart J 1997; 134: 508–513

Attenhofer Jost CH et al. Ebstein's anomaly. Circulation 2007; 115: 277–285

Celermajer DS et al. Outcome in neonates with Ebstein's anomaly. J Am Coll Cardiol 1992; 19: 1041–1046

Cohen LS et al. A reevaluation of risk of in utero exposure to lithium. JAMA 1994; 271: 146–150

Definition

- **Epidemiology**
  Accounts for 7–10% of all congenital heart defects • Predilection for male sex • Most common cyanotic heart defect • Often occurs in Down syndrome, Noonan syndrome, and other chromosome anomalies.
- **Etiology, pathophysiology, pathogenesis**
  Typical findings: Pulmonary stenosis • Ventricular septal defect • Aortic dextroposition (overriding aorta) • Right heart hypertrophy • Always right-to-left shunt • Infundibular right ventricular outflow tract obstruction (severity increases with age) leading to reduced blood ejection of the right ventricle into pulmonary artery with consecutive right-left-shunt via ventricular septal defect • *Pentalogy of Fallot:* in addition to typical findings an atrial septal defect • Reduced pulmonary perfusion can be partially compensated by patent ductus arteriosus or MAPCAs • *Associated anomalies:* Coronary arterial anomalies (10% of cases) • Bicuspid pulmonary valve (49% of cases) • Stenosis of the left pulmonary artery (40% of cases).

Imaging Signs

- **Chest radiograph findings**
  Heart configuration is usually normal in infants • Later classic "boot-shaped" heart (cardiac apex is elevated and rounded) • No pulmonary segment present • Decreased pulmonary vascularity with an increase of lung transparency • Delineation of pulmonary vascular structures later increases due to development of MAPCAs • In 25% of cases right aortic arch with right descending aorta • Blalock–Taussig shunt can be identified on A-P films by its sharp lateral convex margin in the superior mediastinum.
- **Echocardiographic findings**
  Reliable modality for diagnosing the disorder • Visualizes cardiac anomalies • Demonstrates shunt flow.
- **MRI**
  - *ECG-triggered axial T1-weighted SE images:* Preoperative anatomy of the pulmonary artery • Postoperative patency of the Blalock–Taussig shunt.
  - *GE cine and SSFP sequences in short axis:* Right ventricular function.
  - *Phase-contrast MR angiography:* Right ventricular function • regurgitation.
  - *3D contrast-enhanced MR angiography:* Anatomy • MAPCAs • Coronary arteries.
- **Angiographic findings**
  Coronary arterial anatomy • Balloon angioplasty of the pulmonary stenosis • Visualization of MAPCAs.

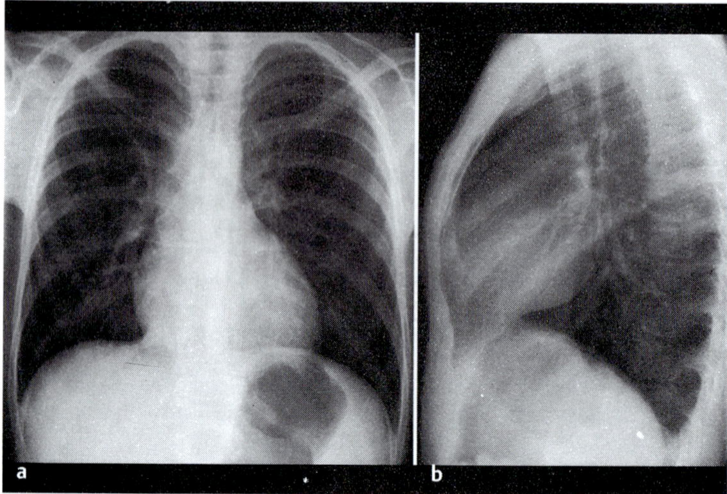

Fig. 2.8 a, b Tetralogy of Fallot. P-A (**a**) and lateral (**b**) chest radiographs. Right ventricular hypertrophy and enlarged retrosternal contact area on the lateral film. Empty pulmonary bay, dextropositioned aortic arch. Central pulmonary vascularity is not much reduced.

Clinical Aspects

- **Typical presentation**

  Postpartum systolic heart murmur • Newborn may not be initially cyanotic • Cyanosis develops after one year at the latest • Impaired exercise tolerance and growth failure may occur • Polycythemia • Clubbing of fingers and toes • Cardiac arrhythmia • Episodic attacks of unconsciousness and seizures • Hypoxemic episodes with squatting posture.

- **Therapeutic options**

  Endocarditis prophylaxis • *Palliative Blalock–Taussig shunt:* End-to-side anastomosis of the subclavian artery to the pulmonary artery • *Palliative modified Blalock–Taussig shunt:* Interposition of a graft • Palliative central aortopulmonary shunt between the ascending aorta and pulmonary artery • *Surgical repair:* Correction of the right ventricular outflow tract obstruction and closure of the ventricular septal defect.

- **Course and prognosis**

  Ten percent of untreated patients survive beyond 20 years of age • Good prognosis after early surgical correction. • Long-term results depend on the degree of right ventricular dysfunction.

▸ **Complications**
Hypoxemic episodes (often cause of death) • Paradoxical embolism (such as in the brain) • Bacterial endocarditis • Right heart insufficiency with heart failure.

Differential Diagnosis

Pulmonary atresia with ventricular septal defect and MAPCAs	– Distinguishable on echocardiography
Tricuspid atresia with ventricular septal defect	– Distinguishable on echocardiography

Tips and Pitfalls

Usually a definitive diagnosis can be made with imaging procedures.

Selected References

Haramati LB et al. MR imaging and CT of vascular anomalies and connections in patients with congenital heart disease: significance in surgical planning. Radiographics 2002; 22: 337–349

Tongsong T et al. Prenatal sonographic diagnosis of tetralogy of Fallot. J Clin Ultrasound 2005; 33: 427–431

Wu ET et al. Balloon Valvuloplasty as an initial palliation in the treatment of newborns and young infants with severely symptomatic tetralogy of Fallot. Cardiology 2005; 105: 52–56

Definition

- **Epidemiology**
  Accounts for 4–6% of all congenital heart defects • Twice as common in boys than in girls.
- **Etiology, pathophysiology, pathogenesis**
  Congenital heart defect with primary cyanosis • During embryonal development incorrect separation of aorta and pulmonary artery from primitive bulbus cordis • Aorta arises from the anatomic right ventricle and the pulmonary artery from the anatomic left ventricle • Atria and ventricles are morphologically normal • The aorta is anterior and usually to the right of the pulmonary artery (the "d" in d-transposition indicates aortic dextroposition) • Pulmonary circulation and systemic circulation are separate • This produces a volume overload on the left ventricle and the right ventricular overload due to the vascular resistance • Postpartum survival is possible only with a shunt as in patent foramen ovale, atrial septal defect (ostium secundum), ventricular septal defect, or patent ductus arteriosus • Often there is a left ventricular outflow tract obstruction (subpulmonary stenosis) • Anomalies of the coronary arteries are often present as well.
  There are three morphological groups:
  - D-transposition with intact ventricular septum (50% of cases).
  - D-transposition with ventricular septal defect (25% of cases).
  - D-transposition with pulmonary stenosis with or without ventricular septal defect (25% of cases).

Imaging Signs

- **Chest radiograph findings**
  A-P radiograph may be normal • Pulmonary artery segment is absent • The superior mediastinum is narrowed • The heart is enlarged (appearing like an "egg on its side") • In ventricular septal defect, pulmonary vascularity is increased • In subpulmonary stenosis, pulmonary vascularity is reduced.
- **Echocardiographic findings**
  Quick and reliable diagnosis.
- **MRI findings**
  ECG-triggered T1-weighted SE images, GE cine and SSFP sequences, and 3D contrast-enhanced MR angiography • Anatomical visualization of the great vessels • Presence of patent foramen ovale, patent ductus arteriosus, and ventricular septal defect • Subpulmonary stenosis may be demonstrated • Especially useful in diagnosing postoperative complications.
- **Angiography**
  Not necessarily indicated preoperatively • May be used to measure pressure • May be useful in palliative procedures (Rashkind procedure).

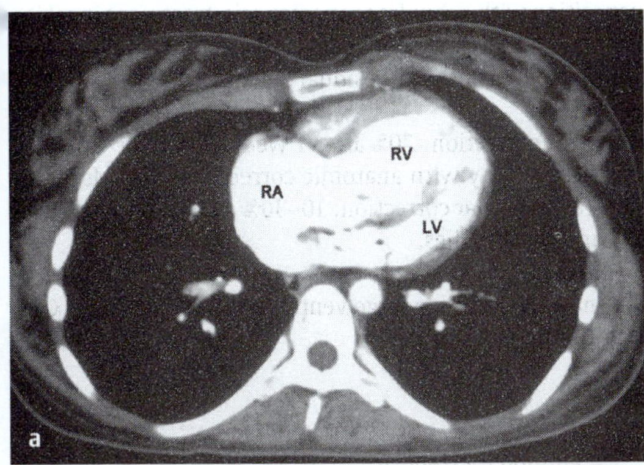

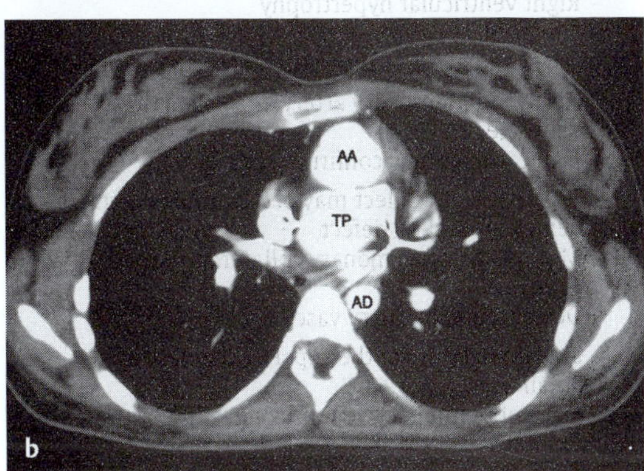

Fig. 2.9 a, b Transposition of the great arteries. Chest CT after contrast administration. Transposition corrected at the atrial level. Hypertrophic right ventricle (RV), from which the aorta arises cranially (AA: ascending aorta, AD: descending aorta). The main pulmonary trunk (TP) arises from the outflow tract of the left ventricle (LV).

Clinical Aspects

- **Typical presentation**

  Severe cyanosis • No improvement with oxygen therapy • Only slight dyspnea.

- **Therapeutic options**

  Palliative: Administering prostaglandin E_1 can delay closure of the ductus arteriosus • Emergency Rashkind atrial septostomy with a balloon catheter under angiographic control.

  Surgical: Anatomic correction ("arterial switch") • Closure of the ventricular septal defect may be indicated • Where right ventricular pressure is markedly below systemic pressure, initial pulmonary banding and a Blalock–Taussig shunt are indicated • Mustard or Senning operation (atrial switch) is indicated where the disorder is diagnosed after the age of 6 months or rarely with complicated coronary

circulation • In d-transposition with subpulmonary stenosis, treatment involves intraventricular correction with a Rastelli right ventricular conduit.
Postoperative: Endocarditis prophylaxis with residual defects.

▸ **Course and prognosis**
Survival rate without surgical correction: 70% after 1 week, 50% after 1 month, 11% after 1 year • Surgical mortality with anatomic correction: 15%. Mortality with atrial switch: 5%. Intraventricular correction: 10–30% • Long-term prognosis depends on coronary artery anomalies.

▸ **Complications**
Right ventricular failure may result from a large ventricular septal defect • Cardiac arrhythmia • Atrial thrombosis.

Differential Diagnosis

Tetralogy of Fallot	– Pulmonary stenosis – Right ventricular hypertrophy – Ventricular septal defect – "Overriding" aorta above the ventricular septal defect
Double outlet right ventricle (DORV)	– Aorta and pulmonary artery arise from the right ventricle – Echocardiography confirms findings
Pulmonary atresia	– Cyanotic heart defect may occur with or without ventricular septal defect – Multiple aortopulmonary collaterals may be visualized – Decreased pulmonary vascularity
Anomalous pulmonary venous connection	– Snowman figure of the superior mediastinum – Small heart – Signs of pulmonary venous congestion

Tips and Pitfalls

Can be confused with other congenital cyanotic heart defects.

Selected References

Donnelly LF et al. Plain-film assessment of the neonate with D-transposition of the great vessels. Pediatr Radiol 1995; 25: 195–197

Gutberlet M et al. Arterial switch procedure for D-transposition of the great arteries: quantitative midterm evaluation of hemodynamic changes with cine MR imaging and phase-shift velocity mapping-initial experience. Radiology 2000; 214: 467–475

Kampmann C et al. Late results after PTCA for coronary stenosis after the arterial switch procedure for transposition of the great arteries. Ann Thorac Surg 2005; 80: 1641–1646

Warnes CA. Transposition of the great arteries. Circulation 2006; 114: 2699–2709

Definition

- **Epidemiology**
  Most common congenital heart disorder (25–30%).
- **Etiology, pathophysiology, pathogenesis**
  - Perimembranous defect (70–80% of cases): in the membranous ventricular septum • The defect borders on the septal cusp of the tricuspid valve and/or aortic valve.
  - Muscular defect: single or multiple ("Swiss cheese" defect) • Bordered by muscle only (mid-ventricular or apical location).
  - "Doubly committed" ventricular septal defect, occurring in the conal septum below the aortic and pulmonary valves.
  - Atrioventricular canal or inlet type, occurring in the inlet septum of the right ventricle.

  Volume overload on the right ventricle and left atrium • In 50% of patients, the ventricular septal defect occurs in combination with other cardiac vascular defects.

Imaging Signs

- **Chest radiograph findings**
  In case of a small ventricular septal defect the findings are normal • Cardiomegaly • Depending on the size of the ventricular septal defect, findings may include increased delineation of the pulmonary vascular structures and a prominent pulmonary artery segment • In pulmonary hypertension, the hilar vessels exhibit an abrupt change in caliber • Heart size decreases again in pulmonary hypertension and Eisenmenger reaction due to diminished shunt flow.
- **Echocardiographic findings**
  Quick and reliable diagnosis • Visualizes the extent and type of the ventricular septal defect • Allows evaluation of valve function.
- **MRI findings**
  ECG-triggered T1-weighted SE images: the septal defect is well demarcated on the four-chamber view • GE cine sequences (with retrospective gating) show valve function and shunt flow (quantifiable with phase-contrast angiography), and flow volume in the aorta and pulmonary artery.
- **Angiography**
  Angiocardiography can verify echocardiographic findings and exclude further anomalies.

Clinical Aspects

- **Typical presentation**
  Typical systolic high-pressure flow sound over the parasternal fourth intercostal space • Precordial murmur may be palpable.

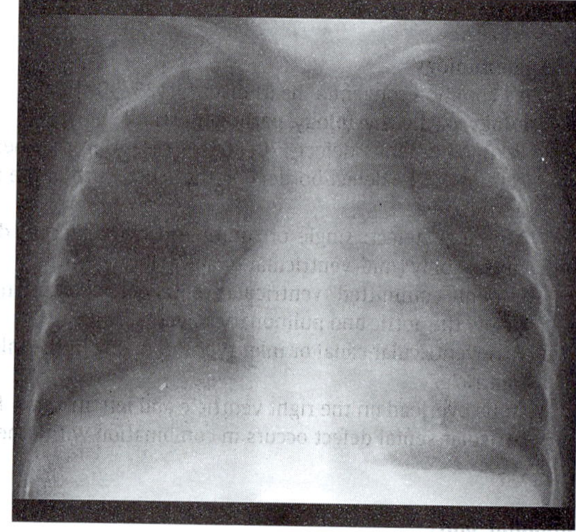

Fig. 2.10 Ventricular septal defect. Chest radiograph shows enlarged heart and markedly increased central pulmonary vascularity. Ventricular septal defect confirmed by echocardiography.

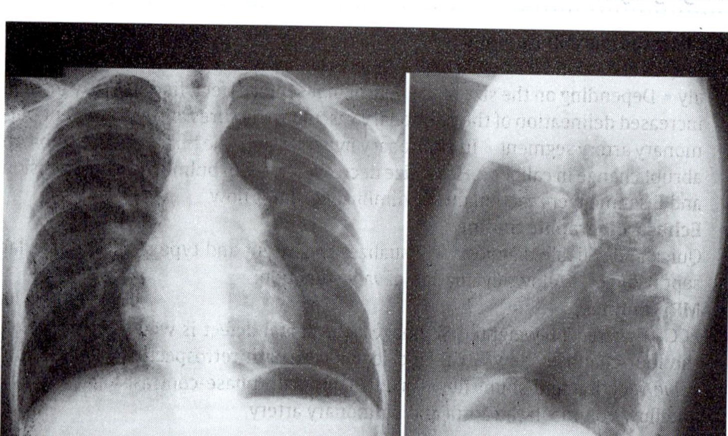

Fig. 2.11 a, b A 16-year-old adolescent with untreated ventricular and atrial septal defects. Chest radiographs in two planes. Reversed shunt (Eisenmenger reaction) confirmed by echocardiography. Decreased central pulmonary vascularity, enlarged pulmonary artery segment, and abrupt change in the caliber of the central pulmonary arteries (hilum amputation) are additional signs of pulmonary arterial hypertension. Retrosternal contact area is markedly enlarged (enlarged right heart).

▸ **Therapeutic options**

Hemodynamically significant defects are closed in angiographic and interventional procedures or open surgical procedures • Uncontrollable cardiac insufficiency is an indication for immediate surgical correction of the ventricular septal defect at any age • Large defects are closed in infancy, medium-sized defects in elective procedures at preschool age • Defects in close proximity to the aortic valve with prolapse of the cusp and aortic insufficiency require repair regardless of the hemodynamic significance of the ventricular septal defect.

▸ **Course and prognosis**

The defect often decreases in size during the first year of life, occasionally closing spontaneously (40% of all lesions in the first 2 years) • Large ventricular septal defects involve a risk of fixed pulmonary hypertension • Patients have a lifelong risk of bacterial endocarditis.

▸ **Complications**

Eisenmenger reaction with reversal of the left-to-right shunt due to chronic pulmonary hypertension (in 10% of large uncorrected defects after 2 years) • Postpericardiotomy syndrome with sterile pericardial and pleural effusion; prognosis is good, etiology unclear.

Differential Diagnosis

Atrial septal defect	– Increased pulmonary vascularity – Cardiomegaly is not necessarily present – Enlarged central pulmonary arteries – Right ventricular enlargement
Patent ductus arteriosus	– Left-to-right shunt – Occurs often in premature infants – Increasing pulmonary opacities in RDS (despite administration of surfactants)

Tips and Pitfalls

Conventional radiographs alone do not allow definitive differentiation of the various left-to-right defects, especially in the early phase.

Selected References

Masura J et al. Percutaneous closure of perimembranous ventricular septal defects with the eccentric Amplatzer device: multicenter follow-up study. Pediatr Cardiol 2005; 26: 216–219

Minette MS et al. Ventricular septal defects. Circulation 2006; 114: 2190–2197

Wang ZJ et al. Cardiovascular shunts: MR imaging evaluation. Radiographics 2003; 23: 181–194

Yoo SJ et al. Magnetic resonance imaging of complex congenital heart disease. Int J Card Imaging 1999; 15: 151–160

Definition

- **Epidemiology**
  The atrial septal defect (ostium secundum) accounts for 8–12% of all congenital heart defects • It occurs three times more often in girls than boys.
- **Etiology, pathophysiology, pathogenesis**
  Often occurs in combination with other heart defects such as pulmonary stenosis • May occur in combination with mitral stenosis (Lutembacher syndrome) • A patent foramen ovale is not a genuine heart defect • However, increased pressure in the right atrium can cause it to develop into a right-to-left shunt.
  Types:
  - Ostium secundum defect (60–70% of cases): 25% of cases occur in combination with partial anomalous pulmonary venous connection to the superior vena cava or right atrium.
  - Sinus venosus defect (5% of cases): 90% of cases occur in combination with partial anomalous pulmonary venous connection to the superior vena cava or right atrium.
  - Ostium primum defect (30% of cases): Component of the atrioventricular septal defect.
  - Hemodynamics: Left-to-right shunt with volume overload on the right ventricle • Pulmonary hypertension with the possibility of an Eisenmenger reaction only occurs in late childhood.

Imaging Signs

- **Chest radiograph findings**
  Increase of retrosternal contact area of the right ventricle • Elevated cardiac apex • Right ventricle later shows a visible left margin as well • Heart size can be normal, depending on the shunt volume • Prominent main pulmonary trunk • Narrow aorta • Pulmonary hyperemia.
- **Echocardiographic findings**
  Location and extent of the defect • Shunt volume • Paradoxical motion of the ventricular septum due to volume load on the right ventricle.
- **MRI findings**
  ECG-triggered T1-weighted SE images: The septal defect is well demarcated on the four-chamber view • GE cine sequences (with retrospective gating): Show valve function and shunt flow (quantifiable with phase-contrast angiography), and flow volume in the aorta and pulmonary artery.
- **Angiography**
  Not necessarily indicated • As an interventional procedure it allows direct repair • Pressure gradient measurement.

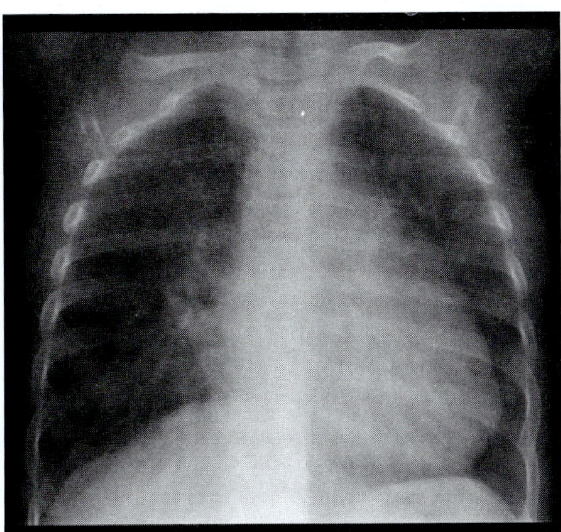

Fig. 2.12 Atrial septal defect (ostium secundum). A-P chest radiograph. Right ventricular heart enlargement, elevated cardiac apex, prominent pulmonary artery segment, and pulmonary hyperemia.

Clinical Aspects

- **Typical presentation**
  Can be asymptomatic • Increased risk for pulmonary infection • Dyspnea with exercise • Signs of cardiac insufficiency (hepatomegaly, failure to thrive, and dyspnea) are rare in newborns and infants • Arrhythmia • Thromboembolic disease (paradoxical embolisms with stroke) • Heart murmur (second heart sound component is discontinuous).
- **Therapeutic options**
  Surgical: Direct repair of the atrial septal defect (larger defects closed with a patch) • *Interventional* (ostium secundum defect): Repair with closure system.
- **Course and prognosis**
  Mortality is 4% up to age 30 • Very good prognosis after repair of the septum defect • Patients have a lifelong risk of bacterial endocarditis.
- **Complications**
  Pulmonary hypertension with Eisenmenger reaction • Paradoxical embolisms, occasionally with cerebral abscesses • Cardiac arrhythmia.

Differential Diagnosis

Ventricular septal defect	– See section on ventricular septal defect
patent ductus arteriosus	– Left-to-right shunt – Occurs often in premature infants – Demonstrates as increasing pulmonary opacities in RDS (despite administration of surfactants)

Tips and Pitfalls

Conventional radiographs alone do not allow definitive differentiation of the various left-to-right defects, especially in the early phase.

Selected References

Beerbaum P et al. Atrial septal defects in pediatric patients: noninvasive sizing with cardiovascular MR imaging. Radiology 2003; 228: 361–369

Fischer G et al. Experience with transcatheter closure of secundum atrial septal defects using the Amplatzer septal occluder: a single centre study in 236 consecutive patients. Heart 2003; 89: 199–204

Hundley WG et al. Assessment of left-to-right intracardiac shunting by velocity-encoded, phase-difference magnetic resonance imaging. A comparison with oximetric and indicator dilution techniques. Circulation 1995; 91: 2955–2960

Definition

▸ **Epidemiology**
Accounts for 10% of all congenital heart defects • Sex predilection: Occurs twice as often in girls than boys.

▸ **Etiology, pathophysiology, pathogenesis**
Persistent sixth branchial arterial arch connecting the left pulmonary artery to the aorta immediately distal to the origin of the left subclavian artery • Physiologic prenatal vascular structure that bypasses the pulmonary circulatory system • Functional obliteration occurs within 48 hours as a result of muscular contraction • Anatomic obliteration occurs as a result of intimal fibrosis and thrombosis • A variable left-to-right shunt is present, depending on the pressure gradient between the pulmonary and systemic circulatory systems and on ductal length and diameter • A patent ductus arteriosus can be crucial for survival in the presence of additional heart defects such as pulmonary artery atresia; prostaglandin E_1 delays closure.

Imaging Signs

▸ **Chest radiograph findings**
Pulmonary segment is enlarged • Increased delineation of central pulmonary vascular structures • Cardiomegaly with prominent left atrium and ventricle • Ascending aorta and aortic arch are enlarged • Shadowing of the aortopulmonary window • Secondary opacification of the lung is seen in RDS.

▸ **Echocardiography**
Visualization of the anatomy • Approximate evaluation of function.

▸ **MRI findings**
ECG-triggered parasagittal T1-weighted SE (black blood) images: Well demarcated patent ductus arteriosus • GE cine and SSFP sequences: Right ventricular function in Eisenmenger reaction with pulmonary hypertension • 3D contrast-enhanced MR angiography: Visualization of the anatomy.

▸ **Angiography**
Not necessarily indicated • Interventional procedure.

Clinical Aspects

▸ **Typical presentation**
Usually asymptomatic • Continuous, systolic-diastolic bruit with maximum intensity over the first and second left parasternal intercostal spaces • In 15% of cases, cardiac insufficiency occurs in infancy with dyspnea and failure to thrive.

▸ **Therapeutic options**
- *Medical:* Indometacin until closure • Endocarditis prophylaxis may be indicated.
- *Surgical:* Where medical or interventional closure of a symptomatic ductus arteriosus is not feasible, surgical transsection is indicated.
- *Interventional:* Coil embolization (risk of recurrence).

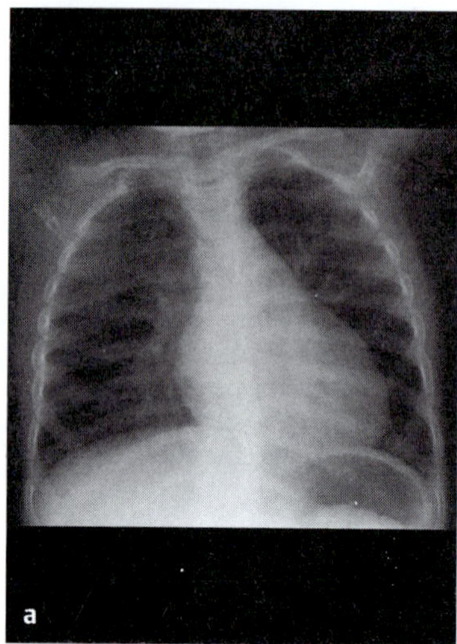

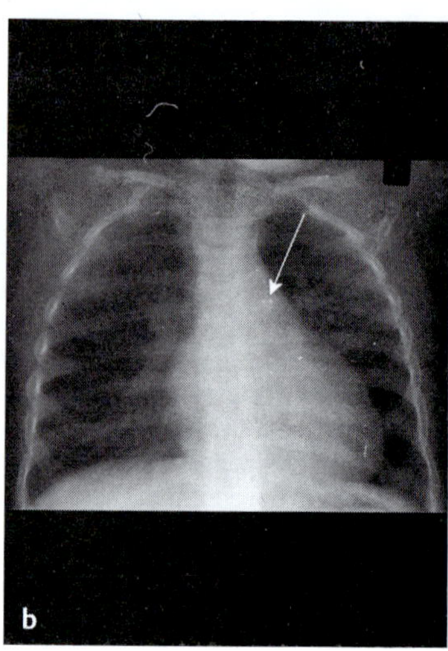

Fig. 2.13 a, b Patent ductus arteriosus. A-P chest radiograph. Moderate cardiomegaly, increased central pulmonary vascularity (**a**). After interventional closure (**b**), radiopaque sealing material is projected on the aortopulmonary window (arrow). The pulmonary hyperemia has abated slightly.

- **Course and prognosis**
  Excellent prognosis after closure • Interventional closure involves a risk or residual or recurrent shunt.
- **Complications**
  Cardiac insufficiency (very rare) • Reversal of the shunt with cyanosis in pulmonary hypertension • Risk of endocarditis.

Differential Diagnosis

Ventricular septal defect	– See section on ventricular septal defects
Atrial septal defect	– Increased pulmonary vascularity – Cardiomegaly is not necessarily present – Enlarged central pulmonary arteries – Right ventricular enlargement

Tips and Pitfalls

Secondary opacification of the lungs in newborns with RDS may be regarded as a primarily pulmonary problem. Always consider a patent ductus arteriosus.

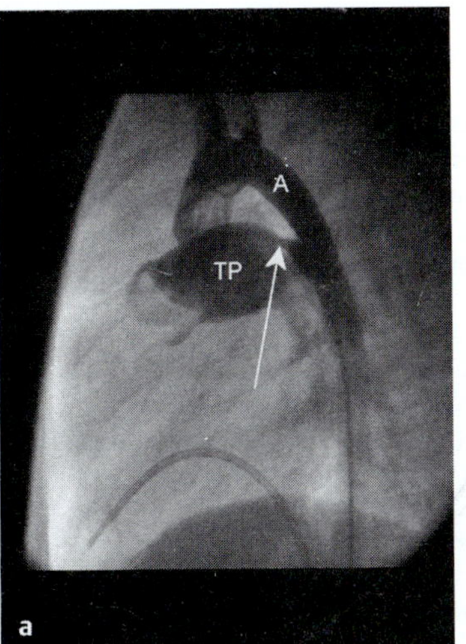

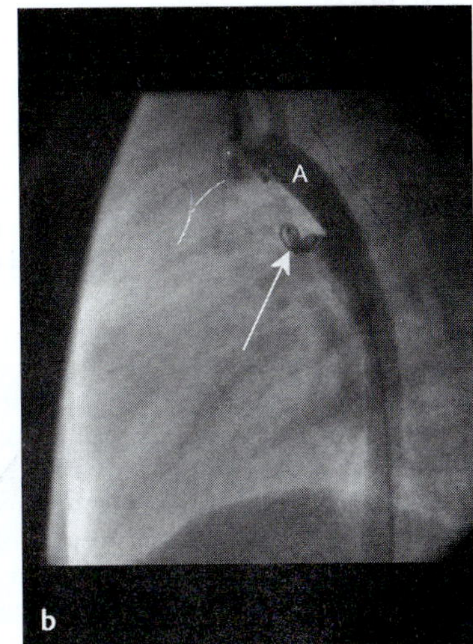

Fig. 2.14 a, b DSA. Typical findings in a patent ductus arteriosus (**a**). The pigtail catheter lies in the thoracic aorta (A). Opacification of the left-to-right shunt and pulmonary trunk (TP) after injection of contrast medium. Postinterventional DSA (**b**) after closure of the ductus arteriosus with metal coils (arrow).

Selected References

Burney K et al. Imaging of implants on chest radiographs: a radiological perspective. Clin Radiol 2007; 62: 204–212

Clyman RI et al. Patent ductus arteriosus: evidence for and against treatment. J Pediatr 2007; 150: 216–219

Dähnert W. Radiology Review Manual. Patent Ducuts Arteriosus. Philadelphia: Lippincott Williams & Wilkins; 2003: 640

Hofbeck M et ai. Safety and efficacy of interventional occlusion of patent ductus arteriosus with detachable coils: a multicenter experience. Eur J Pediatr 2000; 159: 331–337

Definition

- **Epidemiology**
  Accounts for about 1–3% of all congenital heart defects.
- **Etiology, pathophysiology, pathogenesis**
  Total anomalous pulmonary venous connection is a connection between pulmonary veins and major systemic veins • It is associated with other anomalies such as atrial septal defect, patent foramen ovale, and congenital cystic adenomatoid malformation.
  Total anomalous pulmonary venous connection (TAPVC):
  - *Type I:* Supracardiac drainage (50% of cases) into the innominate vein.
  - *Type II:* Cardiac drainage (28% of cases) into the coronary sinus or right atrium.
  - *Type III:* Infradiaphragmatic drainage (17% of cases) into the portal venous system or inferior vena cava via a patent ductus venosus.
  - *Type IV:* Mixed form (5% of cases) involving a combination of types I–III.

  Partial anomalous pulmonary venous connection (PAPVC): Only some of the pulmonary veins drain into systemic venous structures • Others drain normally into the left atrium • Left-to-right shunt with volume overload • Associated with asplenic syndrome (right isomerism).

Imaging Signs

- **Chest radiograph findings**
  Snowman figure (widening of the superior mediastinum due to dilation of the superior vena cava and a left vertical pulmonary vein, type I) • Cardiomegaly (types I and II) • Small heart and pulmonary edema (type III) • Narrow mediastinum (types II and III) • Increased pulmonary vascularity.
- **Echocardiographic findings**
  No venous drainage into the left atrium.
- **CT findings**
  Contrast-enhanced study with appropriate low dosage • Direct visualization of the pulmonary veins • Thickened interlobular septa • Thickening of the bronchial walls • Ground-glass pulmonary opacities.
- **MRI findings**
  Axial and coronal balanced FFE sequence (SSFP) • Direct visualization of venous anatomy • Coronal contrast-enhanced MR angiography provides images with high spatial and temporal resolution using a T1-weighted GE technique with subtraction of individual phases • Phase-contrast angiography.
- **Angiography**
  Rarely indicated • May be useful postoperatively to visualize pulmonary veins and for interventional management of venous stenosis.

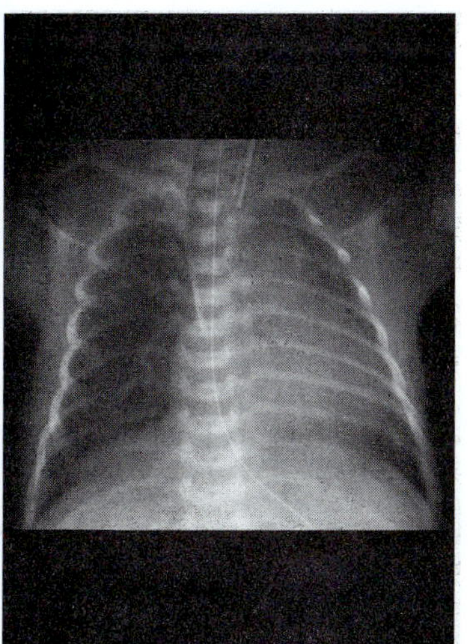

Fig. 2.15 Total anomalous pulmonary venous connection draining into the right atrium (type II, cardiac type), associated atrial septal defect. A-P chest radiograph. Right ventricular heart enlargement and increased central pulmonary vascularity.

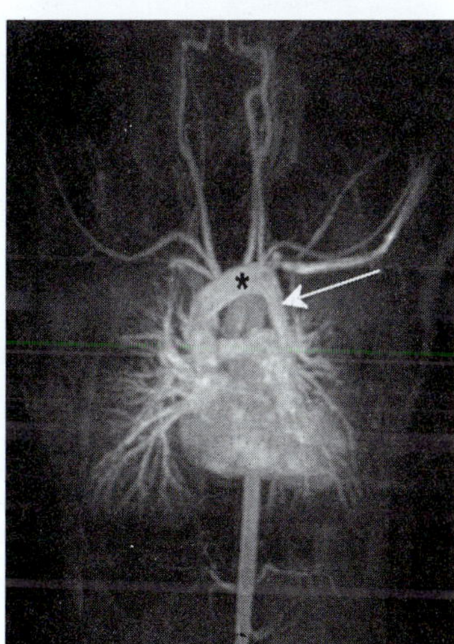

Fig. 2.16 Contrast-enhanced MR image of the chest. Partial anomalous pulmonary venous connection of the left pulmonary veins draining via a vertical vein (arrow) into the innominate vein (*).

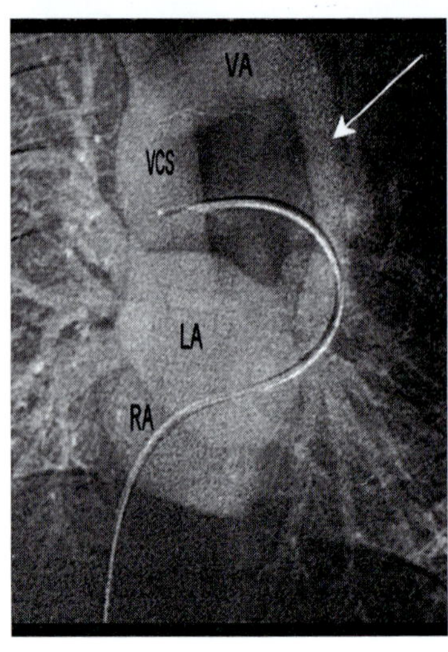

Fig. 2.17 DSA. Contrast medium administration via catheter in the right pulmonary artery. Venous contrast phase. Anomalous left pulmonary venous drainage via a left vertical vein (arrow) into the wide left innominate vein (VA). This then drains via the superior vena cava (VCS) into the right atrium (RA). The right pulmonary veins drain normally into the left atrium (LA).

Clinical Aspects

- **Typical presentation**
  - *Pulmonary venous obstruction:* Acute emergency situation in the first few hours or days of life • cyanosis • dyspnea • pulmonary hypertension.
  - *Without relevant pulmonary venous obstruction:* Increased pulmonary blood flow • Pulmonary hypertension • Tachypnea • Signs of cardiac insufficiency • Dystrophy.
  - Slightly increased pressure in the pulmonary artery may cause only minor symptoms • Cyanosis may be absent or mild.
- **Therapeutic options**
  Obstructive forms require immediate treatment • Nonobstructive forms are treated by elective surgery to connect the pulmonary veins directly to the left atrium.
- **Course and prognosis**
  Obstructive forms are fatal if left untreated.
- **Complications**
  Obstruction at the anastomosis (5–10% of cases).

Differential Diagnosis

Scimitar syndrome	– Hypoplasia of the right lung – Cardiac dextroposition – Hypoplasia of the right pulmonary artery – Arterial supply to the right lower lobe arises from the abdominal aorta – Venous drainage of the right lung is into the inferior vena cava (vein has a typical scimitar shape in the right paracardial region)
Atrial septal defect	– The ostium secundum type in particular cannot be clearly identified on plain radiographs alone
Cor triatriatum	– Septal division of the pulmonary venous connection to the left atrium (with fenestration)

Tips and Pitfalls

Partial anomalous pulmonary venous connections are often asymptomatic.

Selected References

Hyde JAJ et al. Total anomalous pulmonary venous connection: Outcome of surgical correction and management of recurrent venous obstruction. Eur J Cardiothorac Surg 1999; 15: 735–741

Michielon G et al. Total anomalous pulmonary venous connection: Long-term appraisal with evolving technical solutions. Eur J Cardiothor Surg 2002; 22: 184–191

Ricci M et al. Management of pulmonary venous obstruction after correction of TAPVC: risk factors for adverse outcome. Eur J Cardiothorac Surg 2003; 24: 28–36

Definition

- **Epidemiology**
  Usually occurs in newborns with birth trauma (breech presentation, vacuum extraction, forceps delivery) • Frequency < 0.4% of newborns.
- **Etiology, pathophysiology, pathogenesis**
  Traumatic pressure sores and/or impaired venous drainage in the sternocleidomastoid muscle • Muscle edema is initially present • Fibrotic degeneration of muscle fibers subsequently occurs • Usually unilateral • More often on the right (73% of cases) than left (22%).

Imaging Signs

- **Ultrasound findings**
  Focal fusiform or, less often, diffuse swelling of the sternocleidomastoid muscle • Echogenicity ranges from hyperechoic (49% of cases) to hypoechoic • Echo texture is heterogeneous (49% of cases) or homogeneous (51%) • Calcifications occur rarely.
- **CT findings**
  Very rarely indicated • Isodense swelling of the sternocleidomastoid muscle • Adjacent structures are occasionally displaced • No major compression or sheathing.
- **MRI findings**
  Rarely indicated • T2-weighted images show hypointense swelling (fibrosis) of the sternocleidomastoid muscle • Adjacent structures are occasionally displaced • No infiltration.

Clinical Aspects

- **Typical presentation**
  Hard painless swelling in the center of the sternocleidomastoid muscle occurring in the first 2 weeks of life • Can increase in size within 2–4 weeks • Associated with torticollis in 14–20% of cases.
- **Therapeutic options**
  Physical therapy to stretch the neck musculature • Surgical management is very rarely indicated.
- **Course and prognosis**
  Usually resolves spontaneously within 4–8 months.
- **Complications**
  Usually none.

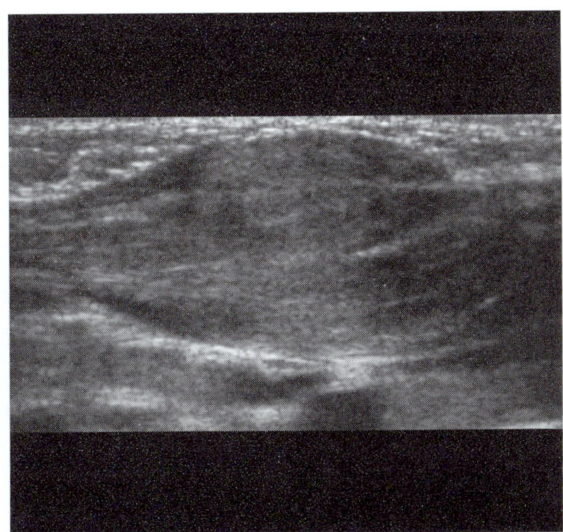

Fig. 3.1 Fibromatosis colli. Ultrasound: Fusiform, primarily hyperechoic swelling of the right sternocleidomastoid muscle.

Differential Diagnosis

Lymphoma	– Masses, enlarged lymph nodes along the cervical neurovascular sheath
Rhabdomyosarcoma	– Solid mass – Often there is infiltration of adjacent structures such as skull base and meninges
Neuroblastoma	– Mass with calcifications and inhomogeneous echo pattern
Cervical cyst	– Lesion anterior to the sternocleidomastoid muscle – Anechoic to echogenic depending on cyst contents – Doppler studies do not show any internal vascularization

Tips and Pitfalls

Can be mistaken for hematoma or solid mass • Aspiration for histologic specimen not indicated.

Selected References

Ablin DS et al. Ultrasound and MR imaging of fibromatosis colli (sternomastoid tumor of infancy). Pediatr Radiol 1998; 28: 230–233

Bedi DG et al. Fibromatosis colli of infancy: variability of sonographic appearance. J Clin Ultrasound 1998; 26: 345–348

Snitzer EL et al. Magnetic resonance imaging appearance of fibromatosis colli. Magn Reson Imaging 1997; 15: 869–871

Vazquez E et al. US, CT, and MR imaging of neck lesions in children. Radiographics 1995; 15: 105–122

Definition

- **Epidemiology**
  Occurs at any age • Predilection for children and adolescents • No sex predilection.
- **Etiology, pathophysiology, pathogenesis**
  - *Median cervical cyst:* Cells of the obliterated thyroglossal duct are activated • There may be a fistula leading to the epidermis • Lies directly in the midline between the foramen cecum at the base of the tongue and the isthmus of the thyroid.
  - *Lateral cervical cyst:* Arises from the second pharyngeal pouch • Lies in the angle of the mandible anterior to the sternocleidomastoid muscle.

Imaging Signs

- **Ultrasound findings**
  Cystic lesion at median location inferior to the hyoid bone (median cervical cyst) or anterior to the sternocleidomastoid muscle (lateral cervical cyst) • Compressible • Anechoic to echogenic internal structure depending on cyst contents • Examination shows location relative to adjacent structures • Cyst can be aspirated where indicated • Duplex ultrasound shows at most marginal vascular structures, no internal vascularization • Posterior echo enhancement • Lateral flexion echoes.
- **CT findings**
  Usually not required.
- **MRI findings**
  Only indicated with equivocal clinical and ultrasound findings • Cyst contents are hyperintense on T2-weighted sequences • No enhancement on T1-weighted images • Moderate marginal enhancement may occur in secondary infections • Most sensitive modality for demonstrating fistulas (fat-suppressed T2-weighted sequence).

Clinical Aspects

- **Typical presentation**
  Spherical cervical swelling • Mobile on palpation • Mobile lesion moves with swallowing • Drainage of secretion may occur where fistula is present.
- **Therapeutic options**
  - *Median cervical cyst:* Treatment invariably involves removal of cyst and fistula including parts of the hyoid bone • Resection of duct as far as the foramen cecum where indicated.
  - *Lateral cervical cyst:* Treatment invariably involves removal of cyst and fistula • Resection of ipsilateral tonsil where indicated.

  Preoperative antibiotic therapy in infection.

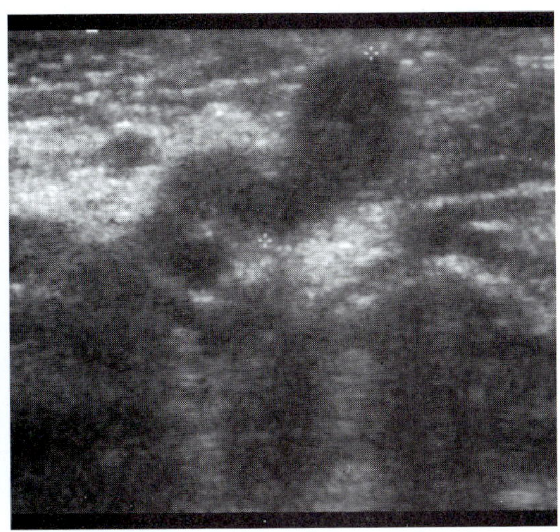

Fig. 3.2 Lateral cervical cyst. Ultrasound. Newborn with small open cutaneous fistula in the neck draining a cloudy fluid. Oval, hypoechoic cystic lesion with isolated small hyperechoic internal echoes.

- **Course and prognosis**
  Usually heals completely after surgery.
- **Complications**
  Cyst can recur • Superinfection • Postoperative complications • Fistula.

Differential Diagnosis

Dermoid cyst	– Occurs in the floor of the mouth
Lymphangioma	– Fluid filled sacs, usually septated occasionally with hemorrhage – Often extensive process without clear median or lateral orientation
Cervical thymic cyst	– Usually lies caudal to the hyoid bone adjacent to the cervical vascular structures – Can occur as isolated lesion – Can occur adjacent to the thymus – Can occur in combination with thymic cysts
Parathyroid cyst	– Usually in adults – Adjacent to thyroid
Cervical bronchogenic cyst	– Cyst up to several centimeters in size – Can displace and compress the trachea
Laryngocele	– Directly adjacent to larynx – Changes size with suction and compression maneuver – Tracheal spot image

Tips and Pitfalls

Can be confused with other disorders considered in differential diagnosis.

Selected References

Benson MT et al. Congenital anomalies of the branchial apparatus: embryology and pathologic anatomy. Radiographics 1992; 12: 943–960

Dähnert W. Radiology review manual. Congenital cystic lesions of neck. Philadelphia: Lippincott Williams & Wilkins; 2003: 355

Mohan PS et al. Thyroglossal duct cysts: a consideration in adults. Am Surg 2005; 71: 508–511

Definition

- **Etiology, pathophysiology, pathogenesis**
  Inflammatory swelling of the cervical lymph nodes due to viral or bacterial infection • Often occurs in children in the setting of upper respiratory infection, tonsillitis, pharyngitis, or pulpitis • Can affect one or more groups of lymph nodes • Unilateral of bilateral • In more than 80% of cases, submandibular lymph nodes and deep cervical lymph nodes along the neurovascular sheath are affected.

Imaging Signs

- **Ultrasound findings**
  Lymph node enlargement exceeding 1.0 cm (axial diameter) • Oval configuration remains • Smooth margin • Hyperechoic hilum and hypoechoic cortex • Necrosis is visualized as a hypoechoic or anechoic center, occasionally with a hyperechoic margin • Doppler ultrasound in necrosis shows a hyperperfused margin (displacement of vascular structures) and a nonperfused area in the area of necrosis.
- **CT findings**
  Contrast-enhanced CT • May be helpful preoperatively in lymph node abscess • Enlarged lymph nodes • Necrosis is visualized as a hypodense mass or ring-enhancing mass isodense to fluid.
- **MRI findings**
  Alternative to CT that avoids the use of ionizing radiation • Morphologic criteria and contrast behavior are identical to CT.

Clinical Aspects

- **Typical presentation**
  Painful, palpable lymph node swelling • Fluctuation in necrosis • Fever • Torticollis may occur in unilateral involvement
- **Therapeutic options**
  Anti-inflammatory and antibiotic treatment • Surgical removal when necrosis has occurred.
- **Course and prognosis**
  Clinical course is usually unproblematic and lesions resolve completely • Abscess formation delays healing.
- **Complications**
  Acute cellulitis • Necrosis • Jugular venous thrombosis • Sepsis.

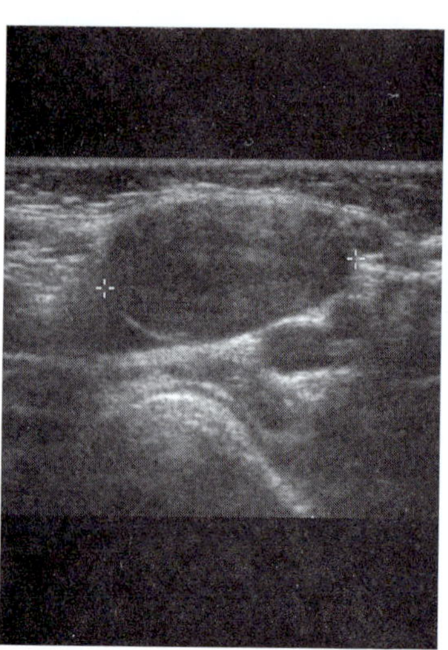

Fig. 3.3 Cervical lymphadenitis. Ultrasound. Oval hypoechoic lymph node in the right neurovascular sheath measuring over 2 cm.

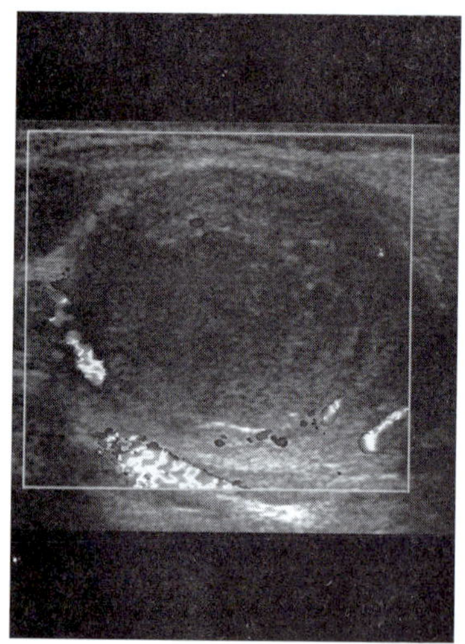

Fig. 3.4 Cervical lymphadenitis with abscess. Doppler ultrasound. Hyperperfused marginal lymph node; nonperfused central necrosis.

Differential Diagnosis

Lymphoma	– Usually painless lymph node swelling – Often a round, very hypoechoic lymph node lacking a hyperechoic lymph node hilum – Lymph node masses, necrosis – Systemic disorder
Tuberculosis, atypical mycobacterial disease	– Usually bilateral lymph node swelling – Necrosis and calcifications – Hardened lymph nodes painful to palpation; nodes can fluctuate where necrosis is present

Tips and Pitfalls

Can be mistaken for malignant systemic disorder.

Selected References

Ahuja AT et al. Sonographic evaluation of cervical lymph nodes. AJR Am J Roentgenol 2005; 184: 1691–1699

Chu WCW et al. Inflammatory lesions of the neck and airways. In: King SJ, Boothroyd AE (eds.) Pediatric ENT Radiology. Medical Radiology. Diagnostic Imaging. Berlin, Heidelberg: Springer; 2002: 245–255

Papakonstantinou O et al. High-resolution and color Doppler ultrasonography of cervical lymphadenopathy in children. Acta Radiol 2001; 42: 470–476

Definition

- **Epidemiology**
  Typically occurs at age 6–12 months.
- **Etiology, pathophysiology, pathogenesis**
  Lymph from the nasopharynx, middle ear, and tonsils drains via retropharyngeal lymph nodes, and infections in these regions can spread to these nodes • Lymphadenitis and abscess of the retropharyngeal lymph nodes secondary to pharyngeal infection • Complicated tonsillitis with peritonsillar abscess • Penetrating injury in intubation or endoluminal procedure.

Imaging Signs

- **Lateral radiograph of the cervical spine**
  Not the modality of choice • Widening of the prevertebral space • Air inclusions may be present.
- **Ultrasound findings**
  Retropharyngeal fluid retention • Diffusely edematous soft tissue with increased echogenicity • Cervical lymphadenitis • Occasionally enlarged tonsil with asymmetry of the pharynx.
- **CT findings**
  Contrast-enhanced CT with late images for visualizing abscess • Peripheral contrast enhancement with hypodense central area nearly isodense to fluid • Demonstrates extent of the process • Asymmetry and thickening of the retropharyngeal soft tissue • Cervical lymphadenitis • Occasionally enlarged tonsil with asymmetry of the pharynx.
- **MRI findings**
  Morphology and contrast behavior are identical to CT • Inflammatory involvement of adjacent structures is better visualized than on CT • Higher soft tissue contrast.

Clinical Aspects

- **Typical presentation**
  Fever • Croup-like cough • Impaired nasal breathing • Dysphagia with regurgitation of food through the nose • Protrusion of the posterior pharyngeal wall • Hoarse speech • Occasionally compensatory head posture in torticollis • Stiffness of the neck • Elevated temperature • Laryngeal edema in progressive distal abscess migration • Cervical lymphadenopathy.
- **Therapeutic options**
  Paramedian incision • Antibiotic therapy.
- **Course and prognosis**
  Prompt diagnosis minimizes complications.
- **Complications**
  Extension of the retropharyngeal abscess to the mediastinum (mediastinitis) • Jugular venous thrombosis • Sepsis.

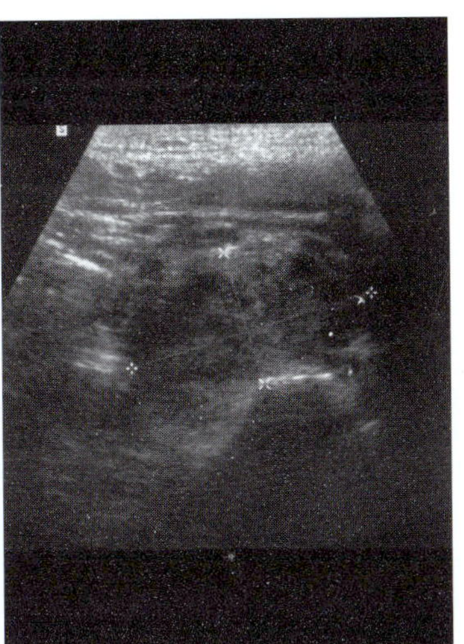

Fig. 3.5 Retropharyngeal abscess. Cervical ultrasound. Enlarged left tonsil with necrosis.

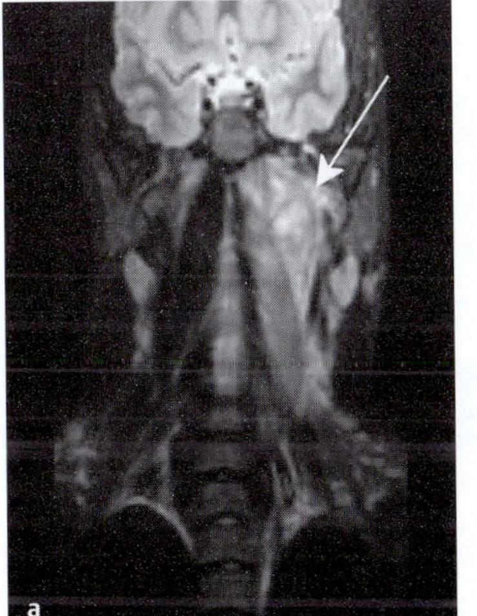

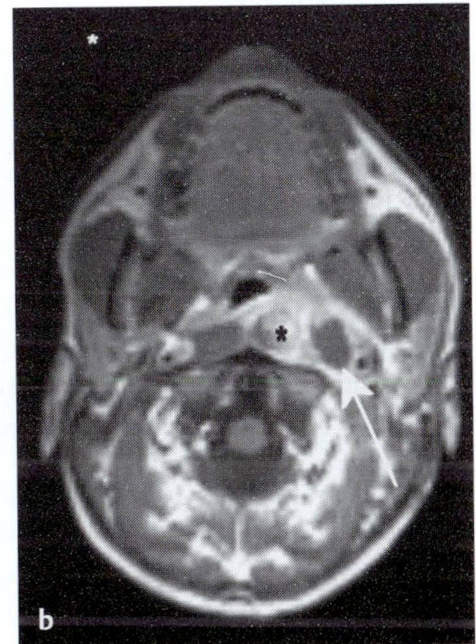

Fig. 3.6 a, b Cervical MR image (coronal STIR image [**a**] and axial T1-weighted SE image after contrast administration [**b**]). Extensive inflammation of the left retropharyngeal space with abscess (arrow) in tonsillitis. Extensive inflammatory reaction in the deep prevertebral musculature as well (*longus colli).

Differential Diagnosis

Diffuse retropharyngeal inflammation	– No abscess
Lymphangioma	– Fluid filled, septated lymphatic sacs – Extent is not usually limited to the retropharyngeal space – Clinical aspects
Epiglottitis	– Enlarged epiglottis – Symmetric subglottic constriction
Cervical cyst	– No cervical lymphadenitis – Clinical aspects – Location of the cystic process is usually median or lateral and subcutaneous

Tips and Pitfalls

Lateral radiograph of the cervical spine on expiration with inclination can mimic expansion of the retropharyngeal space.

Selected References

Al-Sabah B et al. Retropharyngeal abscess in children: 10-year study. J Otolaryngol 2004; 33: 352–355

Craig FW et al. Retropharyngeal abscess in children: clinical presentation, utility of imaging, and current management. Pediatrics 2003; 111: 1394–1398

Philpott CM et al. Paediatric retropharyngeal abscess. J Laryngol Otol 2004; 118: 919–926

Weber AL et al. CT and MR imaging evaluation of neck infections with clinical correlations. Radiol Clin North Am 2000; 38: 941–968

Definition

- **Epidemiology**
  Most common cause of goiter and acquired hypothyroidism in children and adolescents • Usually affects adolescents in puberty • Girls are affected three times as often as boys.
- **Etiology, pathophysiology, pathogenesis**
  Multifactorial and polygenic etiology • Genetic predisposition (HLA DR4, DR5) • Often occurs in Turner syndrome and trisomy 21 • T-cell suppressor defect • Tissue destruction from antibodies against thyroid antigens.

Imaging Signs

- **Ultrasound findings**
  Enlarged thyroid • Finely nodular diffusely hypoechoic pattern from lymphocytic infiltration • *Color Doppler:* Hypervascularization and hyperemia.
- **Nuclear medicine imaging findings**
  Variable findings • Diffuse hyperplasia • Multinodular goiter • Solitary thyroid nodules.

Clinical Aspects

- **Typical presentation**
  Painless goiter • Patient may have difficulty swallowing • Transient hyperthyroid metabolism (Hashimoto toxicosis) may result from production of stimulating antibodies • The primary atrophic form with hypothyroidism leads to slowed growth, delayed development, and limited exercise tolerance • Detection of thyroid antibodies is diagnostic.
- **Therapeutic options**
  L-thyroxine.
- **Course and prognosis**
  In 20% of cases, the disorder is self-limiting with a return to euthyroidism • Course under treatment is usually mild • Decompensation can recur in adults, for example in pregnancy.
- **Complications**
  Encephalopathy • B-cell lymphoma of the thyroid.

Differential Diagnosis

Graves disease	– Enlargement of the thyroid, especially the isthmus – Hypoechoic foci
Acute thyroiditis	– Painful thyroid – Hyperthyroidism – Hypoechoic areas
Diffuse nodular goiter	– Enlarged thyroid with hypoechoic nodules – Cystic lesions and calcifications with regressive changes

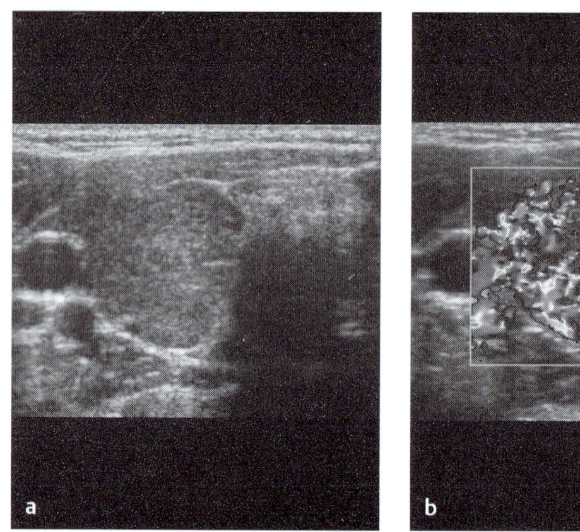

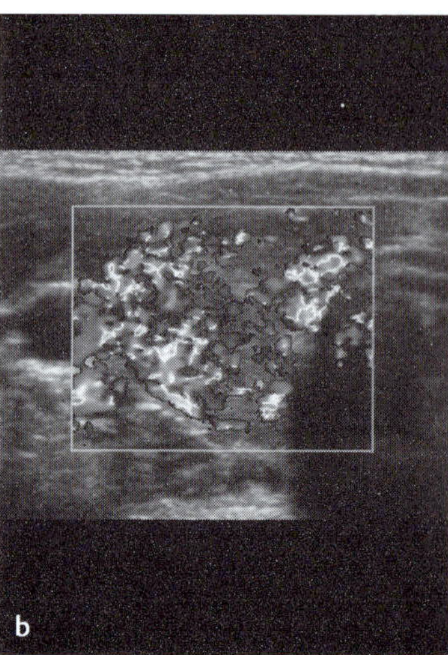

Fig. 3.7 a, b Hashimoto thyroiditis. B-mode ultrasound (**a**) and color Doppler ultrasound (**b**) of the right thyroid lobe. Finely nodular hypoechoic pattern of thyroid parenchyma (**a**), hypervascularity and hyperemia (**b**).

Tips and Pitfalls

Overlooking the finely nodular hypoechoic lymphocytic infiltration • Neglecting to perform color Doppler ultrasound examination • Confusing the disorder with iodine-deficiency goiter.

Selected References

Bennedbaek FN et al. The value of ultrasonography in the diagnosis and follow-up of subacute thyroiditis. Thyroid 1997; 7: 45–50

Roth C et al. Autoimmune thyroiditis in childhood-epidemiology, clinical and laboratory findings in 61 patients. Exp Clin Endocrinol Diabetes 1997; 105 Suppl 4: 66–69

Set PA et al. Sonographic features of Hashimoto thyroiditis in childhood. Clin Radiol 1996; 51: 167–169

Yarman S et al. Scintigraphic varieties in Hashimoto's thyroiditis and comparison with ultrasonography. Nucl Med Commun 1997; 18: 951–956

Definition

- **Epidemiology**
  Usually occurs in premature infants • Less common in term newborns • Associated with maternal diabetes and use of magnesium sulfate by the mother.
- **Etiology, pathophysiology, pathogenesis**
  Neural plexus in the wall of the descending colon is immature • This results in functional colonic obstruction • Transient colonic dysfunction • Disorder is not associated with cystic fibrosis.

Imaging Signs

- **Abdominal radiograph findings**
  Deep-seated ileus • Dilated bowel loops • Ascending and transverse colon filled with meconium.
- **Ultrasound findings**
  Dilated small bowel loops • Right colon is filled with meconium • Alternating normal and reversed peristalsis or absence of peristalsis.
- **Contrast enema**
  Contrast enema outlines a meconium cast • Multiple filling defects are present • Small left colon with narrowed descending colon • Abrupt change in diameter in the splenic flexure • Colon proximal to the obstruction is of normal diameter or dilated.
- **CT**
  Not required.

Clinical Aspects

- **Typical presentation**
  Slight or absent spontaneous passage of meconium in the first 3 days of life • Symptoms of deep intestinal obstruction • Distended abdomen • Visible peristalsis • Vomiting.
- **Therapeutic options**
  Rectal clearance of the obstruction • Contrast enema with water-soluble nonionic contrast agent.
- **Course and prognosis**
  Clearance of the meconium plug is curative.
- **Complications**
  Perforation of the colon with meconium peritonitis • Meconium cyst.

Differential Diagnosis

Meconium ileus	– Microcolon – Obstruction is usually in the terminal ileum – Associated with cystic fibrosis

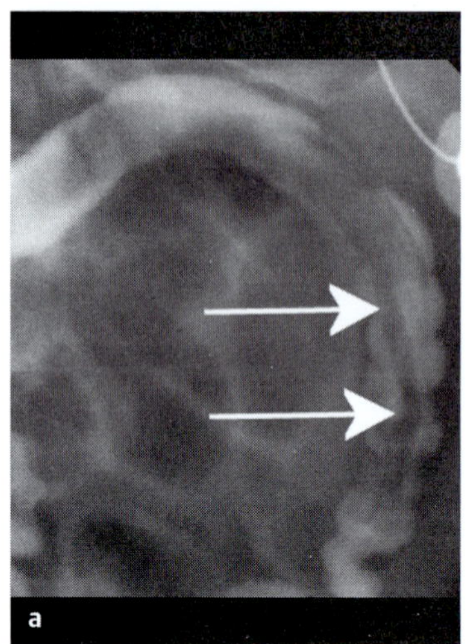

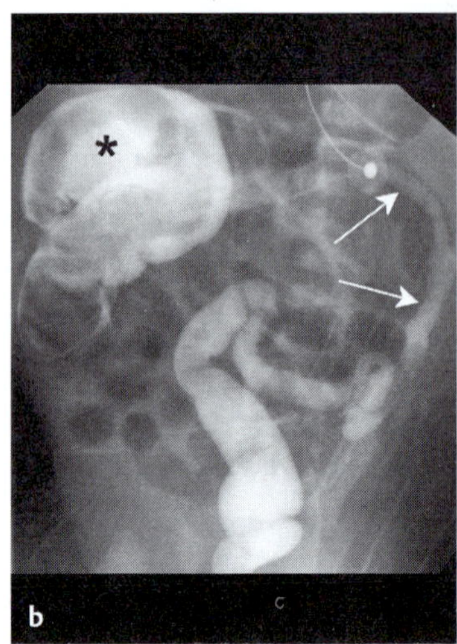

Fig. 4.1 a, b Meconium plug syndrome. Contrast enema. Filling defect (arrows) in the descending colon (meconium cylinder, **a**). The fluoroscopic image (**b**) shows a small left colon (arrows) and a right colon of normal caliber (*).

Hirschsprung disease	– Typical segmental rectosigmoid stenosis – Abrupt change in diameter of the colon with dilated proximal colon
Ileal atresia	– Microcolon – Small bowel loops distal to the atresia are narrowed

Tips and Pitfalls

Digital rectal examination and ultrasound must be performed prior to contrast enema to exclude anorectal malformation • Often the small and large bowels cannot be clearly differentiated on abdominal radiographs in newborns because the typical haustration is not yet detectable • Meconium plugs with air inclusions must not be confused with pneumatosis intestinalis.

Selected References

Burge D et al. Meconium plug obstruction. Pediatr Surg Int 2004; 20: 108–110

Casaccia G et al. The impact of cystic fibrosis on neonatal intestinal obstruction: the need for prenatal/neonatal screening. Pediatr Surg Int 2003; 19: 75–78

Emil S et al. Meconium obstruction in extremely low-birth-weight neonates: guidelines for diagnosis and management. J Pediatr Surg 2004; 39: 731–737

Definition

- **Epidemiology**
  Primarily affects premature infants of low gestational age and birth weight • Rarely affects term newborns with Hirschsprung disease, other bowel obstruction disorders such as atresia, or heart defects.
- **Etiology, pathophysiology, pathogenesis**
  Multifactorial process (stress, asphyxia, hypoxia) • Transient compromise of blood supply to the gastrointestinal tract • This causes mucosal destruction with invasion by pathogenic microorganisms and endotoxins • Disorder affects primarily the terminal ileum and ascending colon • Duodenum is not usually affected as it has separate vascular supply • Immature bowel is damaged by ingested food • Use of indometacin leads to reduced bowel perfusion and increases the risk of necrotizing enterocolitis.

Table 4.1 Common pathogens in necrotizing enterocolitis

Bacteria	Viruses	Fungi
Clostridia	Rotavirus	*Candida* species
Escherichia coli	Cytomegalovirus	
Pseudomonas aeruginosa	Coronavirus	
Klebsiella		
Enterobacter		
Staphylococci		

Imaging Signs

- **Abdominal radiograph findings**
  Patient is supine • Films in a second plane with the patient in a left lateral position or supine with a horizontal beam may be indicated.
  - *First phase:* Generalized dilation of all bowel segments • Distension of only the small bowel (70% of cases) • Small bowel is irregularly distended • Full picture of ileus • Separation of the bowel loops is a sign of bowel wall edema.
  - *Second phase:* Pneumatosis intestinalis (intramural air in two-thirds of the children), appearing initially and most often in the terminal ileum • Subserosal linear lesion • Submucosal cystic lesions, resembling strings of pearls.
  - *Third phase:* Air portogram shows air in typical centrifugal distribution pattern due to absorbed intestinal gas (air in the portal vein).
  - *Fourth phase:* Separation of the bowel loops consistent with ascites and suggesting bowel wall thickening • Loss of the normal bowel wall contour • Distended bowel loops with air–fluid levels consistent with peritonitis • Free intraperitoneal air.

Fig. 4.2 Necrotizing enterocolitis in a premature infant. Plain abdominal radiograph with the patient supine (magnification). Pneumatosis intestinalis (linear type) is apparent, especially in the right colon (large arrows). Air projected on the portal venous system (small arrow).

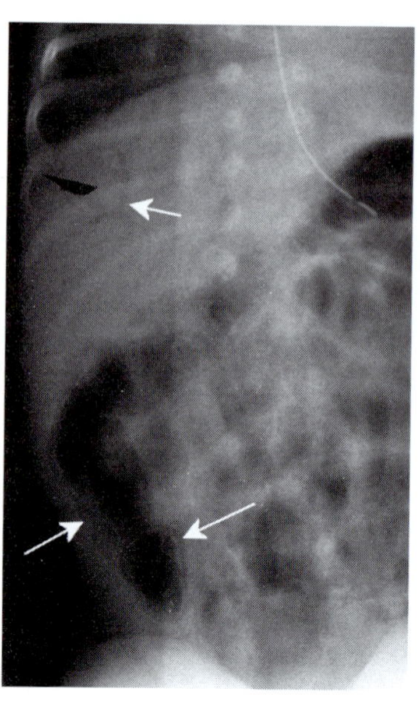

- **Ultrasound findings**
  Thickened bowel walls • Free intraperitoneal fluid • Intramural air in the bowel • Signs of air in the portal vein.
- **Doppler ultrasound findings**
  Characteristic Doppler spectrum with numerous spikes in the portal vein (artifacts from gas bubbles) • Maximum flow velocity in the superior mesenteric artery may be reduced.
- **CT**
  Not required.

Clinical Aspects

- **Typical presentation**
  Onset between 5 and 10 days after birth • Tachycardia • Tachypnea • Anemia • Distended abdomen • Later severe ileus • Bloody stools • Bilious vomiting.
- **Therapeutic options**
  Parenteral nutrition • Antibiotics • Bowel perforation or worsening clinical symptoms require surgical management.
  Prevention of necrotizing enterocolitis: Betamethasone prophylaxis in impending premature delivery • Oral immunoglobulins • Add hydrochloric acid to milk.
- **Course and prognosis**
  Sepsis with bowel perforation • Short bowel syndrome following surgery • Mortality 20–30%.

Complications

Enteroenteric fistulas • Bowel perforation occurs in 12–32% of cases • Bowel stricture occurs after 4–12 weeks in about 10–30% of cases (30% multiple, 80% in descending colon) • Lymphatic hyperplasia and enteric cysts occur rarely.

Differential Diagnosis

Pneumatosis intestinalis from other causes	– Can occur in all ischemic bowel disorders – Can also occur in bowel disorders secondary to insults such as barotrauma or chemotherapy
Meconium ileus	– Minimal or absent passage of meconium – No pneumatosis
Portogram showing air from another cause	– Secondary to catheterization of umbilical vein
Volvulus	– Secondary intestinal ischemia with pneumatosis intestinalis
Neuronal hyperplasia (types A and B)	– Developmental anomaly of the submucosal plexus – Immaturity of the sympathetic nervous system, myenteric plexus, and arteries

Tips and Pitfalls

In necrotizing enterocolitis, even contrast studies with nonionic contrast agents are contraindicated • Pneumatosis intestinalis must not be misinterpreted as a sign of severity of necrotizing enterocolitis • Pneumatosis intestinalis and pneumatosis hepatis are only temporary findings. Therefore, examinations should be performed at frequent intervals where there is clinical suspicion.

Selected References

Dwight P et al. Entero-enteric fistula following mild necrotizing enterocolitis. Eur J Pediatr Surg 2005; 15: 137–139

Halac E et al. Prenatal and postnatal corticosteroid therapy to prevent neonatal necrotizing enterocolitis: a controlled trial. J Pediatr 1990; 117: 132–138

Kim WY et al. Sonographic evaluation of neonates with early-stage necrotizing enterocolitis. Pediatr Radiol 2005; 35: 1056–1061

Neu J. Neonatal necrotizing enterocolitis: an update. Acta Paediatr 2005; 94: 100–105

Tarrado X et al. Comparative study between isolated intestinal perforation and necrotizing enterocolitis. Eur J Pediatr Surg 2005; 15: 88–94

Definition

- **Epidemiology**
  Prevalence 0.2% • Peak frequency is prior to the age of 2 months.
- **Etiology, pathophysiology, pathogenesis**
  Congenital defective rotation of the gut during fetal development • Acute or chronic partial or total obstruction may result • Malrotation can also occur where the colon and root of the mesentery fail to adhere to the posterior wall of the abdomen, placing tension on the mesenteric vascular structures.
  Normal gut rotation: is three 90° counterclockwise rotations (270°) around the superior mesenteric artery (the primitive intestinal loop).
  Nonrotation: is the most common positional anomaly of the gut • Rotational direction is normal but there is only one 90° rotation • The small and large bowels share a common mesentery.
  Malrotation I: Rotational direction is normal but there are only two 90° rotations • The horizontal part of the duodenum rotates behind the axis of the mesenteric vessels • The short root of the mesentery is not fixed • Ladd bands may occur.
  Malrotation II: Change in rotational direction • A normal 90° rotation occurs initially • This is followed by a 90° or 180° inverse rotation • The duodenum lies anterior to the superior mesenteric artery • The cecum and transverse colon lie behind the pedicle of the mesenteric attachment.
  Associated malformations: Congenital diaphragmatic hernia • Omphalocele • Gastroschisis • Duodenal stenosis or atresia or, less often, small bowel atresia • Congenital heart defects • Asplenia or polysplenia syndrome • Situs inversus.

Imaging Signs

- **Abdominal radiograph findings**
  May be normal • "Double bubble" sign in functional obstruction (differential diagnosis should consider duodenal stenosis) • Signs of disruption of intestinal motility • Positional abnormality may be detectable in meteorism.
- **Transit study findings**
  Nonrotation: Duodenojejunal flexure lies to the right of the spine and more distal than the duodenal bulb • The entire small bowel is on the right side • The small bowel exhibits a spiral course.
  Malrotation I: The elevated cecum and ascending colon can compress the duodenum • Cecum may be fixed to the posterior abdominal wall by the Ladd peritoneal bands • This can lead to functional duodenal stenosis.
  Malrotation II: Usually there is no compression of the duodenum • Variable picture depending on the severity of the inverse rotation.
- **Contrast enema findings**
  Nonrotation: Cecum lies anterior to or to the left of the spine • The colon is on the left side.
  Malrotation I: Elevated cecum and ascending colon • Both are slightly to the right of the midline.

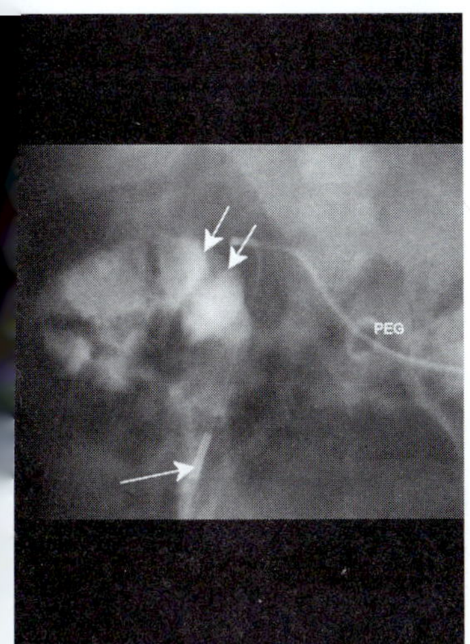

Fig. 4.3 Intestinal nonrotation. Upper gastrointestinal series. A water-soluble nonionic contrast agent is injected into the duodenum via a percutaneous endoscopic cannula (arrow). Atypical position of the duodenojejunal flexure (double arrow) to the right of the spine. The ampulla of Vater lies cranial to the flexure.

Malrotation II: Reversed position of the transverse colon • Filling defect in the transverse colon due to impression by the root of the mesentery • The position of the proximal colon is variable.

- **Color Doppler ultrasound findings**
  Malrotation I: The horizontal part of the duodenum lies posterior to the major mesenteric vessels.
  Malrotation II: Horizontal part of the duodenum lies anterior to the major mesenteric vessels • Anomalous course of the mesenteric vein anterior to or to the left of the superior mesenteric artery (not invariably present).
- **CT findings**
  Useful especially in acute abdomen to demonstrate possible volvulus with ischemia of the bowel.

Clinical Aspects

- **Typical presentation**
  Colic • Bilious vomiting • Malnutrition • Malabsorption where there is congestion in the mesenteric vessels • 25–50% of adolescents do not have any symptoms.
- **Therapeutic options**
  Emergency surgery in volvulus • *Ladd operation:* The Ladd bands are divided to mobilize duodenum • Total correction involves unfolding the mesentery and bringing the vascular structures and bowel into normal position.

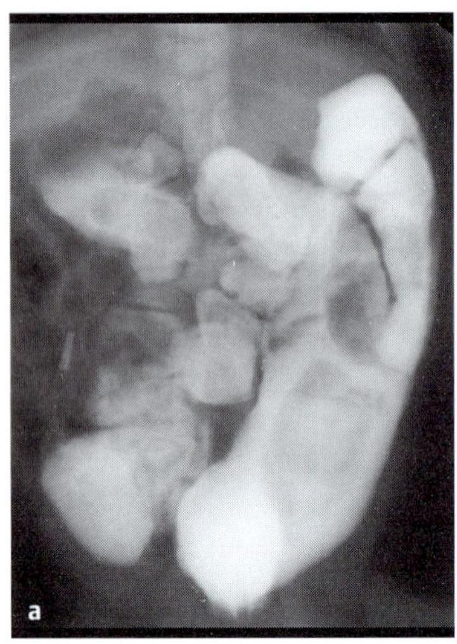

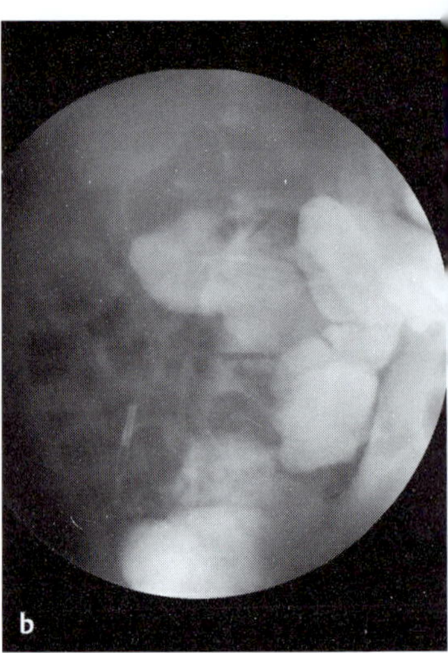

Fig. 4.4 a, b Intestinal nonrotation. Contrast enema. The colon lies mostly in the left half of the abdomen (**a, b**). The inflated small bowel loops are visible in the right half of the abdomen (**b**).

- **Course and prognosis**
  Small bowel volvulus with ischemia and necrosis usually occurs within the first few weeks of life.
- **Complications**
  Intussusception • Chronic appendicitis may go undetected where appendix is in an unusual anatomic location • Ladd bands can exacerbate duodenal stenosis.

Differential Diagnosis

Cecum in the right upper abdomen	– In newborns at physiologic level – Upper gastrointestinal series is diagnostic
Gastroesophageal reflux	– Can be provoked in head down position – Nonbilious vomiting
Duodenal atresia	– No air distal to the duodenum
Duodenal stenosis	– Upper gastrointestinal series demonstrates stenosis and normal position of all other bowel segments – Functional duodenal stenosis can occur in malrotation I
Annular pancreas	– ERCP or MRCP may be indicated to visualize findings – Cross-sectional imaging studies confirm the diagnosis – Normal position of small and large bowel

Tips and Pitfalls

Always consider malrotation where bilious vomiting occurs • Where equivocal obstruction symptoms are present, visualization of the duodenum with precise evaluation of the duodenojejunal flexure is indicated • Where malrotation is suspected, obtain color Doppler ultrasound studies of the mesenteric vascular axis showing the position of the duodenum relative to it • Upper gastrointestinal series is contraindicated in the presence of complete obstruction.

Selected References

Aidlen J et al. Malrotation with midgut volvulus: CT findings of bowel infarction. Pediatr Radiol 2005; 35: 529–531

Applegate KE et al. Intestinal malrotation in children: a problem-solving approach to the upper gastrointestinal series. Radiographics. 2006; 26: 1485–1500

Strouse PJ. Disorders of intestinal rotation and fixation ("malrotation"). Pediatr Radiol 2004; 34: 837–851

Weinberger E et al. Sonographic diagnosis of intestinal malrotation in infants: importance of the relative positions of the superior mesenteric vein and artery. Am J Roentgenol 1992; 159: 825–828

Definition

- **Epidemiology**
  Small bowel volvulus: Usually occurs in newborns and young children • In about 20% of cases, it is associated with other gastrointestinal malformations such as duodenal atresia, duodenal stenosis, or annular pancreas.
  Large bowel volvulus: Is the most common form of volvulus (40% of cases are cecal) • Peak age is between ages 20 and 40 years • Accounts for 10% of large bowel obstructions.
- **Etiology, pathophysiology, pathogenesis**
  Acute mesenteric torsion with strangulation of the mesenteric vascular structures • This leads to ischemia of the bowel and infarction.

Imaging Signs

- **Abdominal radiograph findings**
  Signs of ileus will vary with the level of the obstruction • Massive air filling of the affected bowel segments • Large bowel volvulus creates a typical "coffee bean" sign—inflated dilated bowel segment constricted in the center by the mesenteric attachment • Free air as a sign of perforation • The cecum lies in the right upper abdomen in small bowel volvulus.
- **Ultrasound findings**
  Bowel loops are dilated according to the level of the obstruction • Typical "whirlpool" sign with spiraling course of the bowel • Edematous thickening of the bowel wall • Free intraperitoneal fluid.
- **Color Doppler ultrasound findings**
  The superior mesenteric vein lies to the left of the superior mesenteric artery in intestinal malrotation • In small bowel volvulus, the twisted mesenteric vessels lie in a clockwise spiral within the mesentery.
- **Contrast enema findings**
  This is only rarely indicated to visualize large bowel volvulus at the level of the obstruction • Identifies the position of the cecal pole.
- **CT findings**
  Usually not required • Dilated bowel loops • Spiral course of the involved bowel loops (corkscrew sign in midgut volvulus) • Mesenteric fatty tissue narrows down to the point of torsion • Vascular anatomy is visualized (see color Doppler ultrasound) • Entrapment of mesenteric lymph vessels may lead to formation of lymphoceles.

Clinical Aspects

- **Typical presentation**
  Typical findings include sudden bilious vomiting with shock symptoms ("the deadly vomit") in a previously healthy infant • Intermittent symptoms of obstruction • Bloody stools • Impaired absorption in the small bowel due to mesenteric vascular congestion.

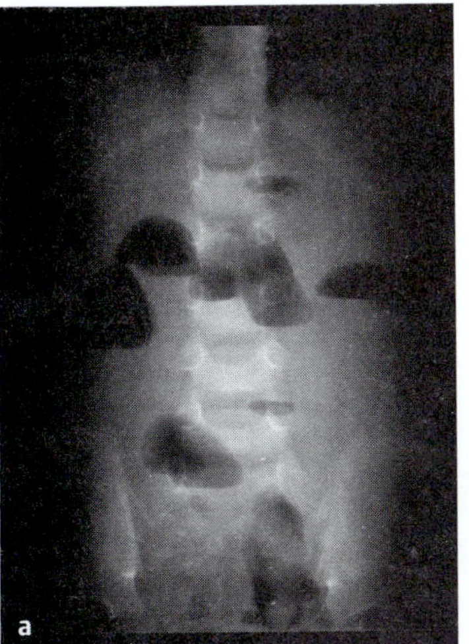

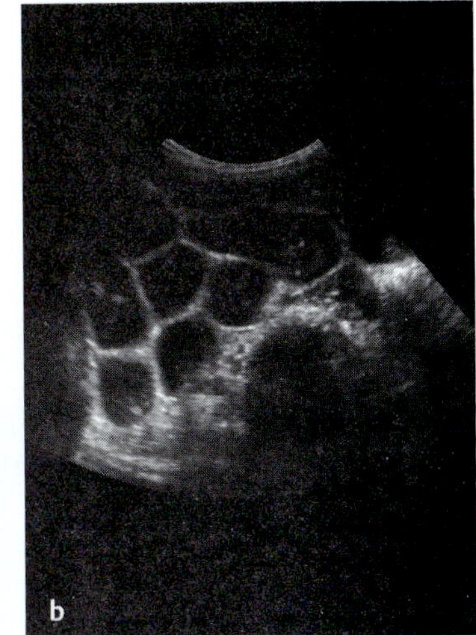

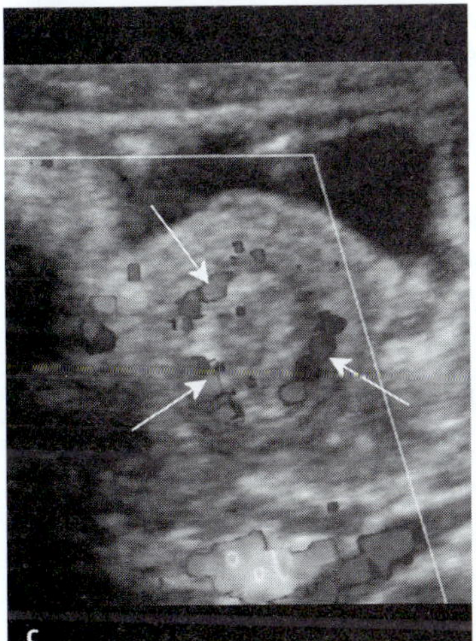

Fig. 4.5 a–c Volvulus. Plain radiograph of the abdomen (**a**). Dilated small bowel loops with air-fluid levels. Ultrasound (**b**). Massively dilated proximal small bowel loops. Color-coded Doppler ultrasound (**c**). "Whirlpool" sign with spiral course of visceral vascular structures (arrows).

- **Therapeutic options**
  Emergency surgery.
- **Course and prognosis**
  Depends on how early the diagnosis is made • Ischemia of the bowel involves a risk of short bowel syndrome.
- **Complications**
  Bowel perforation with peritonitis • Short bowel syndrome.

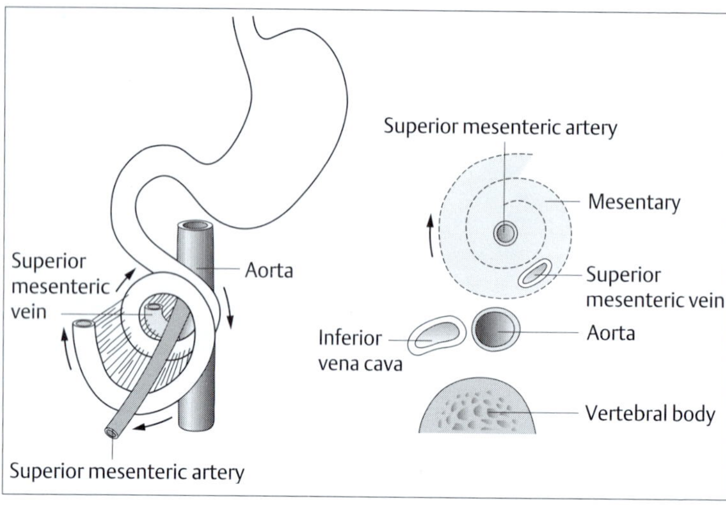

Fig. 4.6 "Whirlpool sign" in volvulus. The small bowel rotates around the root of the mesentery, creating a deformity with the superior mesenteric vein to the left of the superior mesenteric artery (from Benz-Bohm G. Kinderradiologie. Stuttgart: Thieme; 2005).

Differential Diagnosis

Meconium ileus	– Microcolon – Obstruction is usually in the small bowel
Hirschsprung disease	– Typical segmental rectosigmoid stenosis – Abrupt change in diameter of the colon with dilated proximal colon
Ileal atresia	– Microcolon – Small bowel loops distal to the atresia are narrowed
Intestinal Malrotation	– Findings depend on type of malrotation

Tips and Pitfalls

Uncharacteristic or changing symptoms can be misinterpreted as simple gastroenteritis.

Selected References

Buonomo C. Neonatal gastrointestinal emergencies. Radiol Clin North Am 1997; 35: 845–864

McCollough M, Sharieff GQ. Abdominal pain in children. Pediatr Clin North Am 2006; 53: 107–137

Millar AJ et al. Malrotation and volvulus in infancy and childhood. Semin Pediatr Surg 2003; 12: 229–236

Ortiz-Neira CL. The corkscrew sign: midgut volvulus. Radiology 2007; 242: 315–316

Definition

- **Epidemiology**
  Incidence 1:3000–4000 newborns • Increased familial occurrence • Associated with Down syndrome.
- **Etiology, pathophysiology, pathogenesis**
  Defective differentiation of the primitive foregut into esophagus, trachea, and lung in the third to sixth week of embryonal development • Blind ending esophageal pouch, either with a fistula to the trachea (over 90% of cases) or without one, due to defective tracheoesophageal separation • The distal fistula begins slightly superior to the tracheal bifurcation • The H fistula is a special case as there is no discontinuity as in true atresia.
  Classification according to Vogt:
  - *Type I:* Aplasia, esophagus is largely absent (rare).
  - *Type II:* Atresia without a fistula to the trachea (7%).
  - *Type III a:* Atresia with a fistula between trachea and proximal esophageal pouch (1%).
  - *Type III b*: Atresia with a fistula between trachea and distal esophageal pouch (87%).
  - *Type III c:* Atresia with proximal and distal fistulas (2%).
  - *Type IV:* Esophageal fistula, H fistula without atresia (3%).

  VACTERL: Association with additional malformations:
  - V = vertebral: musculoskeletal malformations such as vertebral anomalies (24% of cases).
  - A = anorectal anomalies (20%).
  - C = cardiac, such as atrial or ventricular septal defects and anomalies of the aortic arch (15–39%).
  - TE = tracheoesophageal.
  - R = renal, such as renal agenesis (12%).
  - L = limb, such as malformations of the extremities.

Imaging Signs

- **Chest, abdominal, and skeletal radiograph findings**
  Visualization via gastric tube • After suction aspiration of secretion, the proximal esophageal pouch is insufflated with 1–2 mL of air to visualize the widened, air-filled proximal esophagus • The esophagus may also be visualized with water-soluble contrast agent (approximately 0.5 mL), which should be aspirated by suction immediately after examination • The abdomen will be free of intestinal gas where the distal fistula is absent (types I, II, III a) • Abnormal meteorism occurs in a distal fistula (types III b, III c, IV) • A distal pouch may be detectable because of reflux of air from the stomach (types III b and III c, with gastrostomy types II and III a as well) • Atelectasis • Pneumonia occurs with aspiration • Associated malformations of the spine and extremities may be demonstrated.

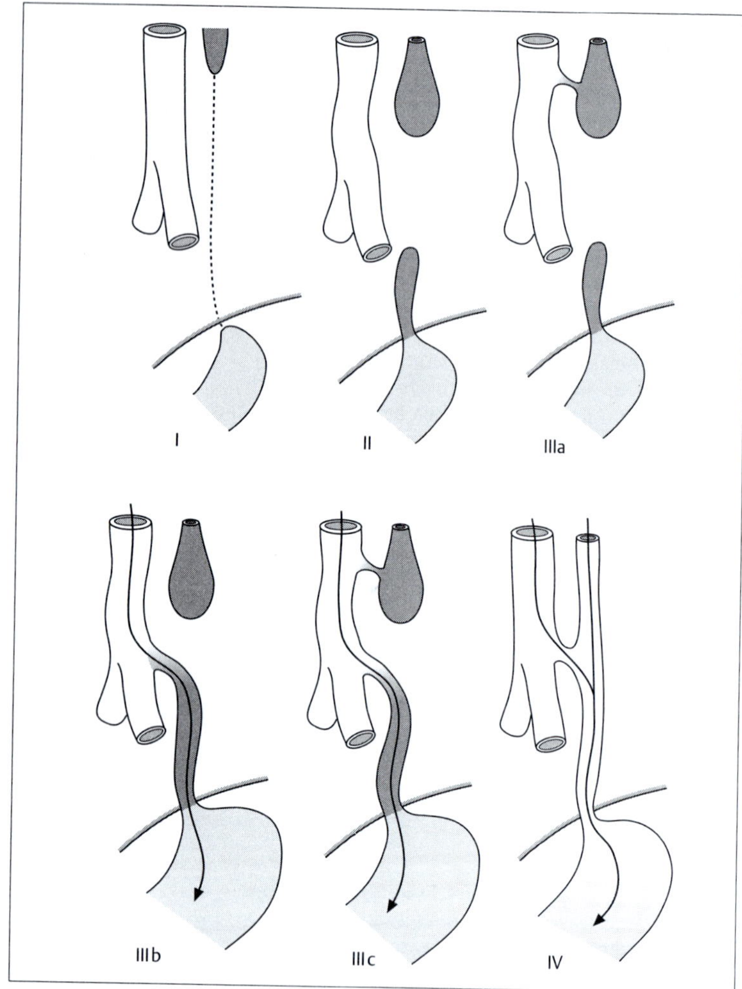

Fig. 4.7 Vogt classification of esophageal atresia. The arrow represents the path of air into the stomach via the tracheoesophageal fistula (from Benz-Bohm G. Kinderradiologie. Stuttgart: Thieme; 2005).

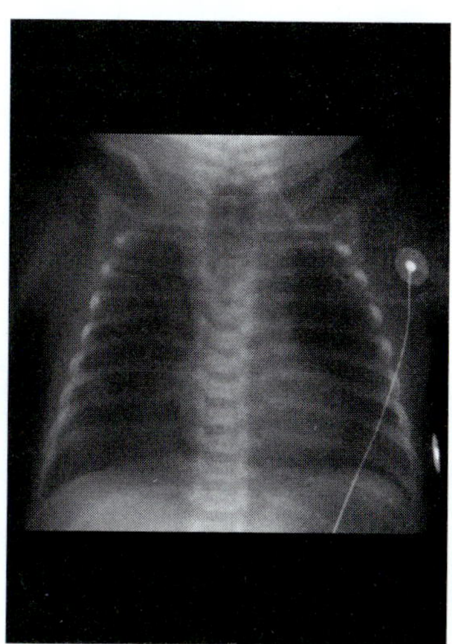

Fig. 4.8 Esophageal atresia—type III b according to Vogt. Chest radiograph. Air-filled proximal esophagus with gastric tube that cannot be advanced further and air in the stomach.

- **Contrast swallow findings**
  A water-soluble nonionic contrast agent is indicated with equivocal findings and in type IV lesions • Fistulas are not always visualized • Fistula extends from the anterior wall of the esophagus obliquely cranially to the trachea and is best demonstrated on a lateral view.
- **Ultrasound findings**
  Stomach cannot be visualized with fluid filling in types I, II, and III a • Reduced bowel filling in types III b and III c.
- **CT**
  Not necessarily indicated to visualize the fistulas.

Clinical Aspects

- **Typical presentation**
  Baby does not drink amniotic fluid, leading to hydramnion • Dyspnea • Cyanosis when saliva from the proximal esophageal pouch enters into the trachea • Foaming at the mouth • Cough • Sunken abdomen where distal fistula is absent • Inflated abdomen where distal fistula is present • Coughing fits during feeding • "Bouncy" resistance is encountered when attempting to place a gastric tube • Gastric juice cannot be aspirated via gastric tube.
  False positive gastric tube probe:
  - Excessively pliable tube will coil up in the pouch without bouncy resistance.
  - Suction aspiration of secretion from the esophageal pouch.
  - Intubation of the stomach via the trachea.

  In these cases endoscopy of the trachea and esophagus may be indicated.

- **Therapeutic options**
  Surgical resection of the fistula • Reconstruction of the esophagus.
- **Course and prognosis**
  Aspiration pneumonia (mortality 25%) • Often accompanied by tracheomalacia.
- **Complications**
  Risk of perforation from gastric tube • Failure of the anastomosis • Esophageal stricture • Impaired contraction • Gastroesophageal reflux • Recurrent fistula (10% of cases).

Differential Diagnosis

Perforation of the pharynx with the gastric tube	– Air insufflation causes pneumomediastinum
Aspiration pneumonia from other causes	– No fistula demonstrated – Gastroesophageal reflux – Foreign body aspiration – Cystic fibrosis – Pulmonary superinfection

Tips and Pitfalls

Diagnosis must be made before the first feeding • Where distal tracheoesophageal fistula is present, obtain a late film (approximately 12 hours postpartum) to demonstrate other possible atresias • The lack of an intestinal stop when placing a gastric tube can delay the diagnosis of an H fistula • Epiglottic passage of contrast medium can lead to misdiagnosis.

Selected References

Benjamin B et al. Diagnosis of H-type tracheoesophageal fistula. J Pediatr Surg 1991; 26: 667–671

Berrocal T et al. Congenital anomalies of the tracheobronchial tree, lung, and mediastinum: embryology, radiology, and pathology. Radiographics 2004; 24: e17

Keckler SJ et al. VACTERL anomalies in patients with esophageal atresia: an updated delineation of the spectrum and review of the literature. Pediatr Surg Int 2007; 23: 309–313

Ratan SK et al. Evaluation of neonates with esophageal atresia using chest CT scan. Pediatr Surg Int 2004; 20: 757–761

Definition

- **Epidemiology**
  Incidence 1:400–1500 • More common in the ileum than jejunum.
- **Etiology, pathophysiology, pathogenesis**
  Atresia is presumably a sequela of ischemia during fetal development • Multiple intestinal atresia is present in 15% of cases • Associated malformations (heart, spine) are rare • Malrotation deformity is also present in 15% of cases • The more distal the air-fluid levels are, the more distal is the obstruction to passage • Proximal atresia produces a "triple bubble" sign • There is no air distal to the atresia • Can be associated with prenatal volvulus or meconium ileus.
  Surgical classification:
  - *Type I:* Membranous occlusion.
  - *Type II:* A fibrous strand interrupts the continuity of the bowel.
  - *Type IIIa:* V-shaped mesenteric defect with missing bowel segment (most common form, 45% of cases).
  - *Type IIIb:* "Apple peel" deformity characterized by absence of the superior mesenteric artery and large parts of the ileum, together with hypoplasia of the mesentery of the small bowel. The small bowel forms a spiral around the vessels of the right colon.
  - *Type IV:* Multiple atresias.

Imaging Signs

- **Chest and abdominal radiograph findings**
  The further distal is the atresia, the more air-fluid levels will be present • Dilated, air-filled proximal small bowel loops • Placing the infant in a head-down position for a long time allows intestinal air to move as far distal as possible • No air in the colon • Sequelae of aspiration may be present • Other malformations may be present.
- **Transit study**
  Usually not required • Can be helpful in detecting additional malrotation.
- **Contrast enema findings**
  Findings include microcolon or normal caliber colon depending on the level of the atresia • Colon is better developed, the higher the atresia is and the later it occurs in fetal development.
- **Ultrasound findings**
  Dilation of bowel loops proximal to the stenosis • Abrupt change in caliber • Other malformations and/or complications may be visualized • Highly active peristalsis or alternating normal and reversed peristalsis in the proximal bowel loops.

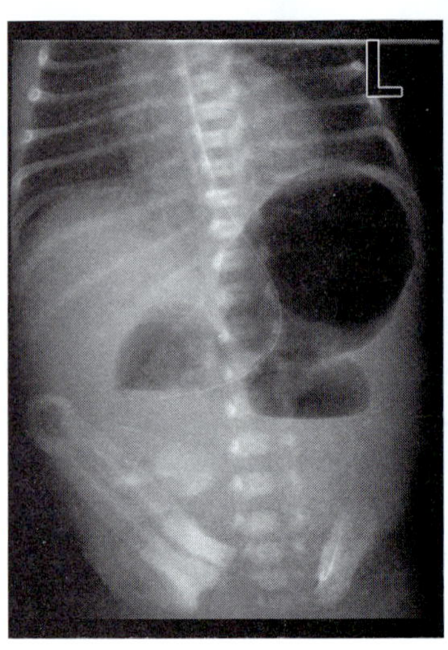

Fig. 4.9 Small bowel atresia directly distal to the ligament of Treitz. Abdominal radiograph. Air-filled stomach, ampulla of Vater, and horizontal/ascending part of the duodenum.

Clinical Aspects

- **Typical presentation**
  Polyhydramnios • Atresia allows normal emptying of meconium but no passage of a normal stool • Signs of obstructed passage with bilious vomiting • Distended abdomen • Onset of symptoms is specific to the level of atresia.
- **Therapeutic options**
  Resection of the affected bowel segment.
- **Course and prognosis**
  Mortality is 10%.
- **Complications**
  Meconium peritonitis after perforation (cystic appearance, calcifications) occurs in 2% of cases • Postoperative short bowel syndrome and disruption of intestinal motility • Strangulation • Anastomotic stenosis.

Differential Diagnosis

Duodenal atresia
- Incidence 1:9000–40000 (common in trisomy 21)
- Three forms (membranous, cordlike with or without a mesenteric defect, complete discontinuity with mesenteric defect)
- Typical "double bubble" sign (air-fluid levels in the stomach and proximal duodenum)
- Examination with patient in left lateral position may be advisable after suction aspiration of gastric juice and air insufflation

Small bowel volvulus
- Usually stool passage is initially normal
- Shock symptoms

Malrotation
- Typical findings on upper gastrointestinal series, contrast enema, and ultrasound

Meconium ileus
- Dilated, meconium-filled small bowel loops
- Usually small-caliber distal ileum
- Both are present in 10% of cases

Meconium plug syndrome
- Contrast enema shows meconium filling defects
- Small left colon
- Proximal colon tends to be dilated rather than small caliber

Hirschsprung disease
- Typical abrupt change in colon caliber in rectosigmoid region
- Megacolon

Tips and Pitfalls

Diagnostic radiology should be postponed until at least 12 hours postpartum • If the abdominal film is obtained too early, the atresia will appear to be more proximal than it actually is • Due to the absence of haustration in newborns, the small bowel is often indistinguishable from the large bowel • Air will be detected in the bowel segments distal to the atresia after rectal enema • Entry of air into the gastrointestinal tract is delayed in these cases:
- Frail premature infants.
- Difficulty swallowing.
- Respiratory dysfunction.
- Vomiting air with stomach contents.
- Parenteral nutrition.

Selected References

Berdon WE et al. Microcolon in newborn infants with intestinal obstruction. Its correlation with the level and time of onset of obstruction. Radiology 1968; 90: 878–885

McAlister WH et al. Emergency gastrointestinal radiology of the newborn. Radiol Clin North Am 1996; 34: 819–844

Sato S et al. Jejunoileal atresia: a 27-year experience. J Pediatr Surg 1998; 33: 1633–1635

Definition

▸ **Epidemiology**
Incidence 1:2500–5000 • Anal atresia in boys most often occurs with a rectourethral fistula • Anal atresia in girls most often occurs with a rectovestibular fistula.

▸ **Etiology, pathophysiology, pathogenesis**
The embryo initially develops a cloaca that is later divided by the urorectal septum • In anal atresia, this septum fails to develop • Fistulas occur in 90% of cases • Rarely vaginal, scrotal, or penile fistulas occur • Associated with numerous additional anomalies (VACTERL), especially of the urogenital tract (approximately 60%), vertebrae (approximately 40%), and gastrointestinal tract (5% of cases have esophageal atresia) • Associated anomalies are twice as common with high lesions than with low lesions.

Table 4.2 Wingspread classification (1984)

Form	Characteristics	Frequency
High lesion	Superior to levator ani	31%
Intermediate lesion	Rectal pouch partially intersects levator sling	13%
Low lesion	Atresia inferior to the levator sling	54%
Other rare anomalies	Cloacal malformation: urethra, vagina, and rectum share a common orifice	2%

Table 4.3 Peña classification of anorectal malformations

High lesion in anal atresia (distance from anal fossa to rectum > 1 cm)
Low lesion in anal atresia (distance from anal fossa to rectum < 1 cm) • Boys and girls: Anal atresia without fistula • rectoperineal fistula • Boys: bladder fistula • urethral bulbar fistula • urethral prostatic fistula • Girls: vestibular fistula
Anal stenosis
Anal membrane
Cloacal malformation in girls

Imaging Signs

▸ **Wangensteen view/Invertography findings**
Requirements: No visible fistula opening • No meconium in vagina or urine • Air can escape through openings, making it difficult to determine the position of the atresia • Perform this examination 12 hours postpartum at the earliest.
Imaging technique: Pelvis is elevated (patient in head down position) • The anal fossa or fissure is marked with radiopaque material such as a lead bead and a lateral projection is used • The position of the rectal pouch is evaluated relative to

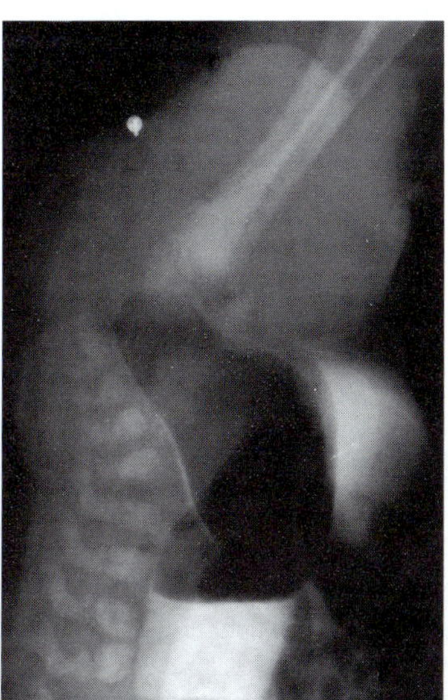

Fig. 4.10 Anal atresia. Wangensteen view (after voiding cystourethrography). The distance between the anal fossa (marked with lead bead) and the rectal air crescent is about 3 cm. Marked filling of the rectum with contrast, with additional rectovesical fistula. Contrast-filled bladder.

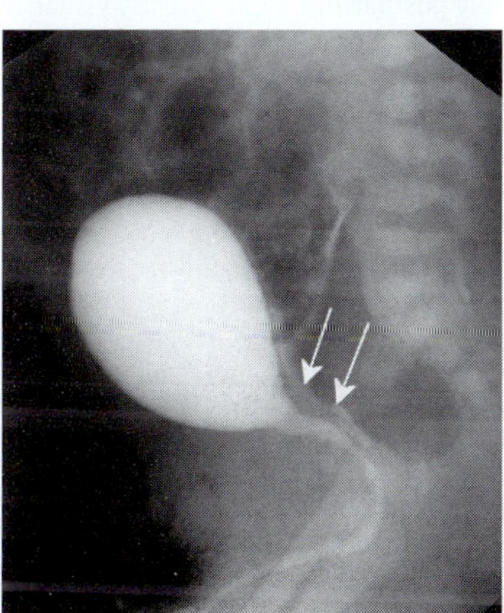

Fig. 4.11 Voiding cystourethrography. Spontaneous micturition reveals a fistula (arrows) from the posterior wall of the bladder to the rectum.

the marking • Spot views on contraction and relaxation may be indicated • The increased intraabdominal pressure or relaxation of the musculature of the pelvic floor shifts the rectal pouch distally.

Interpreting findings: Orientation lines are used to differentiate the three main forms (Wingspread classification, see above):

- *PC line:* Inferior margin of vertebra S5 to the center of the pubic bone.
- *I line:* Parallel to the PC line through the most distal point of the ischium.

- *M line:* Parallel drawn between the PC and I lines defining the floor of the pelvis (levator sling).

Forms of atresia:

- *High lesion:* Rectal pouch lies proximal to the PC line.
- *Intermediate lesion:* Rectal pouch lies within the parallels, distal to the PC line.
- *Low lesion:* Lies below the I line.

Findings: Dilation of the meconium-filled colon • Intraluminal calcifications may be present • Air may be present in the urinary bladder or vagina • Evaluation of the sacrum (absent vertebrae).

► **Contrast enema findings**

Visualization of the distal rectum where there is an external opening that will accept a probe.

► **Abdominal ultrasound findings**

Lower abdomen in longitudinal section: Relationship of rectal pouch to the floor of the bladder (levator sling).

Sagittal perineal ultrasound: Shows the distance between the rectal pouch and anal fossa without compression:

- > 1.5 cm with the rectal pouch cranial to the floor of the bladder: high lesion.
- 1.0–1.5 cm, with the rectal pouch at the level of the floor of the bladder: no clear classification as high or low lesion is possible.
- < 1.0 cm with the rectal pouch caudal to the floor of the bladder: low lesion.

Advantages: Can be performed immediately postpartum • Can directly visualize a fistula or demonstrate air in the bladder • Excludes urogenital anomalies such as hydronephrosis or hydrocolpos.

► **Spinal ultrasound findings**

Visualizes the bony structures of the coccyx • Visualizes the rest of the spine and spinal canal • Excludes a presacral mass.

► **Voiding cystourethrography (VCUG)**

Can exclude fistulas between the rectal pouch and the bladder, urethra, or vagina in high lesions.

► **MRI findings**

T1-weighted SE and T2-weighted TSE sequences in axial and coronal planes with respect to the pelvic floor and in a true sagittal plane • Visualizes the floor of the pelvis, sphincter musculature, and position of the rectal pouch • Sensitive in detecting fistulas (T2-weighted TSE-SPIR and T1-weighted contrast studies) • Visualizes associated malformations and can exclude malformations of the spinal cord, spine, and urogenital tract.

► **Fistula imaging**

Fistulography via fistula opening.

Clinical Aspects

► **Typical presentation**

No normal passage of meconium • Meconium empties via fistulas, urethra, and/or vagina.

- **Therapeutic options**
  Low lesion: Primary proctoperineoplasty • Reconstruction of the sphincter musculature • Reconstruction of sensitive anorectal tissue.
  Other types and lesions with vestibular fistula: Colostomy • Later "pull-through" procedure.
- **Course and prognosis**
  Incontinence, especially where more than two sacral vertebrae are absent.
- **Complications**
  Meconium peritonitis secondary to perforation (cystic appearance, calcifications) • Constipation.

Differential Diagnosis

Meconium ileus	– Insertion of rectal probe and contrast administration possible
Meconium plug syndrome	– Insertion of rectal probe and contrast administration possible – Contrast enema shows meconium filling defect – Small left colon with dilated proximal colon
Hirschsprung disease	– Insertion of rectal probe and contrast administration possible – Typical abrupt change in caliber in rectosigmoid region – Megacolon

Tips and Pitfalls

Diagnostic radiology with invertography should be postponed until at least 12 hours postpartum, otherwise the atresia will appear to be more proximal that it actually is. This influences the choice of surgical procedure with the specific postoperative sequelae it may entail, such as lifelong incontinence. Ultrasound can be performed immediately after delivery • In perineal ultrasound, compression by the transducer can lead to inaccurate measurements • In high and intermediate lesions, a voiding cystourethrography must be obtained to exclude rectourogenital fistulas.

Selected References

Niedzielski JK. Invertography versus ultrasonography and distal colostography for the determination of bowel-skin distance in children with anorectal malformations. Eur J Pediatr Surg 2005; 15: 262–267

Nievelstein RA et al. MR imaging of anorectal malformations and associated anomalies. Eur Radiol 1998; 8: 573–581

Pena A et al. Advances in the management of anorectal malformations. Am J Surg 2000; 180: 370–376

Ratan SK et al. Associated congenital anomalies in patients with anorectal malformations—a need for developing a uniform practical approach. J Pediatr Surg 2004; 39: 1706–1711

Shaul DB et al. Classification of anorectal malformations-initial approach, diagnostic tests and colostomy. Semin Pediatr Surg 1997; 6: 187–195

Hypertrophic Pyloric Stenosis (HPS)

Definition

- **Epidemiology**
  Incidence is as high as 3:1000 • More common in boys than girls by a ratio of 5:1 • Peak frequency: 4–7 weeks of life • Rarely occurs after 12 weeks.
- **Etiology, pathophysiology, pathogenesis**
  Idiopathic hypertrophy and hyperplasia of the circular muscle fibers of the pylorus • Common in firstborn male children • Genetic disposition has been postulated.

Imaging Signs

- **Abdominal radiograph**
  Not required • Can exclude ileus or free intraperitoneal air.
- **Ultrasound findings**
  Longitudinal plane: Pyloric canal length more than 16 mm • Constricted pylorus that does not allow passage of food or air • "Shoulder" sign—thickened musculature projects like a collar into the gastric lumen • Fluid-filled stomach is dilated with hyperperistalsis.
  Axial plane: Muscle layer of one wall is thickened over 3–4 mm • Total diameter of the pylorus is over 8 mm.

Clinical Aspects

- **Typical presentation**
  Projectile nonbilious vomiting immediately after feeding • Dystrophy • Palpably distended pylorus • Positive "tea test" (visible gastric hyperperistalsis after giving the infant tea) • *Laboratory findings:* Metabolic (hypochloremic) alkalosis, hypokalemia, and hyponatremia.
- **Therapeutic options**
  Pyloromyotomy.
- **Course and prognosis**
  Surgery is curative.
- **Complications**
  Metabolic derangement • Dessication • Dystrophy.

Differential Diagnosis

Functional vomiting	– Infection
Proximal duodenal stenosis	– Widened duodenal bulb on ultrasound – No shoulder sign – Vomiting, possibly with bilious component
Roviralta syndrome	– Hypertrophic pyloric stenosis and gastroesophageal reflux – Hiatal hernia

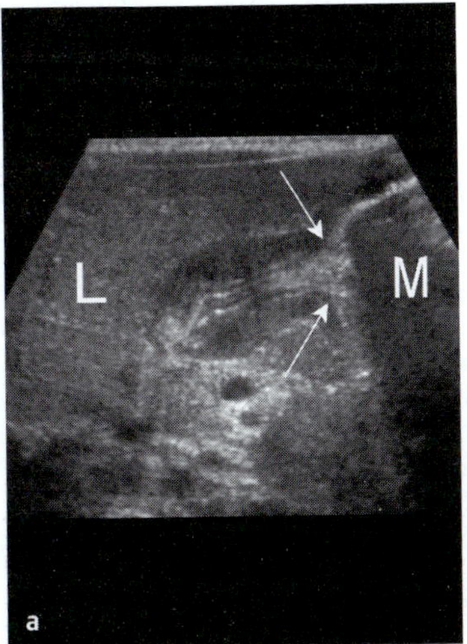

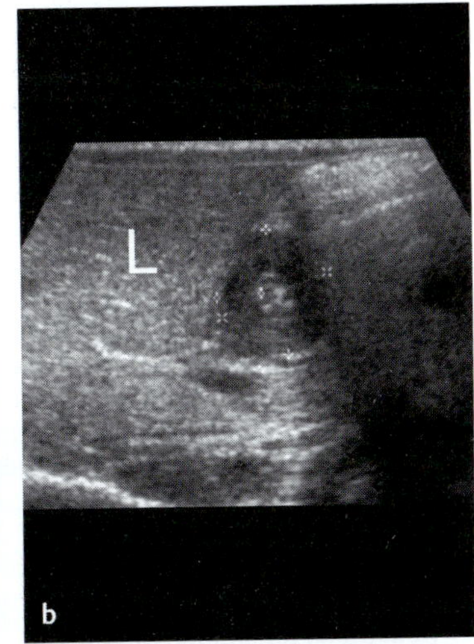

Fig. 4.12 a, b Hypertrophic pyloric stenosis. Longitudinal (**a**) and axial (**b**) ultrasound scan of the upper abdomen. Classic visualization of hypertrophic pyloric stenosis with shoulder sign (arrows) and extended pylorus with thickened wall. The stomach (M) is filled with air. L = liver.

Pylorospasm	– No visibly thickened pylorus (muscle thickness 1.5–2 mm) – Variable width of the antrum – Delayed gastric emptying – Psychogenic causes – No treatment needed

Tips and Pitfalls

With clear clinical and ultrasound findings, there is no differential diagnosis to consider.

Selected References

Gasseling J et al. Hypertrophic pyloric stenosis. Radiol Technol 2004; 75: 314–316

Hall NJ et al. Meta-analysis of laparoscopic versus open pyloromyotomy. Ann Surg 2004; 240: 774–778

Safford SD et al. A study of 11003 patients with hypertrophic pyloric stenosis and the association between surgeon and hospital volume and outcomes. J Pediatr Surg 2005; 40: 967–972

Definition

- **Epidemiology**
  Incidence is about 1:5000 • Occurs four times as often in girls than in boys • Usually occurs sporadically.
- **Etiology, pathophysiology, pathogenesis**
  Defective craniocaudal neuroblast migration prior to the twelfth week of embryonal development • Aplasia of the intramural parasympathetic nerve plexus • Short segment (80% of cases) or long segment without ganglia • Usually occurs in the rectosigmoid region • In extreme cases, the entire colon is affected • Subsequent hyperplasia of the extramural parasympathetic fibers with increased release of acetylcholine and contracture of the ring musculature • Associated with trisomy 21 • Histologic and histochemical studies confirm the diagnosis.
  Rare forms: Short segment aganglionosis • Immature ganglion cells • Neuronal intestinal dysplasia • Unclassifiable ganglion disorders.

Imaging Signs

- **Abdominal radiograph findings**
  There may be signs of distal colonic ileus • In older children the plain radiograph will show a dilated colon with severe fecal impaction • Minimal gas and stool in the rectum.
- **Ultrasound findings**
  Massive fecal impaction with dilation of the colon • Abrupt change in caliber is visualized with minimal stool and gas in the nondilated distal segment of the colon • Findings typical of ileus may be present such as dilated small bowel loops with alternating normal and reversed peristalsis.
- **Contrast enema findings**
  Direct visualization of the abrupt change in colon caliber • Examination is without bowel preparation as the fecal impaction proximal to the stenosis aids in the diagnosis • Supplementary defecography may be helpful • Voiding studies with late images up to 24 hours later demonstrate incomplete passage of contrast agent from the bowel.

Clinical Aspects

- **Typical presentation**
  Therapy-resistant meconium plug syndrome • Distal ileus in newborns • Chronic constipation in older children • Rarely enterocolitis • In 80% of cases, initial symptoms occur in the first few weeks of life.
- **Therapeutic options**
  - *Conservative:* Diet • Laxatives.
  - *Surgical:* Resection of the aganglionic segment.

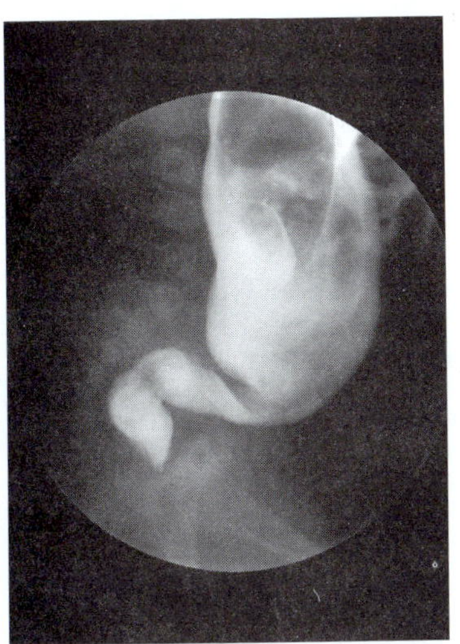

Fig. 4.13 Hirschsprung disease. Lateral view of contrast enema. Pronounced dilation of the sigmoid colon (megacolon), abrupt change in caliber in the rectosigmoid region.

- **Course and prognosis**
  The more extensive the cleansing enemas, the later the megacolon will develop • Complete resection is curative.
- **Complications**
  Necrotizing enterocolitis • Cecal perforation from fecal impaction • Obstructive uropathy due to mass effect of megacolon and compression of the ureters • Postoperative stenosis of the anastomosis • Subtotal resection of the aganglionic segment with recurrent symptoms.

Differential Diagnosis

Anal stenosis	– Diagnosis with biopsy and manometry
Habitual constipation	– Complete voiding of contrast agent – Most common cause of megacolon
Meconium plug syndrome	– Asymptomatic after contrast enema – Visualization of meconium plug – Small left colon
Microcolon	– Without histologic examination, this is indistinguishable from Hirschsprung disease involving the entire colon – Distal small bowel obstruction such as ileal atresia must be excluded

Tips and Pitfalls

A very short aganglionic segment adjacent to the sphincter will escape detection despite defecography (diagnosis is made by anal manometry or biopsy of the bowel wall) • Bowel preparation and rectal examination are contraindicated for 24 hours prior to contrast enema.

Selected References

De Lorijn F et al. Diagnosis of Hirschsprung's disease: a prospective, comparative accuracy study of common tests. J Pediatr 2005; 146: 787–792

Engum SA et al. Long-term results of treatment of Hirschsprung's disease. Semin Pediatr Surg 2004; 13: 273–285

Fotter R. Imaging of constipation in infants and children. Eur Radiol 1998; 8: 248–258

Nofech-Mozes Y et al. Difficulties in making the diagnosis of Hirschsprung disease in early infancy. J Paediatr Child Health 2004; 40: 716–719

Definition

- **Epidemiology**
  Most common cause of occlusive ileus in infants • Peak frequency is at age 3–12 months.
- **Etiology, pathophysiology, pathogenesis**
  Invagination of a proximal bowel segment including the mesentery and vascular structures into the lumen of a distal bowel segment • *Occurrence:* 90% of cases involve the ileocecal region, 6% only the small bowel, and 4% only the large bowel • Usually idiopathic in infants • In older children, it is usually secondary to other disorders (pathologic lead point) such as swollen lymph nodes in infection, Meckel diverticulum, lymphoma, polyp, enteric duplication, hematoma, or cystic fibrosis.

Imaging Signs

- **Ultrasound findings**
  Sensitivity is 100%, specificity 88% • Concentric ring or bull's eye sign on cross-section • Intussusception entirely within the small bowel appearing as a bull's eye measuring < 15 mm in diameter is usually without obstructed passage • Pseudokidney sign (parallel thickened bowel walls) on longitudinal image • No peristalsis or intestinal air in the invaginated area • Enlarged lymph nodes • Thickened bowel wall • Free fluid • Tumors or other causes of intussusception may be present • Bowel segment proximal to the intussusception is dilated, consistent with obstruction.
  Follow-up examination after treatment: Free ileocecal valve • Fluid reflux into the terminal ileum • No residual bull's eye • Findings include thickening of the bowel wall and a swollen ileocecal valve.
- **Doppler ultrasound findings**
  No blood flow signal in the invaginated segment in intramural necrosis.
- **Abdominal radiograph findings**
  Indicated only in patients with poor general health to exclude perforation (free air) and to visualize the ileus • Minimal abdominal gas • A mass isodense to soft tissue may be present as radiographic correlate • Findings are normal in 25% of cases.
- **Contrast enema findings**
  Head of the intussusception appears as a filling defect • Intussusception is resolved by hydrostatic reduction.
- **CT findings**
  Not usually required • Bull's eye can be visualized • Bowel ischemia may be present • Cause may be visualized.

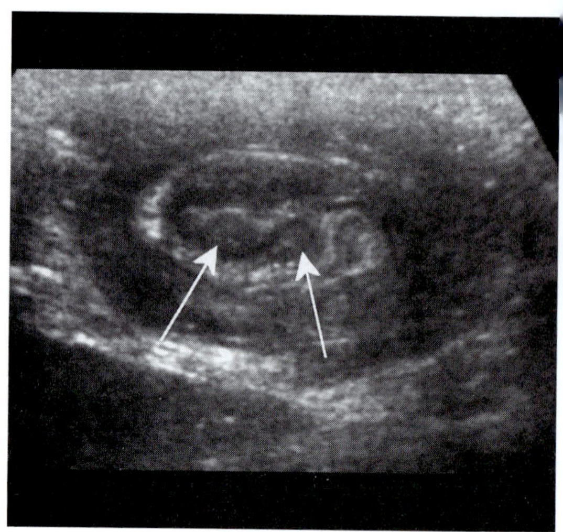

Fig. 4.14 Ultrasound scan of the upper abdomen. Typical subhepatic bull's eye sign in ileocecal intussusception. The lymph nodes are also included in the intussusception (arrows), here clearly visualized embedded in hypoechoic mesenteric fatty tissue.

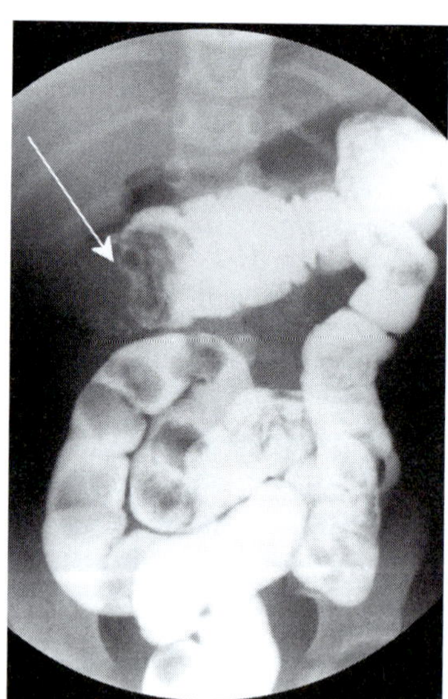

Fig. 4.15 Intussusception. Contrast enema. The head of the invaginated segment is visualized in the hepatic flexure (arrow).

Clinical Aspects

- **Typical presentation**
  Abdominal pain, vomiting, bloody stools, shock, and a palpable abdominal mass • Asymptomatic intervals may occur with spontaneous resolution, particularly in the small bowel.
- **Therapeutic options**
  Hydrostatic reduction (experience has shown that no more than three attempts should be made):
  - Contrast enema with radiopaque, nonionic, water-soluble contrast agent, under fluoroscopy (90–120 cmH_2O).
  - Ultrasound guided contrast enema with physiologic saline solution (90–120 cmH_2O).
  - Controlled-pressure air insufflation under fluoroscopic control (80–120 mmHg).

  Absolute contraindications for hydrostatic reduction:
  - Perforation
  - Signs of peritonitis
  - Shock, dehydration
  - Large quantities of free fluid

  Relative contraindications for hydrostatic reduction:
  - Multiple recurrences
  - Longer history (more than 24 hours)
  - Bloody stools
  - Ileoileal intussusception
  - Suspected tumor
  - Age over 3 years
  - Manifest ileus

  Surgical: Where hydrostatic reduction fails or is contraindicated.
- **Course and prognosis**
  Rate or recurrence is as high as 10% • Usually recurs within 72 hours • Mortality less than 1% where intussusception is reduced within 24 hours.
- **Complications**
  Spontaneous perforation or perforation during reduction (approximately 0.5–3% of cases) • Ileus • Necrosis.

Differential Diagnosis

Antrum	– Resembles a bull's eye when slightly filled
Appendicitis	– Smaller diameter bull's eye – Lies in the right lower abdomen – Inflammatory reaction of adjacent tissue – Pericecal abscess
Gastroenteritis	– Intussusception within the small bowel may occur in gastroenteritis, usually with spontaneous reduction – Fluid-filled small bowel loops – Directional hyperperistalsis – Usually no thickening of the bowel wall – Mesenteric lymphadenitis

Tips and Pitfalls

Ultrasound examination in the presence of conspicuous thickening of the bowel wall and enlarged lymph nodes to exclude malignant lymphoma • Bull's eye in intussusception must not be confused with the bull's eye in severe enterocolitis • Cause of the intussusception must not be misdiagnosed. Therefore a careful ultrasound follow-up examination is always indicated after reduction • Intussusception within the small bowel can be misinterpreted as an ileocecal intussusception.

Selected References

Applegate KE. Clinically suspected intussusception in children: evidence-based review and self-assessment module. Am J Roentgenol 2005; 185(3 Suppl): 175–183

Navarro OM et al. Intussusception: the use of delayed, repeated reduction attempts and the management of intussusceptions due to pathologic lead points in pediatric patients. Am J Roentgenol 2004; 182: 1169–1176

Sorantin E et al. Management of intussusception. Eur Radiol 2004; 14 Suppl 4: L146–154

Definition

- **Epidemiology**
  Most common cause of acute abdomen in children • Peak frequency is at age 12–14 years.
- **Etiology, pathophysiology, pathogenesis**
  Inflammation of the appendix due to obstruction of the lumen (for example by an appendicolith) with accumulation of secretions and superinfection.

Imaging Signs

- **Ultrasound findings**
  Method of choice • Sensitivity 90%, specificity 95% • Longitudinal images show tubular structure with thickened walls, occasionally with fluid accumulations in the lumen • Abnormal, incompressible bull's eye with an axial diameter of over 6 mm (not a reliable finding in patients with cystic fibrosis) • Considerable pain on compression with the transducer • Increased echogenicity of the adjacent mesenteric fatty tissue (due to edema) • Free fluid in the immediate vicinity (early exudate) or in the pouch of Douglas (after perforation) • Appendicolith may be present • Enlarged mesentery lymph nodes • Findings after perforation may include only an irregular soft tissue mass.
  Pericecal abscess: Common sites include the right paracolic region, ileocecal region, posterior to the bladder, subhepatic region (pouch of Morrison), right subphrenic regions, and between the bowel loops.
- **Color Doppler ultrasound findings**
  Increased vascularity due to inflammatory hyperperfusion.
- **Abdominal radiograph findings**
  Usually not required • Can exclude free air • Left convex postural deformity of the lumbar spine • Air and fluid levels in the lower abdomen may occur with abscess • Shadow of the right psoas major is obliterated • Signs of paralytic ileus in peritonitis.
- **CT findings**
  Helpful where other findings are equivocal • Intravenous, oral, and rectal contrast administration • Appendix wall is thickened • Inflammatory involvement of the surrounding fatty tissue and adjacent bowel (small bowel and sigmoid) • Enlarged lymph nodes • Abscess is visualized.

Clinical Aspects

- **Typical presentation**
  Abdominal pain • Nausea • Vomiting • Uncharacteristic gastrointestinal symptoms • Right lower abdomen exhibits tenderness on palpation, pain when tapping, and pain on release of pressure • Fever • Leukocytosis • Elevated C-reactive protein • The younger the patient, the less characteristic the symptoms may be.

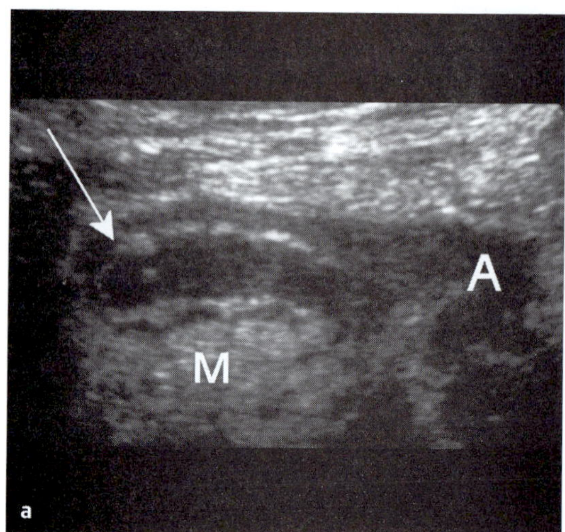

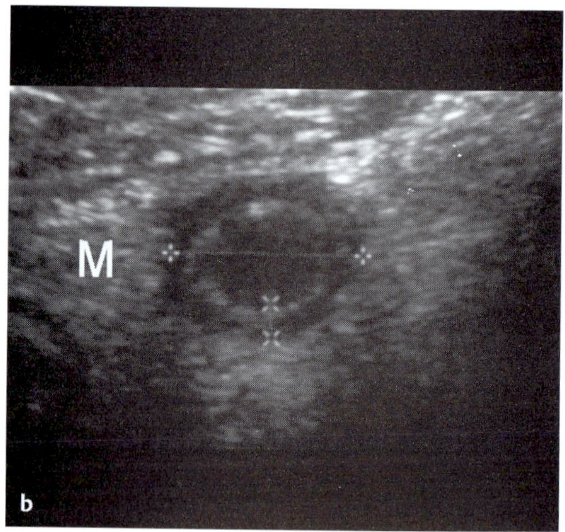

Fig. 4.16 a, b Appendicitis. Ultrasound scan of the right lower abdomen. Typical bull's eye on the longitudinal (**a**) and transverse images (**b**), consistent with a fluid-filled appendix (arrow) with markedly thickened wall. Adjacent inflammatory mesenteric fatty tissue (M) with edema. Fluid retention in adjacent tissue consistent with pericecal abscess (A).

- **Therapeutic options**
  Appendectomy • Perforation is managed with antibiotics, percutaneous abscess drainage, and delayed appendectomy.
- **Course and prognosis**
  Surgery is curative.
- **Complications**
  Covered perforation (pericecal abscess) • Paralytic ileus • Peritonitis.

Differential Diagnosis

Mesenteric lymphadenitis	– Enlarged lymph nodes – Small bowel loops with thickened walls may be associated with a small amount of free fluid between the bowel loops and in the pouch of Douglas
Crohn Disease	– Usually typical history – Clinical aspects – Predilection for the terminal ileum
Lymphoma	– Can also occur as a primary lesion of the bowel wall (MALT lymphoma) – Enlarged mesenteric and retroperitoneal lymph nodes
Torsion of an ovarian cyst	– Hemorrhaging and typical sedimentation may occur – Adjacent to adnexa – Bowel is usually normal
Intussusception	– Typical ultrasound morphology and clinical findings
Meckel diverticulitis	– Clinically indistinguishable – Usually not detectable on ultrasound scans when obscured by intestinal gas

Tips and Pitfalls

Do not look for the appendix only in the typical location in the right lower abdomen; it can also occur in a subhepatic location or posterior to the cecum or bladder • Normal ultrasound findings do not exclude appendicitis.

Selected References

Hernandez JA et al. Imaging of acute appendicitis: US as the primary imaging modality. Pediatr Radiol 2005; 35: 392–395

Keyzer C et al. Comparison of US and unenhanced multi-detector row CT in patients suspected of having acute appendicitis. Radiology 2005; 236: 527–534

Menten R et al. Outer diameter of the vermiform appendix: not a valid sonographic criterion for acute appendicitis in patients with cystic fibrosis. Am J Roentgenol 2005; 184: 1901–1903

Definition

- **Epidemiology**
  Predilection for young adults • 25% of cases begin in childhood or adolescence • No sex predilection.
- **Etiology, pathophysiology, pathogenesis**
  Unknown etiology • Transmural granulomatous inflammation • Can affect the entire gastrointestinal tract—stomach 2–20% of cases, duodenum 4–10%, small bowel 80%, colon 22–55%, rectum 35–50% • Associated with erythema nodosum and pyoderma gangrenosum.
  Extraintestinal manifestations: Fatty degeneration of the liver • Gall stones • Sclerosing cholangitis • Amyloidosis • Sacroiliitis • Ankylosing spondylitis.

Imaging Signs

- **Endoscopy**
  Esophagogastroduodenoscopy • Ileocolonoscopy with biopsy for histologic examination.
- **Ultrasound findings**
  Thickening of the wall in the affected bowel segment • Lack of differentiation in the wall layers • A bull's eye sign may be present • Inflammatory conglomerate mass • Segmental involvement • Terminal ileum is usually affected • Hyperechoic adjacent mesenteric fatty tissue with edema • Reactive lymph node enlargement • Separation of the bowel loops due to mesenteric inflammatory reaction and proliferation of fatty tissue (creeping fat) • Tubular bowel without peristaltic undulations • Complicated clinical course involves abscesses.
- **Color Doppler ultrasound findings**
  Increased vascularity of the bowel wall.
- **Enteroclysis findings**
  Dynamic examination • Coarsening of folds • "Cobblestone relief" • Ulceration • Inflammatory stenosis of the intestinal lumen • Dilation proximal to the stenosis • Antimesenteric pseudodiverticulum • Skip lesions • Fistulas.
- **CT findings**
  May be helpful in imaging fistulas • Demonstrates abscess formation • Guides drain placement.
- **MRI**
  This has largely supplanted enteroclysis.
  Preparation: Involves oral administration of 1 L of a 2.5% mannitol solution over 1 hour • Body weight adapted application of butyl scopolamine • Sequences: True FISP (balanced FFE), T2-weighted TSE-SPIR, fat-suppressed T1-weighted SE sequence after intravenous contrast administration (0.1 mmol/kg of gadolinium-DTPA).

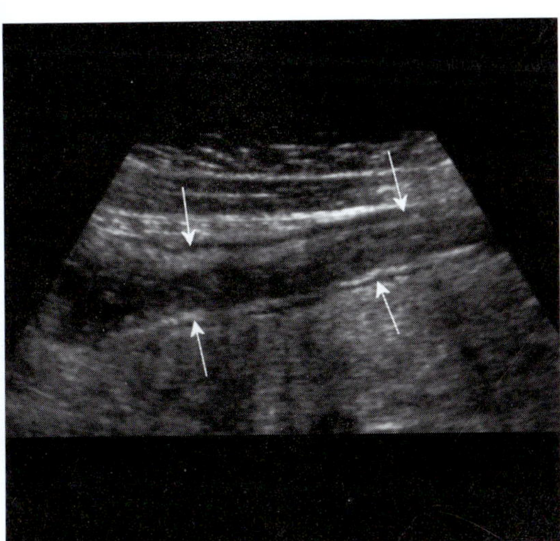

Fig. 4.17 Crohn disease. Ultrasound scan of the right lower abdomen. Long stretch of thickened wall in the terminal ileum (arrows) without peristalsis in the dynamic examination.

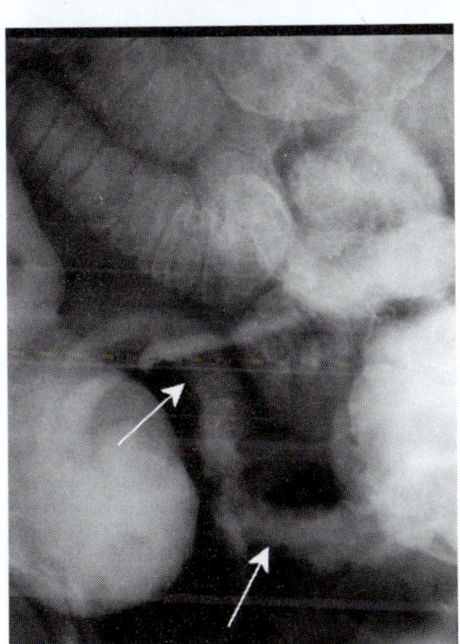

Fig. 4.18 Sellink modified enteroclysis. Long stretch of inflammatory stenosis in the terminal ileum (arrows).

Findings: Include "comb" sign of mesenteric vessels immediately adjacent to the affected bowel segment due to inflammatory hypervascularity • Enlarged lymph nodes • Mesenteric fatty tissue proliferation (creeping fat) with separation of the bowel loops • Fistulas • Abscesses • MR-guided abscess drainage where indicated • Inflammatory stenosis of the bowel lumen.

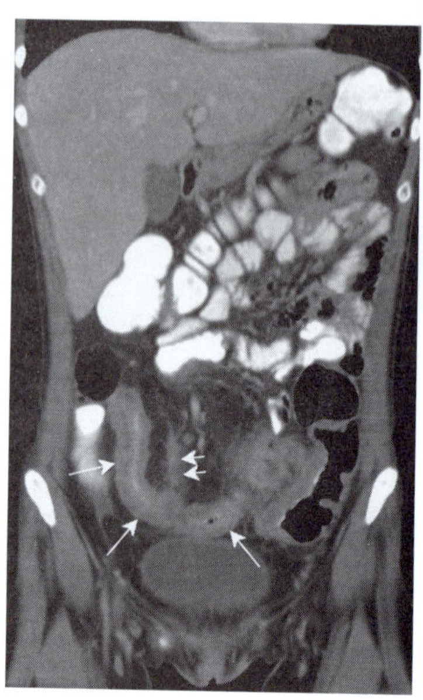

Fig. 4.19 Crohn disease. Contrast-enhanced CT of the abdomen, coronal multiplanar reformation. Massive inflammatory thickening of the wall over a long stretch of the ileum (arrows) and a long fistula in the mesentery (small arrows).

Clinical Aspects

- **Typical presentation**
  Diarrhea, colicky abdominal pain, weight loss, bloody stools, anemia • Perianal abscesses with fistulas (40% of cases) • Malabsorption (30%).
- **Therapeutic options**
  Conservative: Diet • Oral substitution of iron, folic acid, and vitamin B_{12} • 5-amino salicylic acid (sulfasalazine) • Glucocorticoids • Azathioprine • Infliximab • Antibiotics (metronidazole).
  Absolute indications for surgery: Bowel perforation • Intraabdominal and perianal abscesses • Severe intestinal obstruction with recurrent ileus • Acute appendicitis • Acute urinary retention • Toxic megacolon (rare).
- **Course and prognosis**
  Rate of recurrence is as high as 40% following resection, usually within the first 2 years • Mortality is as high as 7% • Surgery is not curative.
- **Complications**
  Deep venous thrombosis in the legs and pelvis • Fistulas (enterocolic, enterocutaneous, perineal, 33% of cases) • Retroperitoneal and intraperitoneal abscesses • Macroscopic perforation • Toxic megacolon • Ileus • Hydronephrosis due to compression of the ureter • Stunted growth • Delayed puberty.

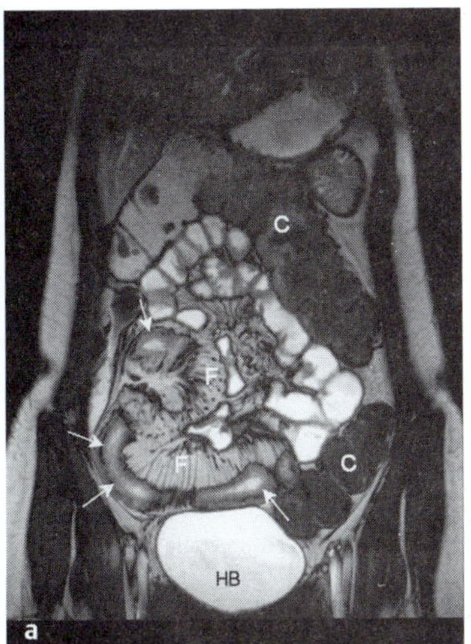

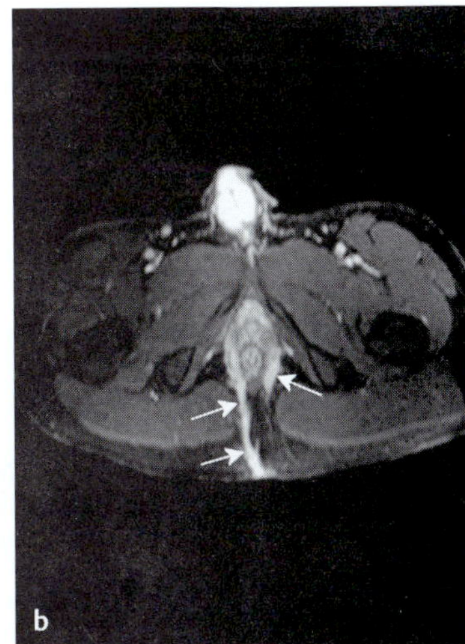

Fig. 4.20 a, b Crohn disease. MR image. The coronal balanced FFE sequence (**a**) allows nearly artifact-free visualization of the small bowel. Multisegmental involvement of the small bowel in Crohn disease (arrows) with proliferation of fatty mesenteric tissue (F) and pronounced mesenteric vascular injection ("comb sign"). The T1-weighted SPIR sequence after contrast administration (**b**) clearly demonstrates bilateral perianal fistulas (arrows). C = colon; HB = bladder.

Differential Diagnosis

Yersiniosis	– Limited to terminal ileum – Severe mesenteric lymphadenopathy – Resolves within 3–4 months – Stool examination
Salmonellosis	– Large bowel is typically involved – Stool findings – Acute onset, watery diarrhea
Tuberculosis	– Cecum is usually involved – Pulmonary involvement – Tuberculosis test
Ulcerative colitis	– Continuous involvement – Colon involved – "Backwash" ileitis
Radiation therapy	– History

Lymphoma	– Bowel stenosis is not typical – No inflammatory reaction in adjacent tissue – No abscess or fistula – Lymphadenopathy in another location
Pseudomembranous colitis	– History of antibiotics use

Tips and Pitfalls

Normal imaging studies cannot reliably exclude a chronic inflammatory bowel disorder • Inflammatory involvement of the appendix in Crohn disease can be misinterpreted as appendicitis.

Selected References

Horsthuis K et al. MRI in Crohn's disease. J Magn Reson Imaging 2005; 22: 1–12

Schmidt T et al. Phase-inversion tissue harmonic imaging compared to fundamental B-mode ultrasound in the evaluation of the pathology of large and small bowel. Eur Radiol 2005; 15: 2021–2030

Scribano M et al. Review article: medical treatment of moderate to severe Crohn's disease. Aliment Pharmacol Ther 2003; 17 Suppl 2: 23–30

Definition

- **Epidemiology**
  Prevalence is 2–3% • Boys are affected three times more often than girls • Usually becomes symptomatic before age 2 years • Only 25–50% of the children have clinically important disease.
- **Etiology, pathophysiology, pathogenesis**
  Persistent proximal end of the vitelline duct • Most common form of persistent duct • Ectopic gastrointestinal mucosa (usually gastric mucosa) develops in 60% of the symptomatic children • Gastrointestinal bleeding occurs in 95% of cases • The diverticulum lies in an antimesenteric location • It usually occurs within the first 80 cm of the small bowel, proximal to the ileocecal valve.

Imaging Signs

- **Ultrasound findings**
  Morphologic findings cannot be clearly distinguished from appendicitis • The lesion is often obscured by superposed intestinal gas.
- **Color Doppler ultrasound**
  Hypervascularity is found in inflammation.
- **CT findings**
  Useful with equivocal findings • CT angiography with intravenous contrast can visualize bleeding (findings are important only with more profuse bleeding) • Oral contrast facilitates localization • Blind-ending pouch with thickening of the wall and fluid retention in the distal ileum • Inflammation of the adjacent mesentery • Occurs in the right lower quadrants, and in the mid-abdomen • Usually close to the midline.
- **Nuclear medicine imaging findings**
  Diagnosis is confirmed with ^{99m}Tc-pertechnetate, which accumulates in the ectopic gastric mucosa • False negative findings occur where gastric mucosa is absent or present in insufficient quantity, and in ischemia secondary to volvulus or intussusception.

Clinical Aspects

- **Typical presentation**
  Usually clinically occult • Recurrent colicky abdominal pain • Bloody stools • Melena • Ileus.
- **Therapeutic options**
  Surgical resection.
- **Course and prognosis**
  Treatment is curative.
- **Complications**
  Diverticular bleeding from peptic ulcers with ectopic gastric mucosa • Perforation • Intussusception • Recurrent inflammation of the diverticulum • Malignant degeneration (rare).

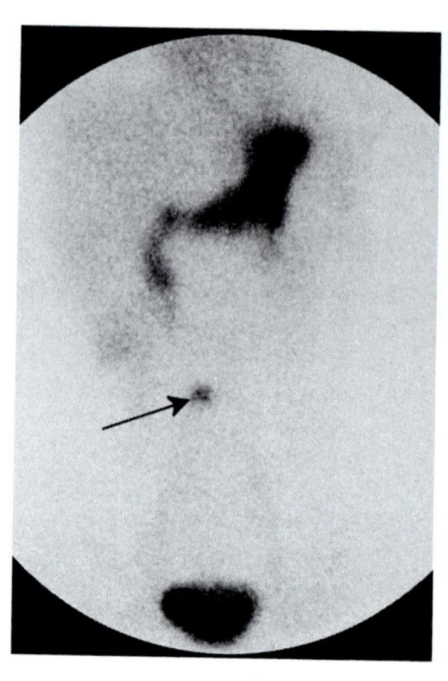

Fig. 4.21 Meckel diverticulum. ^{99m}Tc nuclear medicine image. Increased uptake in the ectopic gastric mucosa (arrow) of the Meckel diverticulum. Bladder is also delineated due to renal excretion of the nuclide.

Differential Diagnosis

Appendicitis	– Clinical and morphologic findings are often indistinguishable
Urachal cyst	– May communicate with the superior aspect of the bladder – Directly in the midline, adjacent to the anterior abdominal wall – Dysuria
Mesenteric cyst	– No direct involvement of the bowel – Usually much larger – No inflammatory reaction of adjacent tissue
Enteric duplication with ectopic gastric mucosa	– Positive nuclear medicine findings

Tips and Pitfalls

Diagnosis may be delayed due to false-negative ultrasound findings.

Selected References

Baldisserotto M et al. Sonographic findings of Meckel's diverticulitis in children. Am J Roentgenol 2003; 180: 425–428

Bennett GL et al. CT of Meckel's diverticulitis in 11 patients. Am J Roentgenol 2004; 182: 625–629

Kumar R et al. Diagnosis of ectopic gastric mucosa using 99Tcm-pertechnetate: spectrum of scintigraphic findings. Br J Radiol 2005; 78: 714–720

Park JJ et al. Meckel diverticulum: the Mayo Clinic experience with 1476 patients (1950–2002). Ann Surg 2005; 241: 529–533

Definition

- **Epidemiology**
  Affects 1–2% of all children • Most common indication for surgery in children • Usually occurs in children less than 1 year old • Frequency among premature infants is particularly high (up to 30%) • Boys are affected five times more often than girls.
- **Etiology, pathophysiology, pathogenesis**
  Displacement of abdominal structures through a congenital or acquired defect • *Hernia sac:* Protrusion of the parietal peritoneum • Hernia contents are surrounded by subcutaneous tissue, skin, or the wall of the scrotum.
  In 90% of all newborns, the processus vaginalis of the peritoneum is patent (not clinically important) • Inguinal hernias in children are nearly invariably congenital indirect hernias (along the inguinal canal) • *Cause:* Patent processus vaginalis or insufficient muscular closure of the inlet to the inguinal canal • Most often occurs on the right (60% of cases), presumably due to the later descent of the right testis • Bilateral hernias occur in 10–20% of cases.

Imaging Signs

- **Ultrasound findings**
  Intestinal air or peristalsis in the inguinal canal • Continuity of the tubular structure into the peritoneal cavity • Ovarian hernia, especially in premature girls • Fluid in the processus vaginalis of the peritoneum • Associated hydrocele.

Clinical Aspects

- **Typical presentation**
  Usually asymptomatic soft reducible inguinal swelling, permanent or intermittent, medial to the inguinal ligament • Can extend into the scrotum (scrotal hernia).
- **Therapeutic options**
  Prompt surgical intervention is indicated in incarceration or ovarian hernia • Observation is indicated in very small premature infants with pulmonary insufficiency in whom there is no incarceration.
- **Course and prognosis**
  Incarceration occurs in 12% of cases • 70% of incarcerations occur within the first year of life.
- **Complications**
  Incarceration with risk of intestinal necrosis • Ileus • Peritonitis • Loss of a testis or ovary.

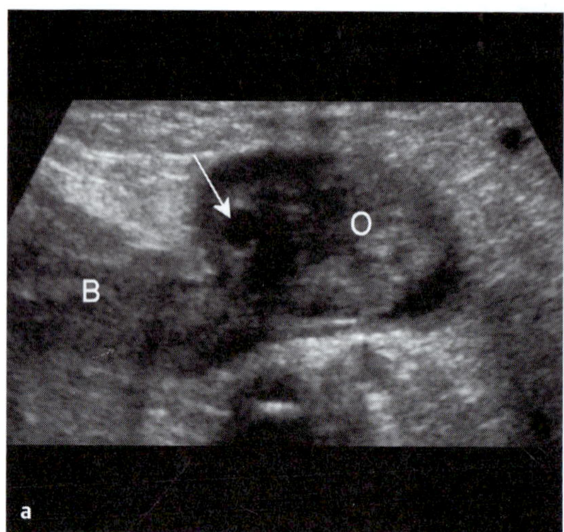

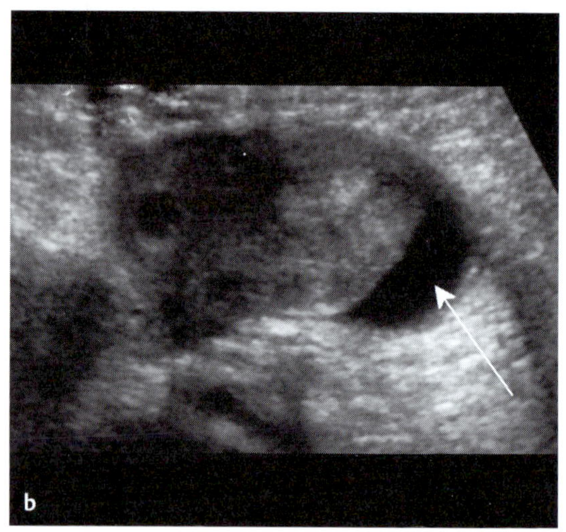

Fig. 4.22 a, b Right inguinal hernia in a 4-week-old girl. Ultrasound of the inguinal region. Ovary (O) exhibiting small follicular cysts (**a**, arrow) is displaced into the inguinal canal. Wide peritoneal defect (B). There is also a small amount of free fluid in the peritoneal hernial sac (**b**, arrow). Findings were confirmed intraoperatively.

Differential Diagnosis

Hydrocele of the testis or spermatic cord	– Fluid in the scrotum or processus vaginalis of the peritoneum, which is closed on the abdominal side – No air or peristalsis in the scrotum
Inguinal undescended testis	– Inguinal testicular tissue with empty ipsilateral scrotal compartment
Lymphadenitis	– Inguinal enlarged lymph nodes with typical ultrasound morphology (central hilar fat sign)
Varicocele	– Color Doppler ultrasound shows varices in the pampiniform plexus – Valsalva maneuver with positive flow reversal

Tips and Pitfalls

Errors include missing an inguinal hernia that contains only mesenteric fatty tissue.

Selected References

Benjamin K. Scrotal and inguinal masses in the newborn period. Adv Neonatal Care 2002; 2: 140–148

Graf JL et al. Pediatric hernias. Semin Ultrasound CT MR 2002; 23: 197–200

Lau ST, Lee YH, Caty MG. Current management of hernias and hydroceles. Semin Pediatr Surg 2007; 16: 50–57

Nicholls E. Inguino-scrotal problems in children. Practitioner 2003; 247: 226–230

Definition

- **Epidemiology**
  Incidence is 1:12 000 • Girls are affected more often than boys.
- **Etiology, pathophysiology, pathogenesis**
  Presumably the same infectious process that is responsible for neonatal hepatitis • Sclerosing cholangitis • Proliferation of the intrahepatic bile ducts into the periportal region • No signs of an extrahepatic duct • 15% of cases are associated with polysplenia or trisomy 18 • Associated with preduodenal portal vein, "interrupted inferior" vena cava, and congenital heart defects.

Imaging Signs

- **Ultrasound findings**
  Sensitivity is 92% • Small gallbladder, longitudinal diameter less than 20 mm • Gallbladder length exceeding 3 cm in a fasting patient excludes atresia • No change in the size of the gallbladder after feeding (30–60 minutes after feeding) • In 75% of cases, the gallbladder is not visualized • Intrahepatic bile ducts are not dilated • Extrahepatic ducts are absent • *Triangular cord sign:* Triangular hyperechoic area near the hilum anterior to the portal vein (fibrotic remnant of the hepatic duct) • Hepatic echo texture can be altered or normal • Hepatomegaly.
- **MRI findings**
  Biliary tree malformation on classic MR cholangiopancreatography sequences.
- **Scintigraphy**
  Sensitivity is as high as 97%, specificity as high as 85% • ^{99m}Tc-bromotrimethyl-IDA (^{99m}Tc-BrIDA) or ^{99m}Tc-mebrofenin (nuclear medicine hepatobiliary imaging) • Normal hepatic uptake • No intestinal uptake after 24 hours is diagnostic • Increased renal tracer excretion.

Clinical Aspects

- **Typical presentation**
  Prolonged jaundice (bilirubin > 2 mg/dL (34.2 µmol/L), bilirubin conjugate > 30% of total bilirubin after 18 days of life) • Biopsy may be indicated.
- **Therapeutic options**
  Surgery (portoenterostomy) • Reanastomosis where the proximal hepatic duct exists • Liver transplantation.
- **Course and prognosis**
  Surgical success rate is about 90% where the child is less than 2 months old at the time of the operation • The older the child at the time of the operation, the poorer the success rate • Definitive healing requires liver transplantation.
- **Complications**
  Biliary cirrhosis with portal hypertension.

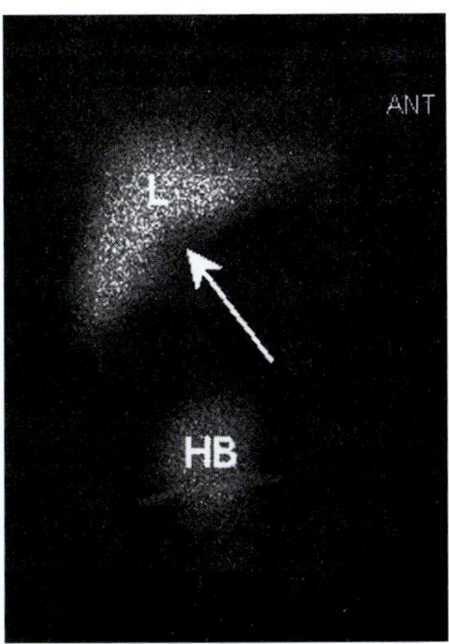

Fig. 4.23 Biliary atresia. A-P hepatobiliary nuclear medicine imaging. Six hours after intravenous contrast injection there is good uptake in the liver (L), but the bile ducts and gallbladder are not visualized (gap, arrow). No uptake in the bowel but the image shows compensatory renal excretion and enhancement of the bladder (HB) (used with the kind permission of Dr. B. Nowak, Department of Nuclear Medicine, Aachen University Medical Center).

Differential Diagnosis

Neonatal hepatitis	– Normal gallbladder size with physiologic postprandial contraction – No triangular cord sign – Delayed but functioning hepatobiliary excretion of the nuclear medicine tracer
Galactosemia	– Normal gallbladder size with physiologic postprandial contraction – No triangular cord sign – Normal nuclear medicine findings – Newborn screening
Choledochal cyst	– Well visualized on ultrasound – Usually manifests later in childhood
Alagille syndrome	– Hypoplasia and/or atrophy of the intrahepatic bile ducts – Typical facies – Cardiovascular anomalies – Butterfly vertebra – Posterior embryotoxon

Tips and Pitfalls

Errors include misinterpreting an absent gallbladder on a postprandial study • Therefore specific visualization of the gallbladder in the fasting child is necessary.

Selected References

Kanegawa K et al. Sonographic diagnosis of biliary atresia in pediatric patients using the "triangular cord" sign versus gallbladder length and contraction. Am J Roentgenol 2003; 181: 1387–1390

Kotb MA et al. Post-portoenterostomy triangular cord sign prognostic value in biliary atresia: a prospective study. Br J Radiol 2005; 78: 884–887

Roca I et al. Hepatobiliary scintigraphy in current pediatric practice. Q J Nucl Med 1998; 42: 113–118

Ryeom HK et al. Biliary atresia: feasibility of mangafodipir trisodium-enhanced MR cholangiography for evaluation. Radiology 2005; 235: 250–258

Definition

- **Epidemiology**

  Incidence is 0.2–0.5 per million • Girls are affected three times more often than boys • Half of cases occur before age 10 years.

- **Etiology, pathophysiology, pathogenesis**

  Congenital segmental and cystic widening of the common bile duct • In up to 90% of cases, the common bile duct is affected • According to the "common channel" theory, the common bile duct and pancreatic duct drain into a common abnormal orifice • This leads to partial digestion of the wall of the common bile duct by pancreatic enzymes • This in turn leads to a fibrous cystic wall without an epithelial lining • Associated with other biliary anomalies such as biliary atresia, gallbladder anomalies, congenital hepatic fibrosis, or carcinoma of the gallbladder or bile ducts • Kehrer and Todani classification.

Table 4.4 Todani classification of choledochal cysts

Type	Characteristics
Ia	Cystic enlargement of the common hepatic duct
Ib	Focal segmental enlargement of the common hepatic duct
Ic	Fusiform enlargement of the common hepatic duct
II	Common bile duct diverticulum
III	Choledochocele affecting only the intraduodenal common hepatic duct
IVa	Multiple cystic enlargements of the intrahepatic and extrahepatic bile ducts
IVb	Multiple cystic enlargements of the extrahepatic bile ducts
V	Caroli disease (multiple cystic enlargements of the intrahepatic bile ducts with cirrhosis of the liver)

Imaging Signs

- **Ultrasound findings**

  Findings include a "second gallbladder," a cystic structure in the porta hepatis • Cystic structure presenting without postprandial contraction • Cyst measures 2–15 cm • May contain stones or sludge • Findings of dilated intrahepatic bile ducts draining into the cyst are diagnostic.

- **CT findings**

  Not necessarily required preoperatively • Unobscured visualization • Distinguishes findings from Caroli disease.

- **MRI findings**

  For precise visualization of ductal anatomy preoperatively recommended • MR cholangiopancreatography: T2-weighted TSE with fat suppression, MIP reconstructions, HASTE or SSFSE sequences.

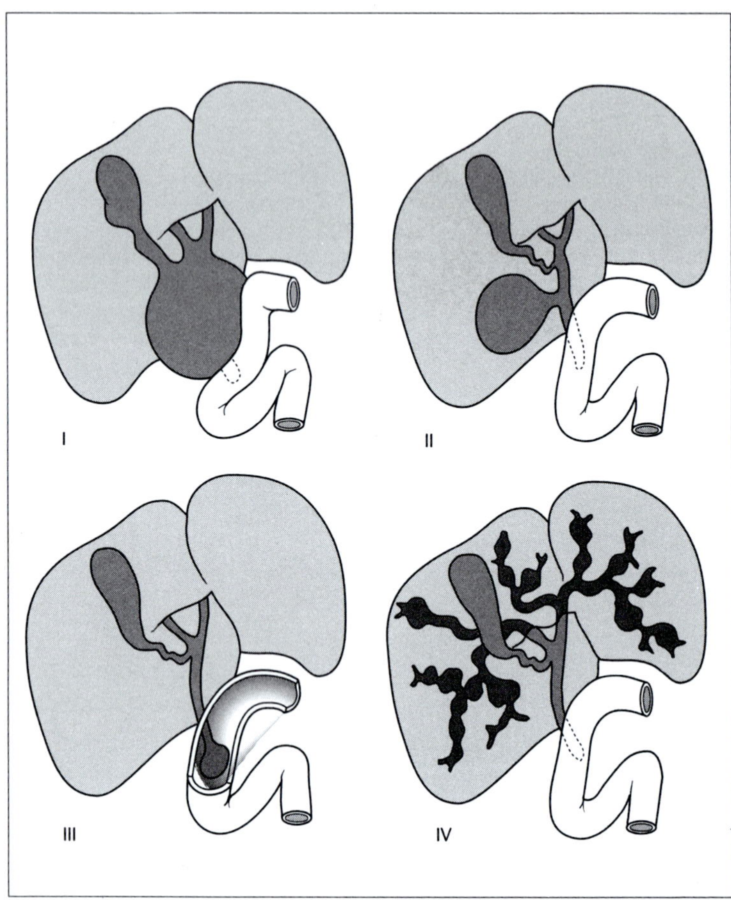

Fig. 4.24 Kehrer classification of choledochal cysts (from Hofmann V. Ultraschalldiagnostik in Pädiatrie und Chirurgie. Stuttgart: Thieme; 2005).

- **Cholangiography**
  ERCP: Risk of pancreatitis • Percutaneous transhepatic technique is used intraoperatively • Intravenous technique is no longer standard.
- **Nuclear medicine imaging findings**
  Hepatobiliary imaging • Late filling of the cyst in cholestasis • Dilation of intrahepatic bile ducts.

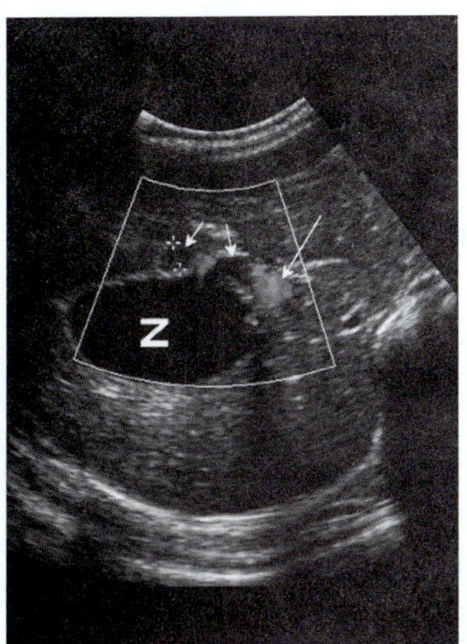

Fig. 4.25 Choledochal cyst. Doppler ultrasound scan of the upper abdomen. Subhepatic cystic mass (Z), "double gall-bladder" sign. The small arrows are indicating the common bile duct, the long arrow is pointing to the portal vein.

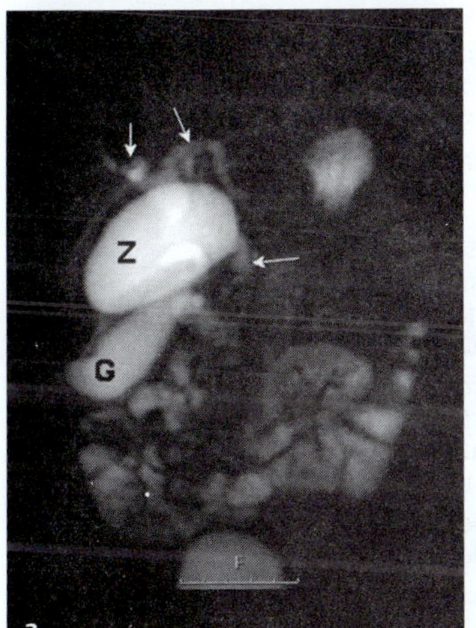

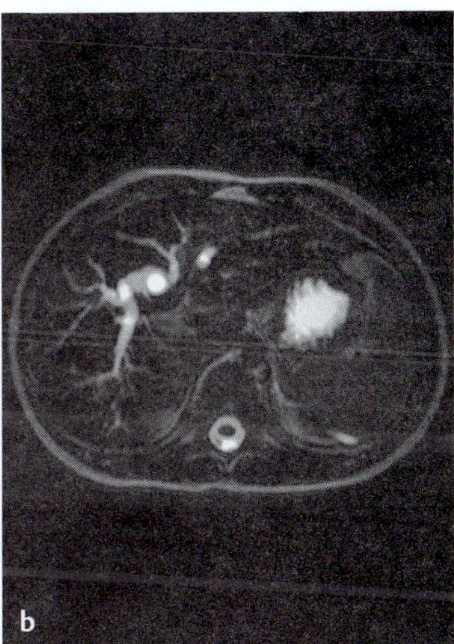

Fig. 4.26 a, b MR cholangiopancreatography. MR image also visualizes the cystic mass (Z) next to the gallbladder (G; **a**). The cyst communicates with the common hepatic duct. Intrahepatic bile duct dilation (**a, b**, arrows).

Clinical Aspects

- **Typical presentation**
  Recurrent abdominal pain • Vomiting • Intermittent jaundice • Palpable swelling in the right upper abdomen • Associated pancreatitis.
- **Therapeutic options**
  Conservative treatment • Where complications occur, cyst excision and ductal anastomosis are indicated.
- **Course and prognosis**
  Can resolve spontaneously.
- **Complications**
  Ascending cholangitis • Biliary cirrhosis • Rupture with biliary peritonitis • Malignant degeneration is rare • Postoperative stricture of the anastomosis, cholelithiasis, cholangitis in secondary infection.

Differential Diagnosis

Hematoma	– History of trauma – Coagulation disorders – Usually exhibit intermediate signal characteristics, not purely cystic
Cystic duodenal duplication	– Directly adjacent to duodenum – Biliary system appears normal – Often incidental finding
Pancreatic pseudocyst	– History of pancreatitis – Localized, walled off collections of pancreatic secretions – Circumscribed pancreatic necrosis
Mesenteric cyst	– Usually lies in the mid and lower abdomen – Directly adjacent to small bowel structures – Normal biliary system
Hepatic cyst	– Intrahepatic location – Dysontogenetic lesion – Normal biliary system – No growth tendency
Biloma	– Intrahepatic or subcapsular location – Iatrogenic lesion, often postoperative
Gallbladder hydrops	– Findings may include stone in the infundibulum of the gallbladder
Duodenal ectasia in annular pancreas	– Passage of food through the ectatic duodenum

Tips and Pitfalls

Avoid direct aspiration of the cyst due to the risk of biliary peritonitis • Postoperative biliary air on ultrasound must not be confused with stones.

Selected References

Babbit DP et al. Choledochal cyst: A concept of etiology. Am J Roentgenol 1973; 199: 57–62

Metreweli C et al. Magnetic resonance cholangiography in children. Br J Radiol 2004; 77: 1059–1064

Nagi B et al. Endoscopic retrograde cholangiopancreatography in the evaluation of anomalous junction of the pancreaticobiliary duct and related disorders. Abdom Imaging 2003; 28: 847–852

Todani T et al. J Hepatobiliary Pancreat Surg 2003; 10: 334–340

Wootton-Gorges SL et al. Giant cystic abdominal masses in children. Pediatr Radiol 2005; 35: 1277–1288

Definition

- **Epidemiology**
  Prevalence 0.1–0.6% in children • Much less common in children than in adults • More often calcified than in adults • Girls are affected more often than boys.
- **Etiology, pathophysiology, pathogenesis**
  Underlying disorders in which stones tend to form:
  - Hemolytic anemia such as thalassemia, sickle cell anemia, Rh and ABO incompatibility.
  - Secondary to massive blood transfusions.
  - After extensive surgery.
  - Protracted immobilization.
  - Chronic inflammatory bowel disease.
  - Protracted parenteral nutrition.
  - Secondary to shock or dehydration.
  - Cystic fibrosis.
  - Biliary anomalies.

Imaging Signs

- **Ultrasound findings**
  Method of choice • Hyperechoic structures in the gallbladder • Stones 3 mm and larger produce acoustic shadows; shadows also vary with mineralization of the stone • Position changes when patient is repositioned ("rolling stone").
- **CT**
  Inferior to ultrasound in diagnosing stones.
- **Cholangiography**
  MR cholangiopancreatography: T2-weighted GE, MIP reconstructions, HASTE or SSFSE sequences.
- **Endoscopy**
  ERCP can be used to extract stones.

Clinical Aspects

- **Typical presentation**
  Often asymptomatic • Often an incidental finding • Colicky abdominal pain.
- **Therapeutic options**
  Asymptomatic patients do not require treatment • Cholecystectomy in symptomatic cases.
- **Course and prognosis**
  Stones can dissolve up to the age of 1 year.
- **Complications**
  Cystic duct stone (gallbladder hydrops without postprandial change in size) • Choledocholithiasis (intrahepatic and/or extrahepatic cholestasis) • Cholecystitis • Cholangitis • Biliary pancreatitis • Choledochoduodenal or cholecystoduodenal fistula.

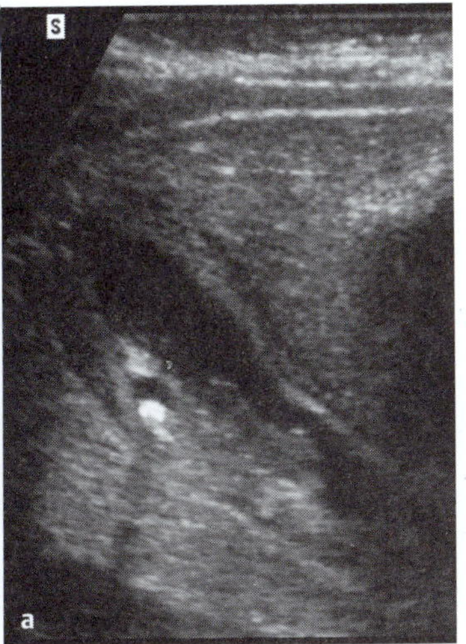

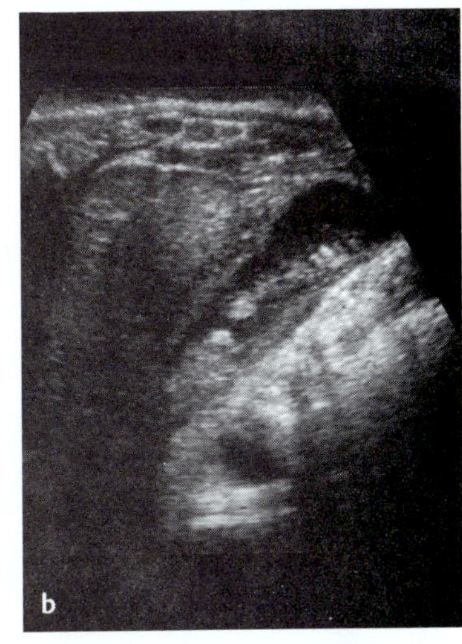

Fig. 4.27 a, b Cholecystolithiasis in a 4-year-old child with severe dehydration and gastrointestinal infection. Ultrasound. Gallbladder sludge (**a**) and a few compact, hyperechoic stones, some with typical acoustic shadows (**b**).

Differential Diagnosis

Gallbladder sludge	– Occurs in cholestasis or protracted parenteral nutrition – Pigment granules and cholesterol crystals – Typical sedimentation phenomenon
Gallbladder polyp	– Does not change position – Gallbladder polyposis is an initial symptom of metachromatic leukodystrophy
"Porcelain" gallbladder	– Gallbladder lumen cannot be identified – Extensive acoustic shadows due to calcification of the gallbladder wall – No intraluminal fluid visualized
Air-filled duodenum	– Typical position – Air artifacts

Tips and Pitfalls

Small gallbladder stones can escape detection in a postprandial examination • Gallbladder stones can be misinterpreted as air in the bowel.

Selected References

Bellows CF et al. Management of gallstones. Am Fam Physician 2005; 72: 637–642

Keller MS et al. Spontaneous resolution of cholelithiasis in infants. Radiology 1985; 157: 345–388

Kratzer W et al. Prevalence of gallstones in sonographic surveys worldwide. J Clin Ultrasound 1999; 27: 1–7

Ure BM et al. Outcome after laparoscopic cholecystotomy and cholecystectomy in children with symptomatic cholecystolithiasis: a preliminary report. Pediatr Surg Int 2001; 17: 396–398

Definition

- **Epidemiology**
  Accounts for 43% of primary pediatric liver tumors • Most common malignant liver tumor and third most common abdominal tumor in children • Peak frequency between the ages of 6 months and 2 years • Affects boys twice as often as girls.
- **Etiology, pathophysiology, pathogenesis**
  Laboratory values: AFP is raised (in up to 90%), thrombocytosis • Rarely occurs in combination with precocious puberty and virilism • Tumor consists of epithelial cells with a pseudocapsule • Can also occur as a multifocal lesion • Typically occurs in the right lobe of the liver • Increased incidence is seen in hemihypertrophy, Beckwith–Wiederman syndrome, familial polyposis, Wilms tumor, and biliary atresia.

Imaging Signs

- **Ultrasound findings**
  Hyperechoic, heterogeneous • Well demarcated • Smoothly marginated • Tumor is usually already a large mass (about 10 cm) when initially detected • Findings include displacement, compression, and encasement of vascular structures • Vascular invasion is a sign of malignancy (portal vein and central hepatic veins are primarily affected) • Coarse calcifications (15–33% of cases) • Calcifications secondary to chemotherapy • Cystic areas are present in tumor necrosis.
- **Color Doppler ultrasound findings**
  Better visualization of the vascular displacement, compression, and invasion • Often there is increased flow in the hepatic artery due to a "steal" mechanism • Hypervascular tumor.
- **CT findings**
  Hypodense, heterogeneous, well demarcated tumor • Peripheral enhancement • There may be vascular invasion • Tumor hemorrhaging or necrosis may be present • Calcifications may occur but are not typical.
- **MRI findings**
  Inhomogeneous • Hypointense on T1-weighted SE sequences with hyperintense areas (hemorrhage) and enhancement • Inhomogeneous, hyperintense on T2-weighted TSE sequences with hypointense areas (fibrous septa).

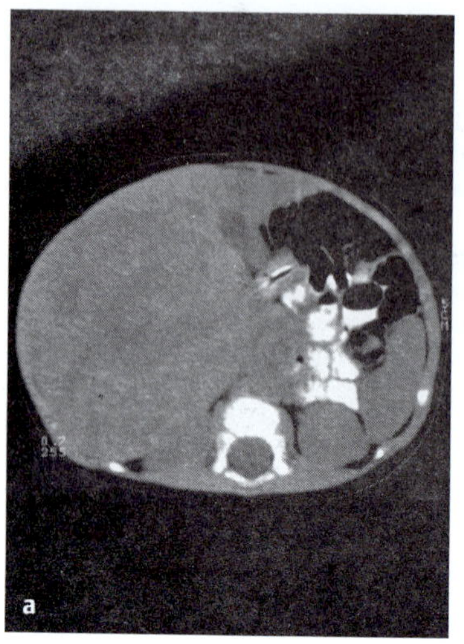

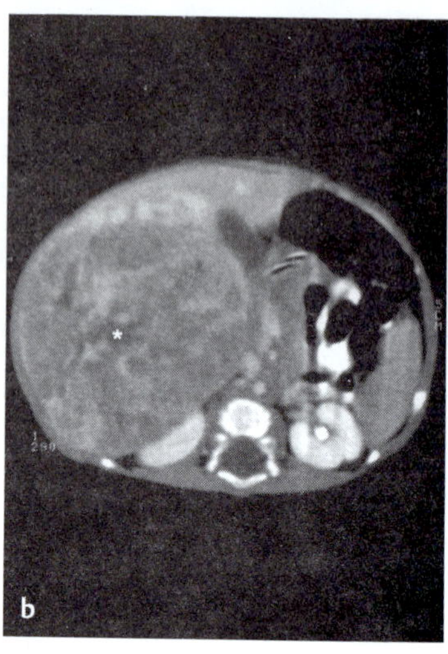

Fig. 4.28 a, b Hepatoblastoma in a 6-month-old infant. Plain CT (**a**) and contrast study (**b**) of the upper abdomen. The large tumor of the right hepatic lobe exhibits small calcifications. Inhomogeneous tumor enhancement with several central areas of necrosis (*).

Clinical Aspects

- **Typical presentation**
  Palpable abdominal tumor • Vomiting • Nausea • Weight loss • Usually painless • Precocious puberty in endocrinologically active tumor.
- **Therapeutic options**
  Resection • Chemotherapy • Liver transplantation.
- **Course and prognosis**
  Sixty percent of tumors are resectable • Overall survival rate is as high as 70%.
- **Complications**
  Tumor hemorrhage • Vascular occlusion • Early metastases.

Differential Diagnosis

Hemangioendothelioma	– Usually before the age of 6 months – AFP is not raised – Thrombocytopenia often present – Granular calcifications – Often associated with cardiac insufficiency
Neuroblastoma metastasis	– Usually multiple lesions or diffuse infiltration
Fibrolamellar hepatocellular carcinoma	– Usually after the age of 5 years, rarely before age 3 – Typical tumor calcifications – AFP is not usually raised
Mesenchymal hamartoma	– Well demarcated lobular tumor with cystic components

Tips and Pitfalls

In large tumors in the right upper abdomen, it is often difficult to clearly identify the organ of origin by ultrasound examination alone.

Selected References

Davies JQ et al. Hepatoblastoma-evolution of management and outcome and significance of histology of the resected tumor. A 31-year experience with 40 cases. J Pediatr Surg 2004; 39: 1321–1327

Emre S et al. Liver tumors in children. Pediatr Transplant 2004; 8: 632–638

Helmberger TK. Pediatric liver neoplasms: a radiologic-pathologic correlation. Eur Radiol 1999; 9: 1339–1347

Powers C et al. Primary liver neoplasms: MR imaging with pathologic correlation. Radiographics 1994; 14: 459–482

Definition

- **Epidemiology**
  Blunt abdominal trauma is rare in children • Affected organs include the kidneys (33% of cases), spleen (24%), pancreas (23%), and liver (10%).
- **Etiology, pathophysiology, pathogenesis**
  These organs are unprotected due to their superficial location and lack of fat • Organs with a high fluid content are less easily compressed • Duodenum and pancreas are pressed against the spine in trauma • The spleen is subjected to external compressive forces transmitted by the elastic ribs • Multiple injuries are present in 18% of cases.
  Mechanism of injury and typical organ injuries:
  - Traffic accident: Spine, kidneys, retroperitoneum, spleen.
  - Trauma in pedestrian run over by a vehicle: Bowel, bladder.
  - Fall from a bicycle, kick in the abdomen (abuse): Pancreas, duodenum, liver.
  - Fall onto the upper abdomen: Liver, spleen, pancreas.
  - Fall on the left side: Spleen, kidney.

Imaging Signs

- **Ultrasound findings**
  Free fluid (blood), anechoic to hyperechoic • Hematoma is often present posterior to the bladder, in the hepatorenal and/or splenorenal regions, or within the bowel • Acute hematomas are hyperechoic, chronic hematomas hypoechoic • Sensitivity for spleen injuries is 90% • Contusion and laceration causes organ enlargement • Lacerations or intraparenchymal hematoma appear as parenchymal inhomogeneities or linear structures • Abnormal organ surface • Mobility of the organ with respiration is limited or absent • Subcapsular hematoma may occur in liver and spleen • Perirenal hematoma • Blood clots in the renal pelvis or bladder • Retroperitoneal hematoma • Urinoma may occur when there is involvement of the renal pelvis or ureter.
- **Color Doppler ultrasound findings**
  Visualize the vascular structures supplying and draining the area to exclude vascular injury such as avulsion of the renal pedicle • Exclude intraparenchymal perfusion defects.
- **CT findings**
  Indicated with any discrepancy between ultrasound findings and clinical condition • Especially in multiple trauma or craniocerebral trauma • Normally single phase CT will be sufficient—exceptions include injury to the renal pelvis, ureter, or bladder • Unenhanced CT is not suitable • CT may be able to better visualize the extent of injury and associated musculoskeletal injuries.
- **Abdominal radiograph**
  To exclude bowel perforation (where CT is not performed) and visualize free air.

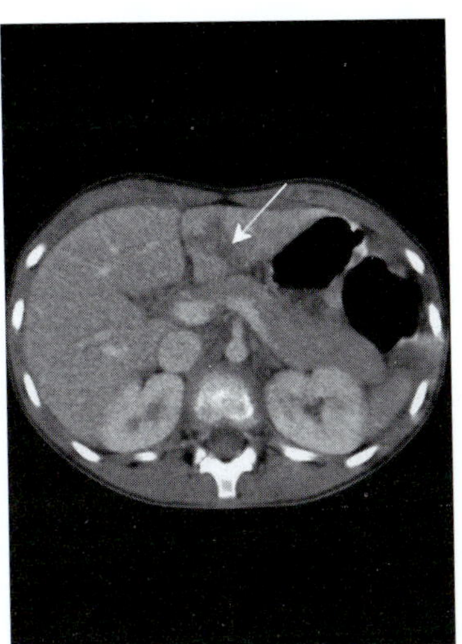

Fig. 4.29 Ruptured liver. Contrast-enhanced CT of the upper abdomen. Intraparenchymal injury to the left hepatic lobe (arrow) with associated hematoma. The parenchymal laceration extends to the surface of the liver.

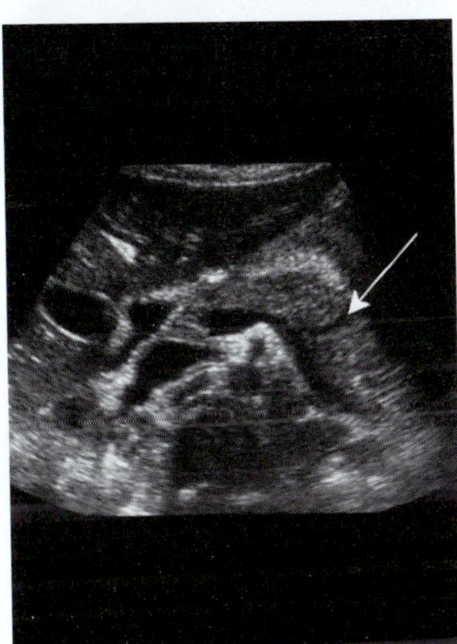

Fig. 4.30 Ruptured pancreas. Ultrasound. Parenchymal laceration (arrow) in the body of the pancreas.

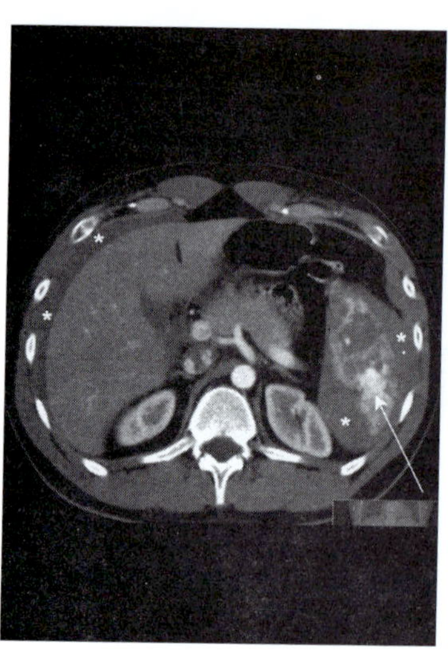

Fig. 4.31 Ruptured spleen. Multiphase CT of the abdomen. The early arterial phase clearly demonstrates peracute splenic bleeding (arrow) with considerable laceration of the spleen. Pronounced hematoma around the spleen (*) and subcapsular hematoma in the liver (*).

Clinical Aspects

- **Typical presentation**
  History of trauma • External injuries such as contusion marks are present • Abdominal pain • There may be an asymptomatic interval with shock • Defensive muscular tension.
- **Therapeutic options**
  Conservative treatment and/or surgery (8–15% of cases) may be required depending on the extent of injury and specific findings • Treatment should invariably strive to preserve the organ.
- **Course and prognosis**
  Mortality in blunt abdominal trauma is 5–30%.
- **Complications**
  Biloma • Urinoma • Pancreatic pseudocyst • Biliary peritonitis • Delayed rupture of the spleen • Acute pancreatitis (trauma is the most common cause in children) • Overwhelming post-splenectomy infection syndrome (50% mortality).

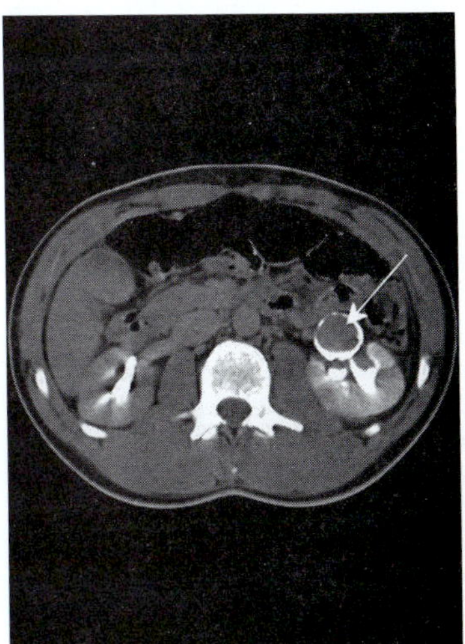

Fig. 4.32 Ruptured kidney. Urographic contrast phase of CT of the upper abdomen: Kidney laceration with blood clots (arrow) in the renal pelvis. Findings suggest involvement of the renal pelvis.

Differential Diagnosis

Free fluid from other causes	– Gastroenteritis – A small quantity of free fluid in the pouch of Douglas is normal in girls – Cardiac insufficiency

Tips and Pitfalls

An ultrasound scan that fails to demonstrate free fluid is not cause for relief because free fluid is absent in 37% of organ injuries • The location of the free fluid may depend on patient positioning (in a patient in right lateral position with splenic rupture, free fluid will be accumulated on the right side) • Be alert to the possibility of a delayed rupture of the spleen; ultrasound follow-up within 24 hours is indicated • Ultrasound evaluation of the retroperitoneum is hampered by overlying intestinal gas.

Selected References

Bakker J et al. Sonography as the primary screening method in evaluating blunt abdominal trauma. J Clin Ultrasound 2005; 33: 155–163

Deluca JA et al. Injuries associated with pediatric liver trauma. Am Surg 2007; 73: 37–41

Fenton SJ et al. CT scan and the pediatric trauma patient—are we overdoing it? J Pediatr Surg 2004; 39: 1877–1881

Definition

- **Epidemiology**
  Prevalence is 1–2% • Increased incidence in siblings (25%) • Girls are affected considerably more often than boys.
- **Etiology, pathophysiology, pathogenesis**
  Retrograde flow of urine from the bladder into the ureters and renal pelvis.
  Primary vesicoureteral reflux (90% of all cases): Congenital malformation of the ureterovesical junction • Hypoplasia of the trigone of the bladder with laterally displaced, abnormal ureteric orifice (shaped like a horseshoe or golf hole) • Short intramural ureter segment such as occurs with a malpositioned ureterovesical junction • Periureteric vesical diverticulum (Hutch diverticulum) in congenital insufficiency of the ureteric hiatus • Ureterocele.
  Secondary vesicoureteral reflux (10% of all cases): Infravesical obstruction such as a urethral valve • Neurogenic bladder • Passing calculi.
  Risk factors: Ureteropelvic junction obstruction (37% of all cases) • Single kidney (37%) • Reflux in immediate relatives (32%) • Multicystic or dysplastic degeneration of the kidney (28%).

Table 5.1 Grading (International Reflux Study Group)

Grade	Findings
I	Reflux in the ureter only
II	Reflux in the ureter and renal pelvis without dilation
III	Beginning dilation and increased tortuosity of the ureter with slight or moderate dilation of the renal pelvis and mild blunting of the calyces
IV	Increasing dilation and tortuosity of the ureter with moderate dilation of the renal pelvis and calyces and moderate blunting of the calyces. The impressions of the renal papillae are still detectable.
V	Severe dilation and significant tortuosity of the ureter with severe dilation of the entire renal pelvis. The impressions of the renal papillae are no longer detectable

Imaging Signs

- **B-mode ultrasound findings**
  Dilation of the renal pelvis • Dilation of the ureter proximal to the bladder • Thinning of the renal parenchyma • Shrinkage of the kidney • Renal scarring • Thickening of the wall of the ureter and/or renal pelvis • Thickening of the bladder wall • Trabeculation of the bladder wall • Urine retention • Vesical diverticulum.
- **Ultrasound evaluation of reflux**
  Intravesical injection of air or contrast agent such as Levovist • Conventional B-mode ultrasound • Findings at rest and during voiding include contrast agent or

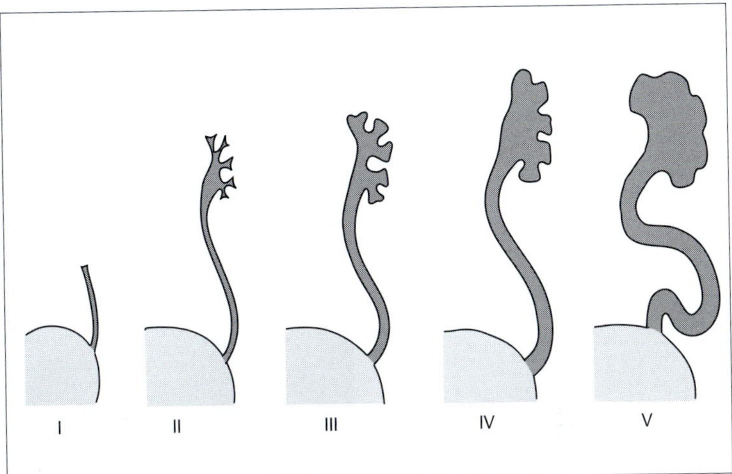

Fig. 5.1 Grading of vesicoureteral reflux (from Benz-Bohm G. Kinderradiologie. Stuttgart: Thieme; 2005).

air in the distal ureter or renal pelvis • Sensitivity is 60–70% • Suitable for follow-up of reflux in asymptomatic children at increased risk of reflux.

- **Color Doppler ultrasound findings**
  May be useful in differentiating the renal pelvis and renal vein.
- **Voiding cystourethrography (VCUG)**
  Technique: Performed under antibiotic cover after treatment of urinary tract infection • Transurethral or suprapubic infusion of contrast medium into the bladder at rate of about 10–20 mL/min • Images are obtained at maximum bladder filling and during voiding (micturition two to three times)
  Findings: In boys, a lateral oblique view ensures unobstructed visualization of the urethra • Unobstructed visualization of the ureterovesical junction is important in reflux • Next both kidneys are documented • In vesicoureteral reflux, there will be contrast in the ureter and/or renal pelvis • Possible causes may be visualized, such as an anomalous ureterovesical junction, urethral valve in boys or meatal stenosis in girls.
- **Nuclear medicine imaging findings**
  Tracer: ^{99m}Tc-MAG3 • To evaluate decreased renal function • Examination should be delayed until after the age of 6 weeks as renal function can be limited before then • *Direct radionuclide cystography:* A minimal increase in uptake in the renal pelvis at rest and during voiding is diagnostic of vesicoureteral reflux • This study is thought to be more sensitive than a VCUG • Not routinely used.
- **MR urography**
  May be used as a supplementary study to visualize reflux nephropathy.

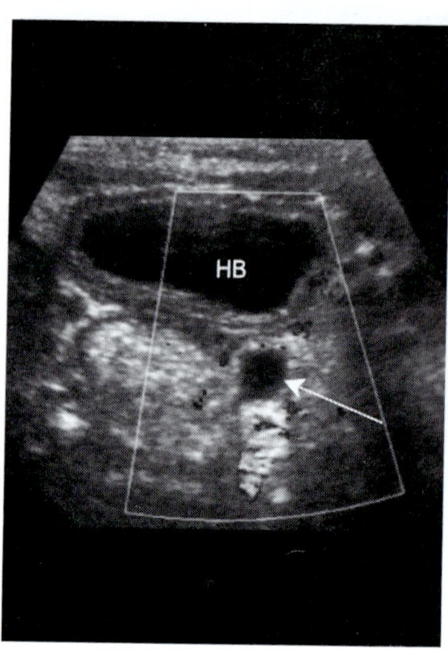

Fig. 5.2 Vesicoureteral reflux. Transverse lower abdominal color-coded Doppler ultrasound. Distal left ureter (arrow) is dilated during micturition, an indirect sign of vesicoureteric reflux. The bladder (HB) is only moderately filled.

Clinical Aspects

- **Typical presentation**
  Recurrent urinary tract infections.
- **Therapeutic options**
  Conservative treatment with antibiotic prophylaxis • Endoscopic periureteric injection of dextranomer/hyaluronic acid copolymer (Deflux) • Ureteral reimplantation is indicated for higher-grade reflux.
- **Course and prognosis**
  Spontaneous resolution of vesicoureteric reflux occurs in 80% of cases by puberty • The prognosis depends on the grade and severity of the reflux, the time at which the diagnosis is made, and the severity of pyelonephritis and scarring.
- **Complications**
  Pyelonephritis • Reflux nephropathy • Compromised renal function • Renal hypertension.

Differential Diagnosis

Primary megaureter	– With or without obstruction (MAG3) – Ectopic or orthotopic ureterovesical junction (ultrasound or MRI) – With or without reflux (VCUG)

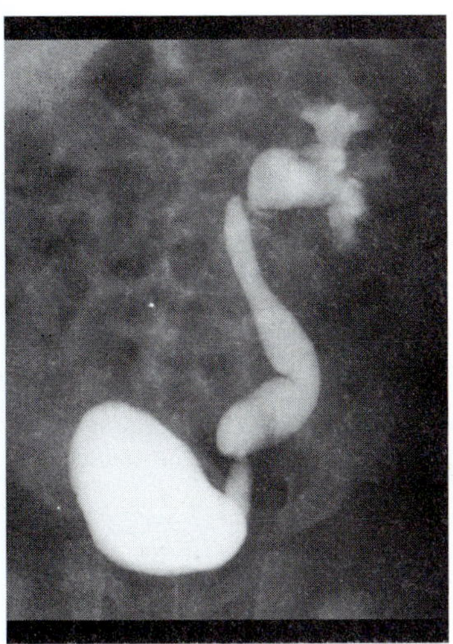

Fig. 5.3 VCUG. There is grade IV vesicoureteric reflux in the left ureter.

Tips and Pitfalls

Bowel wall or superimposed bone can mimic contrast agent on VCUG. Resolved by obtaining image in a second plane • Calcifications in the renal pelvis can also mimic vesicoureteric reflux on ultrasound • Ultrasound evaluation of reflux will fail to detect urethral valves, small bladder diverticula, or periurethral diverticula • Urethral valves can escape detection on VCUG with a catheter in situ (boys should also be examined without a catheter in situ) • Influx of contrast into the vagina must not be confused with vesicoureteral reflux • Failure of ultrasound to visualize a dilated renal pelvis or ureter does not exclude high-grade reflux (especially with an empty bladder).

Selected References

Avni EF et al. Can careful ultrasound examination of the urinary tract exclude vesicoureteric reflux in the neonate? Br J Radiol 1997; 70: 977–982

Darge K et al. Current status of vesicoureteral reflux diagnosis. World J Urol 2004; 22: 88–95

Darge K et al. Diagnosis of vesicoureteric reflux with low-dose contrast-enhanced harmonic ultrasound imaging. Pediatr Radiol 2005; 35: 73–78

Smellie JM et al. Childhood reflux and urinary infection: a follow-up of 10–41 years in 226 adults. Pediatr Nephrol 1998; 12: 727–736

Yu RN et al. Renal ultrasound studies after endoscopic injection of dextranomer/hyaluronic acid copolymer for vesicoureteral reflux. Urology 2006; 68: 866–868

Definition

▸ **Epidemiology**
Most common cause of uropathy with dilation • Affects boys five times as often as girls • Higher incidence in multicystic dysplastic kidneys • In 27% of cases, it is associated with other urogenital anomalies such as vesicoureteric reflux, obstructive megaureter, or renal agenesis.

▸ **Etiology, pathophysiology, pathogenesis**
Intrinsic obstruction: Some of the muscle fibers of the ureteropelvic junction are replaced by fibrous tissue • Abnormal composition and course of the ureteropelvic muscle fibers.
Extrinsic obstruction: Aberrant vascular structures such as the renal vessels • Masses that constrict ureteropelvic junction externally (renal cysts or aneurysms) • Horseshoe kidney or malrotation with compression of the ureter.

Imaging Signs

▸ **Ultrasound findings**
Dilated renal pelvis • Caliceal necks are thickened • Renal pelvis is rounded and the ureteropelvic junction is not clearly delineated • The width of the central intrarenal collecting system is usually more than 10 mm • Parenchymal narrowing with increased echogenicity • Findings in severe cases include a hydronephrotic kidney • Enlarged kidney • Ureter cannot be clearly delineated over its entire length • Bladder and ureteric orifices appear normal • The ureter may also be dilated where there is associated distal ureteric obstruction.

▸ **Diuresis ultrasound findings**
Particularly useful in distinguishing compensated and uncompensated ureteropelvic junction obstruction • Intravenous injection of furosemide 0.5 mg/kg • Allows evaluation of the width of the renal pelvis • In compensated ureteropelvic junction obstruction, the dilation will resolve within 20 minutes of the furosemide injection • Patients with decompensated ureteropelvic junction obstruction will show more pronounced and persistent dilation of the renal pelvis.

▸ **Colour Doppler ultrasound**
May be used to visualize aberrant vascular anatomy.

▸ **MRI findings**
MR urography directly visualizes the renal pelvis • HASTE, RARE, True-FISP • T1-weighted 3D GE sequence is used after injection of gadolinium and low-dose furosemide • Static and dynamic MR urography is used to evaluate renal function • MR angiography is used to visualize aberrant vascular anatomy • Unobstructed visualization of both kidneys and their adjacent structures • Dilation of the renal pelvis can be distinguished from parapelvic cysts.

▸ **Nuclear medicine imaging findings**
^{99m}Tc-MAG3 • Used to evaluate compromised renal function • Visualizes obstructive components (furosemide test).

▸ **Voiding cystourethrography (VCUG)**
Used to exclude associated vesicoureteric reflux.

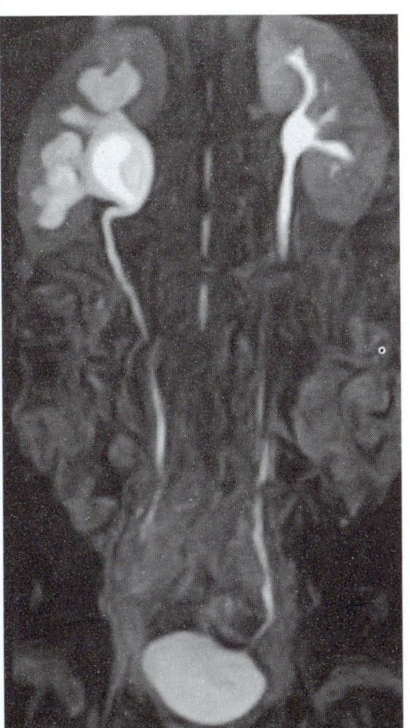

Fig. 5.4 Right ureteropelvic junction obstruction. MIP reconstruction of T1-weighted MR urography. Dilated right pelvicaliceal system, normal caliber ureter. Kinking immediately distal to the origin of the ureter caused by a lower polar vessel.

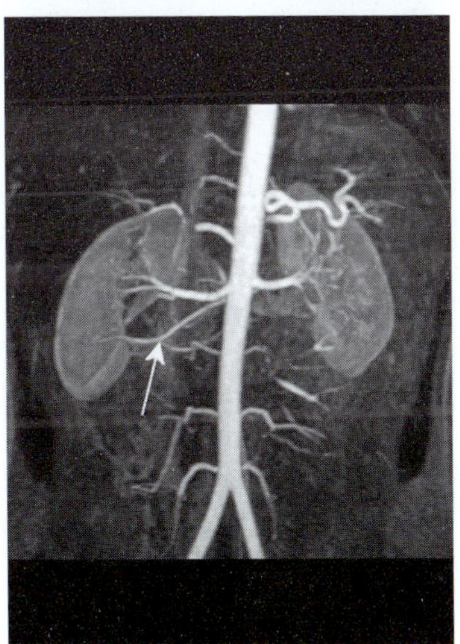

Fig. 5.5 T1-weighted MR angiogram after contrast administration. MIP reconstruction. Dilated right renal pelvis, right lower polar vessel (arrow) compressing the ureteropelvic junction.

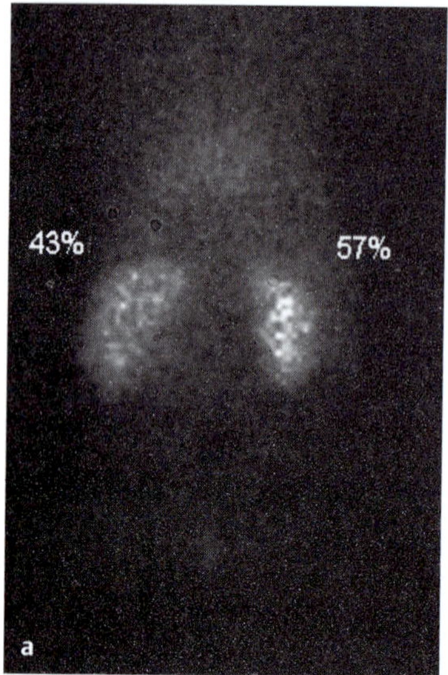

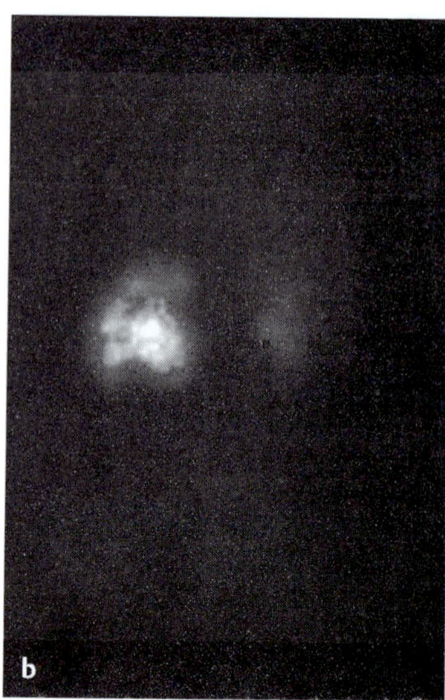

Fig. 5.6 a, b Left ureteropelvic junction obstruction: ^{99m}Tc MAG3 nuclear medicine imaging (posterior view).The summation image of the first three minutes (**a**) shows nearly symmetric uptake on both sides. The summation image of minutes 24–30 (**b**) shows largely complete excretion on the right and congestion on the left (used with the kind permission of Dr. B. Nowak, Department of Nuclear Medicine, Aachen University Medical Center).

Clinical Aspects

- **Typical presentation**
  Usually clinically occult • Tentative diagnosis is usually made during prenatal screening examination • Can be the cause of a urinary tract infection • Abdominal pain • Hematuria.
- **Therapeutic options**
  Conservative treatment is indicated where dilation does not increase during diuresis examination.
  Surgical treatment of obstruction and compromised renal function:
  - *Anderson–Hynes pyeloplasty:* Resection of the stenotic segment.
  - *Endopyelotomy:* Endoscopic incision.
  - Nephroureterectomy when renal function is less than 10%.
  - Percutaneous nephrostomy in infection.

- **Course and prognosis**
  Excellent when renal function was not reduced • Surgery in infants does not lead to an improvement in renal function; it only prevents subsequent worsening of renal function.
- **Complications**
  Urosepsis • Pyonephrosis.

Differential Diagnosis

Isolated ureteric stenosis	– Funnel-shaped junction between renal pelvis and ureter – Proximal ureter dilated
Multicystic dysplastic kidney	– Ultrasound does not demonstrate any connection between cysts and renal pelvis – Pathologic findings on nuclear medicine imaging and MR urography

Tips and Pitfalls

The dilation of the caliceal neck can persist for several years even after surgery. This must not be misinterpreted as recurrent obstruction on follow-up studies where the affected kidney shows normal increase in size and findings on nuclear medicine imaging are normal • An extrarenal ampullary renal pelvis must not be confused with a dilated renal caliceal system.

Selected References

Dähnert W. Ureteropelvic junction obstruction. In: Dähnert W. Radiology Review Manual. Baltimore: Williams & Wilkins; 1991: 476

McDaniel BB et al. Dynamic contrast-enhanced MR urography in the evaluation of pediatric hydronephrosis: Part 2, anatomic and functional assessment of uteropelvic junction obstruction. AJR Am J Roentgenol 2005; 185: 1608–1614

Rohrschneider WK et al. Functional and morphologic evaluation of congenital urinary tract dilatation by using combined static-dynamic MR urography: findings in kidneys with a single collecting system. Radiology 2002; 224: 683–694

Rooks VJ et al. Extrinsic ureteropelvic junction obstruction from a crossing renal vessel: demography and imaging. Pediatr Radiol 2001; 31: 120–124

Definition

- **Epidemiology**
  Most common cystic disorder of the kidney in children • Incidence is 1:4300 live births • Boys are affected twice as often as girls.
- **Etiology, pathophysiology, pathogenesis**
  Occurs sporadically • No genetic defect has been demonstrated • Increased familial incidence • Unilateral; bilateral involvement is incompatible with life • Presumably attributable to intrauterine obstruction of the ureter or the ureteropelvic junction • Dysplastic renal parenchyma with multiple cysts of variable size • *Pelvoinfundibular type:* Atresia of ureter and renal pelvis • *Hydronephrotic type:* Only atretic segment of ureter • No renal function • Atretic ipsilateral ureter.
  Associated malformations (40–50% of cases): Cystic dysplasia of the rete testis or seminal vesicles • Atresia in the gastrointestinal tract • Heart defects • Meningomyelocele • Vesicoureteric reflux (20% of cases) • Contralateral ureteropelvic junction obstruction.
  Associated syndromes include chromosomal aberrations and VACTERL syndrome.

Imaging Signs

- **Ultrasound findings**
  Multiple, thin-walled cysts of varying size • No communication between the cysts • Renal caliceal system is absent • Minimal or absent hyperechoic parenchyma • Compensatory hypertrophy of the contralateral kidney.
- **MRI**
  MR urography • HASTE, RARE, true FISP: Clusters of cysts resembling bunches of grapes • T1-weighted 3D-GE sequence after injection of contrast agent and low-dose furosemide: Visualization of the contralateral side with associated malformations • Static and dynamic MR urography is used to evaluate renal function of the contralateral side.
- **Nuclear medicine imaging**
  No renal function on the affected side.
- **Voiding cystourethrography (VCUG)**
  Used to confirm or exclude associated vesicoureteric reflux.

Clinical Aspects

- **Typical presentation**
  Usually detected during prenatal screening • Palpable abdominal mass • Hypertension.
- **Therapeutic options**
  Watch and wait for spontaneous resolution • Management of associated malformations and complications • Surgical resection is indicated in the absence of spontaneous resolution and in complications with mass effect.

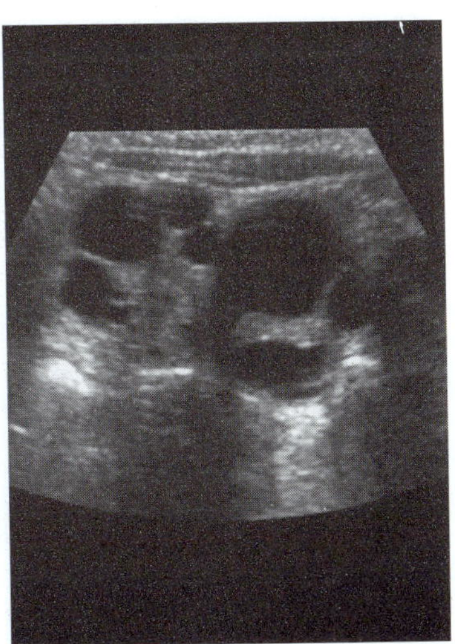

Fig. 5.7 Multicystic dysplastic kidney. Ultrasound. Multiple cysts of varying size interspersed with hyperechoic dysplastic renal tissue.

- **Course and prognosis**
  Spontaneous resolution may occur up to the age of 1 year • Resection is curative • Associated complications may lead to renal insufficiency.
- **Complications**
  Compression of adjacent structures • Infection • Hemorrhage • Renal insufficiency accompanied by compromised renal function on the contralateral side.

Differential Diagnosis

Ureteropelvic junction obstruction	– Dilated renal caliceal system – Ureter is present – Bladder and ureteric orifice are normal – Renal function is usually preserved
Autosomal recessive polycystic kidney disease	– Bilateral hyperechoic kidney enlargement – Loss of corticomedullary differentiation – Multiple small cysts (1–2 mm)
Megacalicosis	– Increased number of calices – Slight decrease in parenchymal tissue – Renal function is not compromised
Medullary sponge kidney	– Cystic dilation of the tubules in the medullary pyramids – Usually bilateral – Greatly enlarged hypoechoic kidney – Loss of corticomedullary differentiation – Nephrocalcinosis

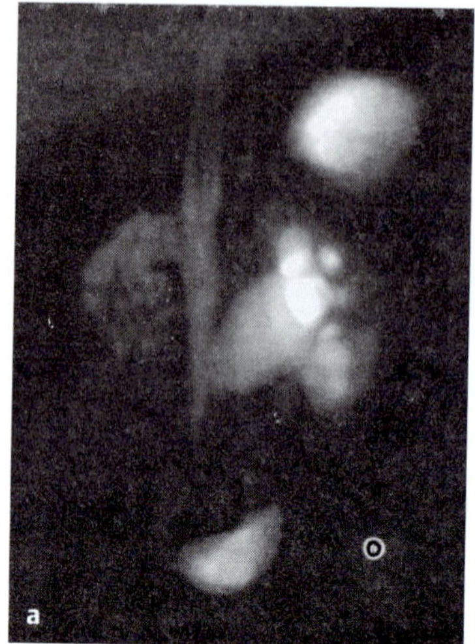

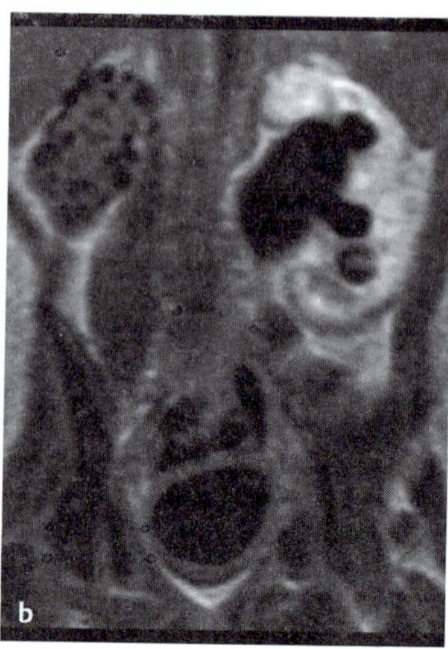

Fig. 5.8 a, b Right multicystic dysplastic kidney and left ureteropelvic junction obstruction. HASTE (**a**) and T1-weighted MR urography (**b**). Clusters of multiple cysts on the right, hyperintense on HASTE (T2-weighted) and hypointense on T1-weighted images. The decompensated ureteropelvic junction obstruction causes greatly delayed contrast excretion into the dilated left renal pelvis.

Tips and Pitfalls

Can be confused with other cystic disorders of the kidney.

Selected References

Kaneko K et al. Abnormal contralateral kidney in unilateral multicystic dysplastic kidney disease. Pediatr Radiol 1995; 25: 275–277

Mercado-Deane MG et al. US of renal insufficiency in neonates. Radiographics 2002; 22: 1429–1438

Rudnik-Schoneborn S et al. Clinical features of unilateral multicystic renal dysplasia in children. Eur J Pediatr 1998; 157: 666–672

Shaheen IS et al. Multicystic dysplastic kidney and pelviureteric junction obstruction. Pediatr Surg Int 2005; 21: 282–284

Thompson HS et al. Renal cystic diseases. Eur Radiol 1997; 7: 1267–1275

Definition

- **Epidemiology**
  Duplex anomalies of the renal pelvis and ureter are among the most common malformations of the urogenital tract.
- **Etiology, pathophysiology, pathogenesis**
  Embryonal developmental anomaly • The collecting system in a duplex kidney can be either obstructed (ureterocele) or refluxing (malformed junction with the trigone of the bladder) • Malformation of the renal parenchyma.
  Bifid ureter: Premature division of the ureteric bud • Two ureters arise from the duplex kidney and drain into a distal ureter.
  Double ureter: Arises from two ureteric buds • *Meyer–Weigert rule:* The ureter entering the bladder caudally arises from the upper moiety of the duplex kidney and the ureter entering the bladder cranially arises from the lower moiety • Associated with ureteropelvic junction obstruction (usually the lower moiety is affected).
  Both ureters can have orthotopic and ectopic junctions:
  - Lower moiety with ectopic junction: usually refluxing.
  - Upper moiety with ectopic junction: often associated with ureterocele (obstructed).
  - Ectopic ureteric junction with the urethra or vagina may also occur (constant drip of urine.)

Imaging Signs

- **Ultrasound findings**
  Isolated duplex kidneys are usually an incidental finding • The longitudinal axis of the kidney is elongated • The central echo reflection is interrupted by a parenchymal bridge • Usually the axes of the two moieties are offset from each other on dynamic ultrasound studies • The renal pelvis is dilated where there is reflux or obstruction • Megaureter may be present • *Ureterocele:* Typical "cobra head" cystic mass in the bladder • There may be an ectopic ureterovesical junction.
- **Doppler ultrasound findings**
  Findings may include duplicated renal arterial supply.
- **Voiding cystourethrography (VCUG)**
  Absolutely indicated in dilation of the renal caliceal system to exclude or confirm refluxing moiety in a duplex system • Ureterocele is visualized as a filling defect within the contrast-filled bladder.
- **MRI**
  HASTE and RARE sequences are used to visualize a dilated collecting system and nonfunctioning moieties • T1-weighted 3D GE sequence after injection of contrast and low-dose furosemide is used in a nondilated collecting systems • Dynamic T1-weighted GE after contrast administration is used to evaluate renal function • Anatomy of the collecting system is precisely visualized, occasionally with an ectopic ureteric orifice.

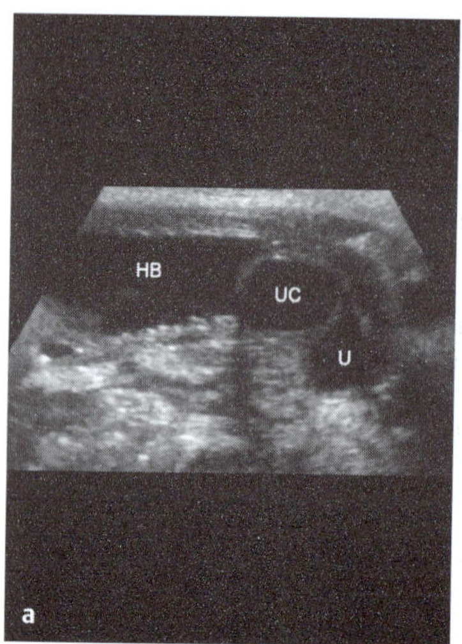

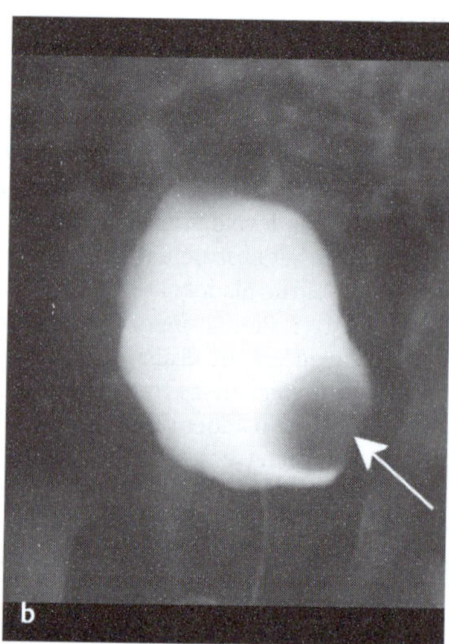

Fig. 5.9 a, b Ureterocele. Ultrasound (**a**) and VCUG (**b**). Typical ultrasound ureterocele (UC), protruding into the bladder lumen (HB) and obstructing the ureter (U). Conventional radiograph of contrast-filled bladder (**b**) shows a typical filling defect caused by the ureterocele (arrow).

- **Nuclear medicine renal imaging**
  Tracer: ^{99m}Tc-MAG3 • Used to evaluate compromised renal function • Visualizes obstructed components (furosemide test).

Clinical Aspects

- **Typical presentation**
  Isolated duplex kidneys are usually asymptomatic and are discovered as incidental findings • Malformations of the collecting system may lead to urinary tract infection, disturbed micturition, hematuria, and compromised renal function.
- **Therapeutic options**
  The goal is to preserve as much functional renal parenchyma as possible • Reimplantation of the ureter • Incision of ureterocele • Partial nephroureterectomy of the nonfunctional moiety in a duplex system • Temporary supravesical urine drainage where renal function is jeopardized.
- **Course and prognosis**
  Prognosis is good in the absence of a refluxing or obstructed ureter • Prognosis varies with the timepoint of the diagnosis and degree of compromised renal function.

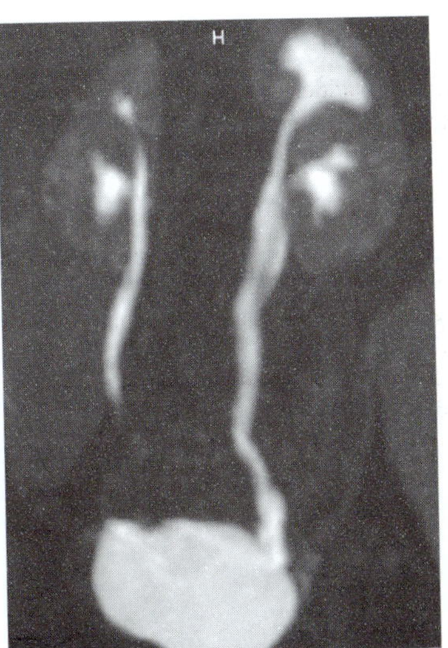

Fig. 5.10 Duplex kidney in a 1-year-old girl. Contrast-enhanced T1-weighted MR urography (MIP). Bilateral duplex kidneys with right fissured ureter and left double ureter.

▸ **Complications**

Large ureteroceles can compress the second ipsilateral ureter and the contralateral ureter, compromising urinary drainage • In extremely rare cases the ureterocele can prolapse into the urethra, leading to disturbed micturition • Ascending urinary tract infections with pyelonephritis (with abscess formation) can occur • Total loss of renal function can occur.

Differential Diagnosis

▸ **Ureterocele**

Bladder mass	– Such as rhabdomyosarcoma of the bladder or hematoma in the bladder – Distinguishable on ultrasound
Hutch diverticulum	– Rarely protrudes into the bladder lumen – Can be visualized separately from the ureter on ultrasound – Predisposed to vesicoureteric reflux

▸ **Duplex kidney**

Simple parenchymal bridge (hypertrophic renal column)	– Renal pelvis is not completely separated – No associated malformations of the collecting system – Visualization of renal arterial supply on Doppler ultrasound
Renal tumor	– Abnormal parenchymal structure – Loss of corticomedullary differentiation – Inhomogeneous mass – Tumor vascular supply

Tips and Pitfalls

An ureterocele can escape detection when the bladder is empty • The picture of ureteropelvic junction obstruction can also occur where a duplex kidney is associated with other urinary tract anomalies.

Selected References

Avni FE et al. The role of MR imaging for the assessment of complicated duplex kidneys in children: preliminary report. Pediatr Radiol 2001; 31: 215–223

Riccabona M et al. Feasibility of MR urography in neonates and infants with anomalies of the upper urinary tract. Eur Radiol 2002; 12: 1442–1450

Staatz G et al. Magnetic resonance urography in children: Evaluation of suspected ureteral ectopia in duplex systems. J Urol 2001; 166: 2346–2350

Definition

- **Epidemiology**
  The most common cause of congenital infravesical obstruction • Affects only boys.
- **Etiology, pathophysiology, pathogenesis**
  Congenital folds that lie in the posterior segment of the urethra (prostatic urethra and membranous portion) distal to the verumontanum • There are three types classified according to position and size.

Imaging Signs

- **Ultrasound findings**
  Thickened bladder wall with trabeculation (note that a thickened wall can lead to secondary stenosis of the intramural ureters) • Bladder wall thickness with moderate filling > 4 mm • Bladder wall thickness with nearly empty bladder > 7 mm • Urine retention • Dilation of the ureters and renal pelvis, usually bilateral • Dilation of the prostatic urethra, especially during micturition is a variable finding • Kidneys often exhibit dysplastic changes such as total or partial loss of corticomedullary differentiation • Direct perineal visualization of the urethra during micturition after filling the bladder with ultrasound contrast agent.
- **Voiding cystourethrography (VCUG)**
  The urethral valve causing obstruction is directly visualized as a linear filling defect • Dilation is seen proximal to the stenosis, usually in the prostatic urethra, with an abrupt change in caliber to the penile urethra • Trabeculation of the bladder wall • Urine retention • Vesicoureteric reflux (usually on the left) • Retrograde visualization of the ductus deferens.
- **Nuclear medicine imaging**
  Tracer: ^{99m}Tc-MAG3 • Compromised renal function • Visualizes obstructed components (furosemide test).

Clinical Aspects

- **Typical presentation**
  Oligohydramnios with pulmonary hypoplasia • Urinary tract infections (36% of cases) • Signs of obstruction (enuresis, continual wetness) • Palpable bladder and kidneys in newborns • Failure to thrive (13%) • Hematuria (5%) • Abnormal uroflowmeter results.
- **Therapeutic options**
  Incision of the urethral valve.
- **Course and prognosis**
  Prognosis varies with the time of the diagnosis • Prognosis is good with early detection and treatment.

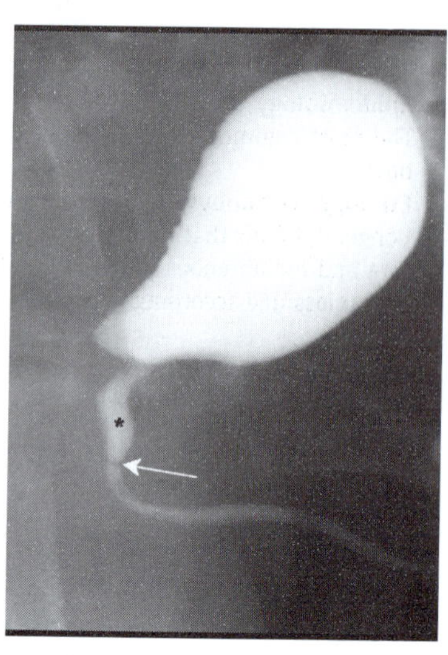

Fig. 5.11 Urethral valve. VCUG. The urethral valve (arrow) is visualized as a linear filling defect. Dilation of the prostatic urethra (*) and detrusor hypertrophy with trabeculation of the bladder wall, indirect signs of infravesical obstruction.

▸ **Complications**

Associated vesicoureteric reflux (usually on the left) • Bladder rupture (usually intrauterine with urinary ascites) • Urinoma • Urothorax • Urosepsis • Renal insufficiency.

Differential Diagnosis

Ureteropelvic junction obstruction	– Dilated pelvicaliceal system – No dilation of the ureter – Normal bladder and urethra
Primary megaureter	– Obstructed or refluxing – Not obstructed or refluxing – Normal bladder and urethra
Neurogenic bladder	– For example, in a meningomyelocele in spina bifida (ultrasound examination of the spinal canal is always indicated) – Normal urethra
Prolapsed ureterocele	– Prolapse of a ureterocele into the urethra during micturition – Secondary infravesical obstruction – Ureterocele can be visualized on ultrasound

Tips and Pitfalls

Urethral valves can escape detection on a VCUG with a catheter in situ (boys should also be examined without a catheter in situ) • Can be misinterpreted as an urethral stricture with an urethral valve • Be alert to changes in the anterior urethra • Where the urethral valve cannot be directly visualized, be alert to indirect signs of an existing infravesical obstruction.

Selected References

Berrocal T et al. Vesicoureteral reflux: can the urethra be adequately assessed by using contrast-enhanced voiding US of the bladder? Radiology 2005; 234: 235–241

Chertin B et al. Long-term results of primary avulsion of posterior urethral valves using a Fogarty balloon catheter. J Urol 2002; 168: 1841–1843

Cremin BJ. A review of the ultrasonic appearances of posterior urethral valve and ureteroceles. Pediatr Radiol 1986; 16: 357–364

Sty JR et al. Genitourinary imaging techniques. Pediatr Clin North Am 2006; 53: 339–361

Definition

- **Epidemiology**
  Most common bacterial infection in children • Incidence up to age 15 is higher in girls than in boys (5% in girls, less then 1% in boys) • In boys, incidence is highest during the first year of life.
- **Etiology, pathophysiology, pathogenesis**
  Most often caused by congenital urinary tract anomalies • In girls, the short urethra is conducive to urinary tract infections • Usually hematogenous in newborns • Less often the infection is iatrogenic, such as secondary to VCUG • Kidney swelling in infants is usually bilateral and more severe • The pathogen is usually *Escherichia coli.*
  Risk factors:
  - Urinary obstruction such as ureterocele, stone, urethral valve, phimosis, or megaureter.
  - Duplex kidney.
  - Other renal anomalies.
  - Vesicoureteric reflux (in about a third of cases).

Imaging Signs

- **Ultrasound findings**
  Unilaterally or bilaterally enlarged kidneys (volumetric measurement) • Corticomedullary differentiation is diminished • Reduced renal echogenicity • Thickening of the renal pelvis wall • Bladder wall may also be thickened in cystitis • Abscesses may be present • Hydronephrosis • Pyonephrosis (echogenic material in the renal pelvis).
- **Color Doppler ultrasound findings**
  Reduced perfusion of the inflamed parts of the kidney • Wedge-shaped nonperfused areas.
- **CT findings**
  Enlarged kidney • *Microabscesses:* Hypodense areas in the renal cortex measuring 1–5 mm without a mass effect • Postcontrast images in the parenchymal phase show a typical radial pattern of renal parenchyma with segmental hypodensity of the renal cortex • Delayed and reduced renal contrast enhancement and excretion • Wedge-shaped nonperfused areas • Increased density in perirenal fatty tissue consistent with inflammatory edema.
- **MRI findings**
  MR urography: Visualization of the renal caliceal system and the urinary tract • *MRI of the kidney:* Visualization of renal morphology • Perfusion • Abscess.
- **Nuclear medicine imaging**
  Nuclear medicine imaging with DMSA • Very sensitive in detecting parenchymal lesions such as scars and in visualizing renal function • Wedge-shaped nonperfused areas • MRI may be used in place of this study.
- **Voiding cystourethrography (VCUG)**
  In recurrent urinary infections with fever to exclude vesicoureteric reflux.

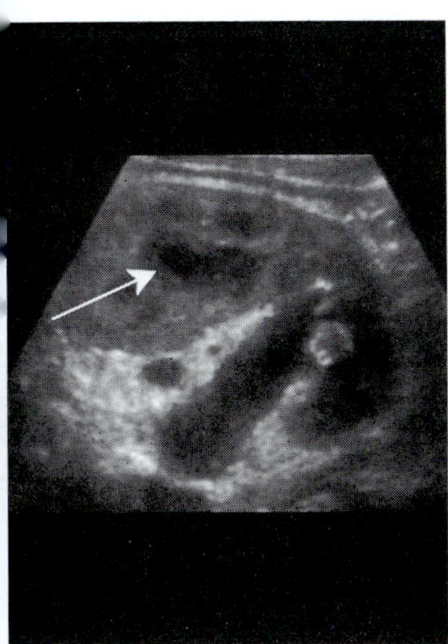

Fig. 5.12 Acute pyelonephritis. Ultrasound. Inflammatory thickening of the wall of the renal pelvis (arrow) in acute pyelonephritis. Findings also include diminished corticomedullary differentiation.

Clinical Aspects

- **Typical presentation**
  Fever • Abdominal pain • Vomiting • Loss of appetite • Dysuria, pollakiuria, hematuria • Enuresis • Leukocytosis • Elevated C-reactive protein • Abnormal urine findings (bacteria, leukocytes, nitrite, or hematuria).
- **Therapeutic options**
  Initially parenteral antibiotics, later orally • Drainage may be indicated in hydronephrosis • Percutaneous drainage is indicated where abscess occurs.
- **Course and prognosis**
  Renal swelling persists up to 6 weeks • Prognosis is good with prompt onset of treatment and elimination of the underlying cause • Disorder recurs within one year in 30% of cases • 5-year recurrence rate is 50% • Recurrence is twice as common in girls than in boys.
- **Complications**
  Renal abscess • Perirenal abscess • Pyonephrosis • Scarring • Shrunken kidney • Urosepsis.

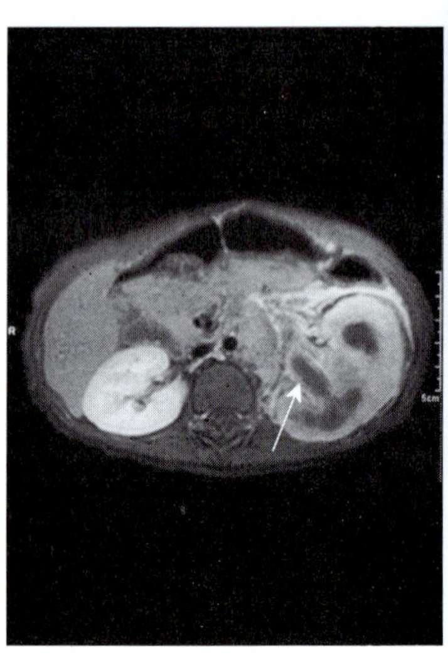

Fig. 5.13 MR image, contrast-enhanced T1-weighted TSE SPIR. Inflammatory enlarged left kidney showing less enhancement than the contralateral kidney. The wall of the renal pelvis is thickened (arrow).

Differential Diagnosis

Compensatory hypertrophy of the kidney	– Small contralateral kidney – Multicystic dysplastic contralateral kidney – Unilaterally compromised renal function – Secondary to nephrectomy or where a single kidney is present
Wilms tumor	– Focal swelling in pyelonephritis can mimic a tumor (focal interstitial nephritis) – Clinical and laboratory findings, follow-up
Renal infarction	– Wedge-shaped nonperfused area – Possible known underlying disorder such as arrhythmia – Clinical and laboratory findings, follow-up
Glomerulonephritis	– Diminished corticomedullary differentiation – No detectable focal lesion – Bilaterally enlarged kidneys – Histologic examination is required to confirm the diagnosis

Tips and Pitfalls

Normal renal ultrasound findings do not exclude pyelonephritis • In recurrent pyelonephritis, the examiner should look for vesicoureteric reflux or other urogenital anomalies.

Selected References

Kraus SJ et al. Genitourinary imaging in children. Pediatr Clin North Am 2001; 48: 1381–1424

Lavocat MP et al. Imaging of pyelonephritis. Pediatr Radiol 1997; 27: 159–165

Paterson A et al. Urinary tract infection: an update on imaging strategies. Eur Radiol 2004; 14 Suppl 4: L89–100

Sakarya ME et al. The role of power Doppler ultrasonography in the diagnosis of acute pyelonephritis. Br J Urol 1998; 81: 360–363

Definition

- **Epidemiology**
  Increased incidence in newborns.
- **Etiology, pathophysiology, pathogenesis**
  Medullary form:
  - Renal hypercalciuria: Renal tubular acidosis • Medullary sponge kidney.
  - Drug-induced hypercalciuria: Furosemide • Steroids • ACTH.
  - Alimentary hypercalciuria: Hypervitaminosis D • Calcium or phosphate substitution.
  - Endocrine hypercalciuria: Hyperparathyroidism • Cushing syndrome • Diabetes insipidus • Hyperthyroidism.
  - Idiopathic hypercalciuria.
  - Hyperoxaluria: Primary hereditary form • Secondary enteric form.
  - Hyperuricemia: Renal gout • Lesch–Nyhan syndrome.
  - Papillary necrosis.

  Cortical form: Renal cortical necrosis • Chronic glomerulonephritis • Alport syndrome • Congenital oxalosis.

Imaging Signs

- **Ultrasound**
  Most sensitive method.
  Three main forms:
  - Cortical nephrocalcinosis (5% of cases).
  - Medullary nephrocalcinosis (95%).
  - Global nephrocalcinosis (affecting cortex and medullary).

  Classification of medullary nephrocalcinosis:
  - *Grade I:* Loss of corticomedullary differentiation or increased echogenicity in the apices of the renal pyramids.
  - *Grade II A (garland type):* Perimedullary increase in echogenicity except for the central portions of the renal pyramids.
  - *Grade II B:* Diffuse increase in echogenicity in the entire renal pyramid.
  - *Grade III:* Grade II and posterior acoustic shadow.

Clinical Aspects

- **Typical presentation**
  Usually an incidental finding in premature infants and newborns • Clinically asymptomatic • Diagnosis can only be made where there are appropriate clinical findings.
- **Therapeutic options**
  Treatment and observation of the underlying disorder.
- **Course and prognosis**
  Prognosis varies greatly depending on the cause and severity • May resolve completely.

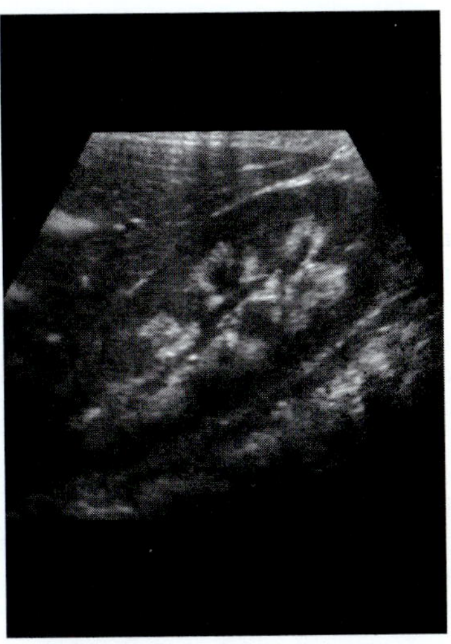

Fig. 5.14 Nephrocalcinosis in a premature infant. Ultrasound. Grade IIA-B medullary nephrocalcinosis

- **Complications**
  This depends on the underlying disorder.

Differential Diagnosis

Autosomal recessive polycystic kidney disease	– Enlarged hyperechoic kidney – Loss of corticomedullary differentiation – Cysts may not be detectable
Tamm-Horsfall protein	– Increased echogenicity in the renal pyramids – Usually disappears spontaneously and quickly

Tips and Pitfalls

Morphologic findings alone are of questionable clinical significance where they do not correlate with clinical findings and the picture of the underlying disorder • Most cases of nephrocalcinosis do not exhibit a typical acoustic shadow.

Selected References

Dähnert W. Nephrocalcinosis. In: Dähnert W. Radiology Review Manual. Baltimore: Williams & Wilkins; 1991; 454

Dick PT et al. Observer reliability in grading nephrocalcinosis on ultrasound examinations in children. Pediatr Radiol 1999; 29: 68–72

Hein G et al. Development of nephrocalcinosis in very low birth weight infants. Pediatr Nephrol 2004; 19: 616–620

Definition

- **Epidemiology**

  Most common renal tumor in children • Accounts for 10–12% of all pediatric malignancies • Peak age between 2 and 4 years • Incidence is 1:100 000 • No sex predilection.

- **Etiology, pathophysiology, pathogenesis**

  Arises from undifferentiated metanephrogenic embryonic tissue • Usually unilateral • Bilateral in 5–10% of cases • About 15% of cases are associated with other congenital malformations—hemihypertrophy, sporadic aniridia, cerebral gigantism, Beckwith–Wiedemann syndrome, pseudohermaphroditism, neurofibromatosis, renal anomalies such as horseshoe and duplex kidney.

  Staging: (according to SIOP):
  - *Stage I:* Tumor is limited to the kidney and is completely excised.
  - *Stage II:* Tumor extends beyond the kidney but is completely excised.
  - *Stage III:* Residual tumor without hematogenous metastases, abdominal lymph node metastases, or preoperative or intraoperative tumor rupture.
  - *Stage IV:* Hematogenous distant metastases, extraabdominal lymph node metastases.
  - *Stage V:* Bilateral renal tumors.

  Histologic subtypes: of primary pediatric renal tumors:

  I. *Favorable histology* (low malignancy, 10% of lesions):
  - Congenital mesoblastic nephroma
  - Multilocular cystic nephroma
  - Fibroadenomatous nephroblastoma

  II. *Standard histology* (moderate malignancy, 80%):
  - Mixed type of nephroblastoma
  - Blastemic form of nephroblastoma
  - Epithelial form of nephroblastoma
  - Stromal tumors, including fetal rhabdomyomatous nephroblastoma

  III. *Unfavorable histology* (high malignancy, < 10%):
  - Nephroblastoma with focal or diffuse anaplasia
  - Clear cell sarcoma of the kidney
  - Rhabdoid tumor of the kidney

Imaging Signs

- **Ultrasound findings**

  Modality of choice for follow-up • Highly heterogeneous tumor, usually isoechoic to liver tissue • Ultrasound morphology varies with the size and stage of the tumor • Pseudocapsule • Often the tumor is large when first diagnosed (12 cm on average) • Central tumor necrosis is hypoechoic • Tumor calcifications are rare (about 10% of cases) • Small cystic tumor components (focal hemorrhages and necrosis) are present in about 50% of cases • The rest of the kidney is displaced • Renal pelvis may be dilated or compressed • Large tumors may lead to

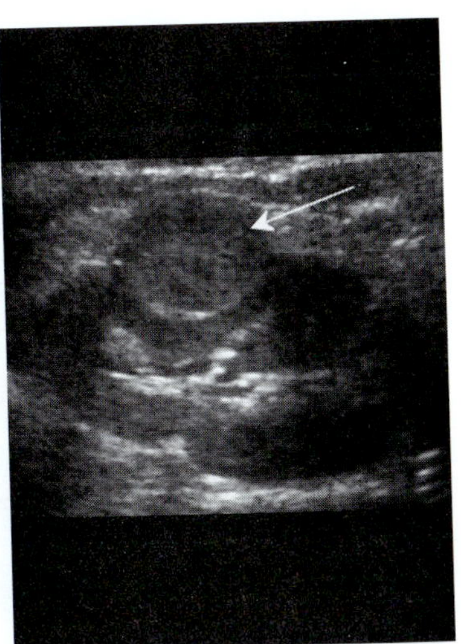

Fig. 5.15 Three-year-old child with hemihypertrophy and histologically proven nephroblastoma. Ultrasound of the left kidney. Kidney tumor on the lateral cortex with homogeneous echo pattern isoechoic to liver tissue (arrow).

complete loss of normal renal architecture • Lymph node or liver metastases (usually hypoechoic).

▸ **Color Doppler ultrasound findings**
Hypervascular tumor • Tumor thrombus in the renal vein, inferior vena cava, and/or right atrium • Renal vascular pedicle is visualized • Large abdominal vessels are displaced; tumor encasement is atypical.

▸ **CT findings**
Inhomogeneous enhancement • Indispensable study for excluding pulmonary metastases (in 20% of cases at initial diagnosis) • Penetration of pseudocapsule into the renal pelvis • Infiltration of adjacent structures • Invasion or displacement of vascular structures • Lymph node and/or liver metastases.

▸ **MRI findings**
Allows measurement of tumor volume • Inhomogeneous signal intensity • Usually hypointense on T1-weighted images, hyperintense on T2-weighted images • Necrosis and hemorrhage are readily identifiable • The pseudocapsule is markedly hypointense on T1-weighted images and shows significant enhancement (typical of nephroblastoma) • Vascular anatomy and invasion are visualized • Well suited for follow-up studies in patients under chemotherapy • Suitable for diagnosis and follow-up of predisposing nephroblastomatosis.

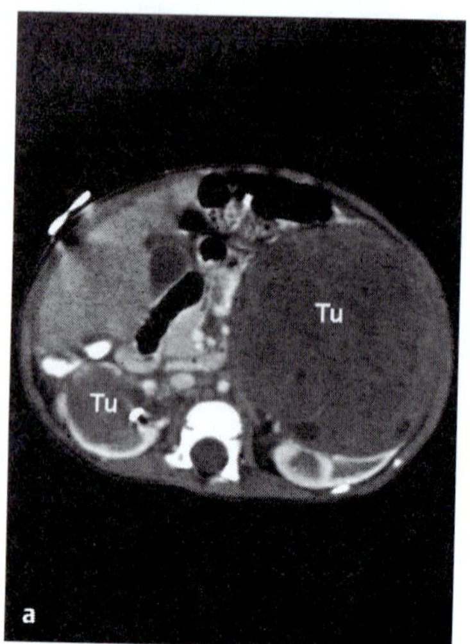

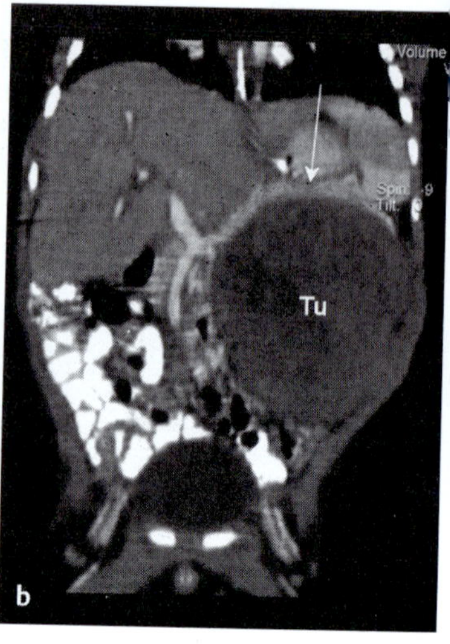

Fig. 5.16 a, b Bilateral Wilms tumors (Tu), larger on the left than the right. Contrast-enhanced CT of the abdomen with coronal reconstruction. Findings include multiple hypodense areas within the tumor (necrosis), especially on the left (**a**). The left nephroblastoma has markedly displaced the splenic vein (**b**, arrow).

Clinical Aspects

- **Typical presentation**
  Painless abdominal swelling (60–90% of cases) • Hematuria (7–25%) • Arterial hypertension (50–60%) • Abdominal pain (25%) • Fever (15%).
- **Therapeutic options**
  Combination of preoperative chemotherapy and surgery, supplemented by radiation therapy in high-risk patients.
- **Course and prognosis**
  Depends greatly on the histologic subtype • Overall cure rate is as high as 90% (clear cell sarcomas and rhabdoid tumors).
- **Complications**
  Abdominal trauma can lead to tumor rupture • Early vascular invasion and distant metastases (12% of cases at initial diagnosis).

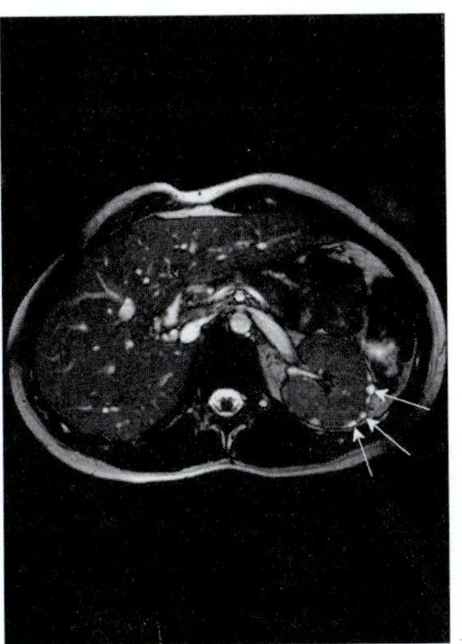

Fig. 5.17 Nephroblastomatosis. MR image, balanced FFE unenhanced sequence. Typical well-demarcated subcortical nodular structures (arrows).

Differential Diagnosis

Neuroblastoma	– More pronounced tumor calcifications – On the surface of the kidney – Renal architecture is preserved – Tumor typically encases vessels; displacement and compression are rare
Xanthogranulomatous pyelonephritis	– Both global and segmental – Echo pattern is isoechoic to liver tissue – Cysts with internal echoes – Cast of the renal pelvis may be present – Thickening of the renal pelvic wall – Often complete destruction of the kidney
Clear cell sarcoma of the kidney	– Morphologic findings are indistinguishable from nephroblastoma – Formerly regarded as aggressive subtype of nephroblastoma – Diagnosed later, between ages 3 and 5 years – Osteolytic and osteoblastic metastases (nuclear medicine skeletal imaging is indicated)
Rhabdoid tumor of the kidney	– Morphologic findings are indistinguishable from nephroblastoma – Formerly regarded as aggressive subtype of nephroblastoma – Infants (younger than 1 year old)

Multilocular cystic nephroma	– Synonym: multicystic or polycystic nephroblastoma – Kidney is irregularly permeated with cystic areas – Kidney tissue is intact, especially marginal tissue – Cysts within cysts are visualized – Nephrectomy is curative
Congenital mesoblastic nephroma	– Primary lesion is benign although infiltrative growth is possible – Primarily cystic – Loss of function in affected kidney – Most common renal tumor in infants below the age of 6 months
Nephroblastomatosis	– Nodular nephroblastomatosis lesions are usually subcortical – Often difficult to detect on ultrasound – Normally resolve spontaneously – Can degenerate into nephroblastoma – Ultrasound follow-up scans every 3 months – Slight contrast enhancement on CT and MR image

Tips and Pitfalls

The rare xanthogranulomatous pyelonephritis can be misinterpreted as a renal tumor • Tumor size is often underestimated on ultrasound scans • Vascular structures are not visualized in detail • Large tumors with calcifications can be misinterpreted as a neuroblastoma in the absence of well-defined organ margins • On single-phase CT, the extensions of the tumor in the veins draining the region are often missed where venous contrast is not adequate.

Selected References

Glick RD et al. Renal tumors in infants less than 6 months of age. Pediatr Surg 2004; 39: 522–525

Riccabona M. Imaging of renal tumours in infancy and childhood. Eur Radiol 2003; 13 Suppl 4: L116–129

McHugh K. Renal and adrenal tumours in children. Cancer Imaging 2007; 7: 41–51

Meyer JS et al. Imaging of neuroblastoma and Wilms' tumor. Magn Reson Imaging Clin North Am 2002; 10: 275–302

Definition

- **Epidemiology**
  Most common adrenal mass in newborns (incidence 1.7:1000 newborns) • Right side in 70% of cases • Bilateral in 5–10% • Can occur as a prenatal or postnatal lesion • Occurs more often in large for gestational age newborns.
- **Etiology, pathophysiology, pathogenesis**
  Birth trauma such as forceps delivery • Neonatal asphyxia, hypoxia, and hypotension • Newborn sepsis—meningococcal sepsis for example leads to Waterhouse–Friderichsen syndrome with adrenal hemorrhage and disseminated intravascular coagulation • Systemic disorders • Renal venous thrombosis • Thrombosis of the inferior vena cava • Congenital asplenia • Traumatic adrenal hemorrhage in children is very rare, usually occurring in combination with liver or spleen injuries • Progresses to final stage within about one year.

Imaging Signs

- **Ultrasound findings**
  Homogeneous, hyperechoic mass in the adrenal glands, later becoming inhomogeneous to hypoechoic • Loss of typical corticomedullary differentiation • In the late stages, a purely cystic lesion may be present • Caudal displacement of the kidney • Size of the lesion decreases over time • Hyperechoic capsule • In the final stage, the lesion is a small solid partially calcified mass.
- **Color Doppler ultrasound findings**
  Evaluation of the renal veins and inferior vena cava • No detectable tumor vascularization.
- **Plain abdominal radiograph findings**
  Adrenal calcification in the late stage.
- **CT**
  Usually not required to evaluate the adrenal glands in newborns and infants.
- **MRI findings**
  Signal characteristics vary with the stage of the hemorrhage • Chronic hematomas exhibit a hemosiderin ring • Thrombosis of the renal vein or inferior vena cava may be identifiable as the cause of the hemorrhage (balanced FFE sequence) • This study is indicated to exclude a neuroblastoma.

Clinical Aspects

- **Typical presentation**
  Palpable tumor • Anemia • Acute decrease in hemoglobin • Jaundice • Usually an incidental finding on ultrasound.
- **Therapeutic options**
  Follow-up studies are indicated • Temporary corticosteroid substitution where there is adrenal insufficiency.
- **Course and prognosis**
  Unilateral hemorrhages are usually uncomplicated.

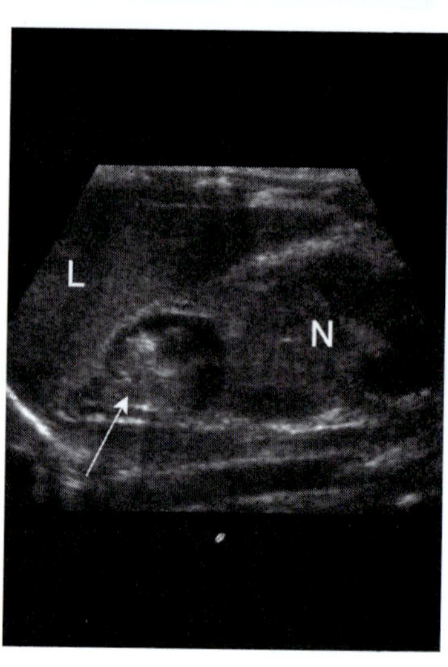

Fig. 5.18 Adrenal hemorrhage in a newborn with perinatal asphyxia. Ultrasound. Acute hemorrhage in the right adrenal gland (arrow). The hemorrhage shows a hyperechoic inhomogeneous echo pattern. L = liver, N = right kidney.

- **Complications**
  Adrenal dysfunction in Addison disease, especially with bilateral adrenal hemorrhages • Superinfection with abscess formation.

Differential Diagnosis

Neuroblastoma	– Rare in newborns – Tumor calcifications typically occur – Abnormal pattern of vascularization – Increased urinary excretion of catecholamine metabolic products
Multicystic nephroblastoma	– Directly adjacent to kidney – Normal imaging findings in the adrenal gland
Congenital adrenal hyperplasia	– Bilaterally enlarged adrenal glands – Normal corticomedullary differentiation
Wolman disease	– Inherited autosomal recessive storage disorder associated with xanthomatosis, leading to abdominal and central nervous system lipid deposits and adrenal calcifications – Leads to symptoms of Niemann–Pick disease

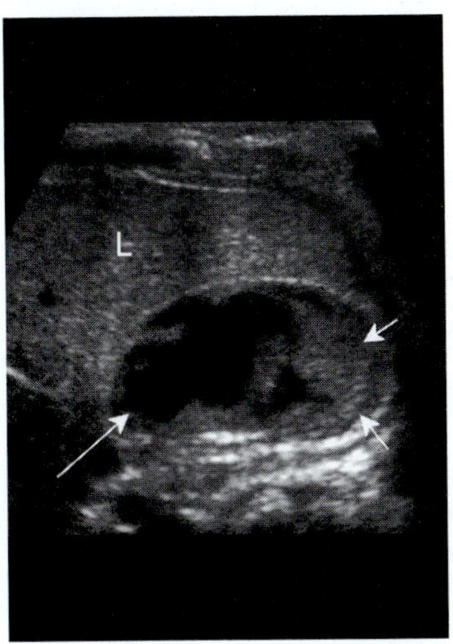

Fig. 5.19 Ultrasound scan of the upper abdomen in another newborn born of a diabetic mother, showing chronic adrenal hemorrhage. Findings include cystic areas (large arrow) in addition to solid components (small arrows). L = liver, M = spleen.

Tips and Pitfalls

A malignant tumor should be considered where the typical change in the ultrasound picture fails to occur and the size of the adrenal mass remains constant over 4 weeks • Adrenal hemorrhage must invariably be excluded as a possible cause of any scrotal hematoma • However, the scrotal hematoma can also be associated with a neuroblastoma.

Selected References

Desa DJ et al. Hemorrhagic necrosis of the adrenal gland in perinatal infants: A clinicopathological study. J Pathol 1972; 106: 133–149

Duman N et al. Scrotal hematoma due to neonatal adrenal hemorrhage. Pediatr Int 2004; 46: 360–362

Noviello C et al. Neonatal adrenal hemorrhage presenting as contralateral scrotal hematoma. Minerva Pediatr 2007; 59: 157–159

Velaphi SC et al. Neonatal adrenal hemorrhage: clinical and abdominal sonographic findings. Clin Pediatr (Phila) 2001; 40: 545–548

Definition

- **Epidemiology**
  Most common abdominal tumor in infants (accounts for about 12% of all perinatal tumors) • Third most common malignant tumor in infants (after leukemia and central nervous system tumors) • 90% of all neuroblastomas are diagnosed before age 5 years.
- **Etiology, pathophysiology, pathogenesis**
  Malignant tumor of the neural crest of sympathetic nerve tissue • One-third of all lesions arise from the sympathetic chain, two-thirds from the adrenal gland • 70% are retroperitoneal tumors, 20% mediastinal • Increased levels of catecholamine products are present (in 75–90% of cases) • Genetic factors include N-myc oncogene amplification and loss of heterozygosity in chromosome 1 p.
  Staging: (according to Brodeur):
  - *Stage I:* Tumor is limited to its region of origin • Total macroscopic resection with or without microscopic residual tumor • No lymph node involvement.
  - *Stage II A:* Unilateral tumor • Subtotal macroscopic resection • No lymph node involvement.
  - *Stage II B:* Unilateral tumor • Total or subtotal macroscopic resection • Involvement of ipsilateral regional lymph nodes.
  - *Stage III:* Tumor extends across the midline with or without involvement of regional lymph nodes.

  Or: Unilateral tumor with contralateral regional lymph node involvement.
  Or: Midline tumor with bilateral involvement of regional lymph nodes.
  - *Stage IV:* Metastases in remote lymph nodes, bone, bone marrow, liver, and/or other organs (except those whose involvement defines stage IV S).
  - *Stage IVS:* Local primary tumor according to the definition of stage I or II with metastases in the liver, skin, and/or bone marrow (< 10% of cases), limited to infants.

Imaging Signs

- **Ultrasound findings**
  Well demarcated, hyperechoic, inhomogeneous tumor (be alert to cystic neuroblastoma and ganglioneuroblastoma) • Lateral and caudal displacement of the kidney • Invasion of the kidney occurs in advanced stages of tumor growth • Small calcifications are typically present • Tumor encases vascular structures; typically growing along the posterior aspect of the aorta and/or vena cava • Liver and lymph node metastases are visualized in advanced stages.
- **Color Doppler ultrasound findings**
  Adjacent vascular structures are visualized (vascular compression or invasion) • Tumor vascularization.
- **CT findings**
  Used for staging where MRI is unavailable • Sensitive in detecting tumor calcifications • Tumor growth posterior to the aorta and/or vena cava is typical • Modality is indicated especially in thoracic imaging.

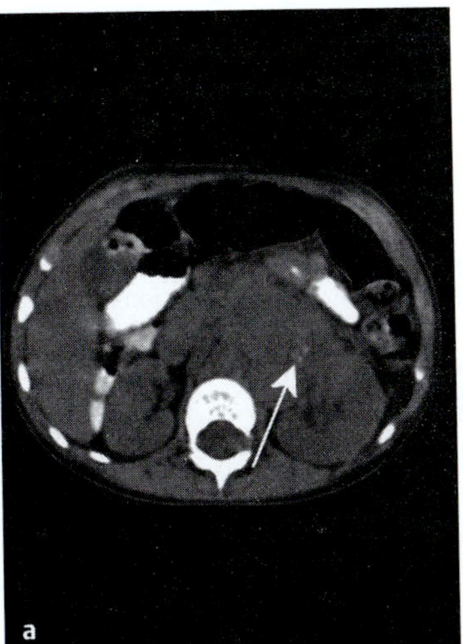

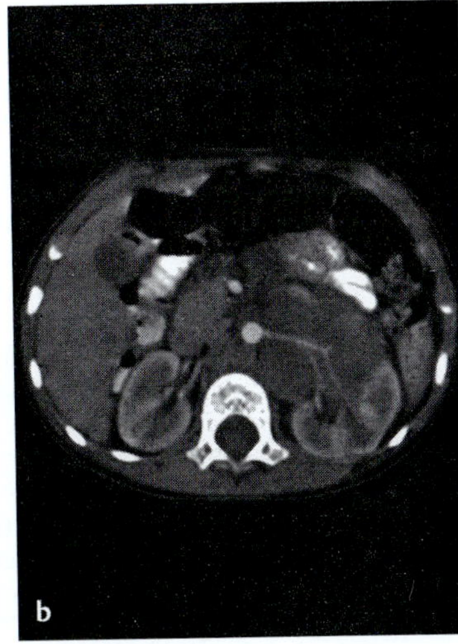

Fig. 5.20 a, b Neuroblastoma. Plain CT (**a**) and contrast study (**b**) of the abdomen. Large left retroperitoneal mass exhibiting small central calcifications (**a**, arrow) and encasing the left renal artery (**b**).

- **MRI**
  Initial staging • Follow-up in patients undergoing chemotherapy • Usually hypointense on T1-weighted images and hyperintense on T2-weighted images • Marked enhancement • Used to exclude or confirm tumor invasion into the spinal canal • Findings may include bone marrow metastases.
- **Nuclear medicine imaging**
  MIBG scintigraphy • For specific marking of the primary tumor and metastases.

Clinical Aspects

- **Typical presentation**
  Palpable tumor • Fever • Diarrhea from vasoactive intestinal peptide production • Bone pain, especially in the legs • Cerebellar ataxia • Nystagmus • periorbital edema and ecchymosis of the upper lid in retrobulbar neuroblastoma • Hypertension • Flush symptoms • Tachycardia • Headache • Failure to thrive • Horner syndrome.
  Laboratory values: Catecholamine metabolites in serum and urine (vanillylmandelic acid, homovanillic acid, dopamine) and the neuron-specific enolase are tumor markers • Unspecific findings include elevated lactate dehydrogenase and ferritin.

▸ **Therapeutic options**
Treatment depends on the tumor stage • In stage I, surgical resection of the tumor alone is sufficient • In higher stages, preoperative chemotherapy is indicated • Stage IV requires additional radiation therapy.

▸ **Course and prognosis**
Prognosis depends on the stage of the tumor, hormone activity, and age • Small tumor size, young age of the child, and hormone activity are factors that favorably influence the prognosis • 5-year survival rate for all stages is about 55%, stages I–III about 80%, stage IV less than 20% • Spontaneous remission can occur.

▸ **Complications**
Paraplegia can occur with intraforaminal and intraspinal invasion by an extra-adrenal neuroblastoma • Distant metastases.

Differential Diagnosis

Wilms tumor	– Less pronounced tumor vascularization – Slight contrast media enhancement – Arises from the renal parenchyma – Tumor calcifications are rare – Tumor does not grow posterior to the aorta and/or vena cava – Tumor thrombus in renal vein
Adrenal hemorrhage	– Typical ultrasound morphology with varying echotexture depending on time progress – Decreasing size – No vascularization
Retroperitoneal teratoma	– Contains fat as well as calcifications – Sharply demarcated tumor without signs of malignant growth – Less pronounced vascularization – Negative MIBG scintigraphy

Tips and Pitfalls

CT cannot ensure sufficient evaluation of intraspinal tumor growth; where there is spinal involvement, MRI of the entire spinal canal is indicated • Where there is cerebral involvement, dural invasion must be excluded.

Selected References

Dähnert W. Neuroblastoma. In: Dähnert W. Radiology Review Manual. Baltimore: Williams & Wilkins; 1991: 455–456

Lonergam GJ et al. Neuroblastoma, ganglioneuroblastoma, and ganglioneuroma: radiologic-pathologic correlation. Radiographics 2002; 22: 911–934

McHugh K. Renal and adrenal tumours in children. Cancer Imaging 2007; 7: 41–51

Papaioannou G et al. Neuroblastoma in childhood: review and radiological findings. Cancer Imaging 2005; 5: 116–127

Siegel MJ et al. Staging of neuroblastoma at imaging: report of the radiology diagnostic oncology group. Radiology 2002; 223: 168–175

Definition

- **Epidemiology**

  Most common soft tissue tumor in children • Incidence is 4–8% of all malignant tumors in children under age 15 • Accounts for 10–25% of all sarcomas • Peak frequency is between the ages of 2 and 6 years • Boys are affected twice as often as girls.

- **Etiology, pathophysiology, pathogenesis**

  Rhabdomyosarcoma most often occurs in the head and neck • Second most common origin is from the pelvic organs • Tumor shows a predilection for the uterus and vagina in girls, and the bladder and prostate in boys.

  - *Bladder:* Usually arises from the neck and trigone of the bladder • Invades the bladder wall.
  - *Prostate:* Usually invades the neck of the bladder, posterior urethra, and perirectal soft tissue.

  Less common locations: Uterine cervix • Urethra • Pelvic wall • Seminal vesicles • Ductus deferens.

  Initial extensive tumor growth • Lymphatic and hematogenous metastases to the lungs, bone, and liver • Types include embryonal rhabdomyosarcoma (with botryoid and spindle-cell variants, accounting for two-thirds of cases) and alveolar rhabdomyosarcoma (with the solid alveolar variant).

Table 5.2 Staging of rhabdomyosarcoma

Stage	Findings
1	Location: • Eye • Sex organs • Bladder • Head and neck
2	• Tumor location other than in stage 1 • Unilocular • Diameter less than 5 cm • No lymphatic metastases
3	• Tumor location other than in stage 1 • Unilocular • Diameter of 5 cm or more • Metastases to local and regional lymph nodes
4	Distant metastases at the time of diagnosis

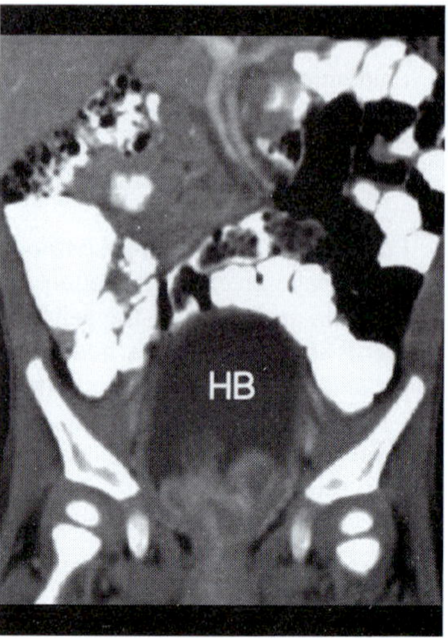

Fig. 5.21 Rhabdomyosarcoma of the bladder (HB) in a 16-month-old girl. Coronal multiplanar reconstruction of an abdominal CT obtained with intravenous, oral, and rectal contrast media.

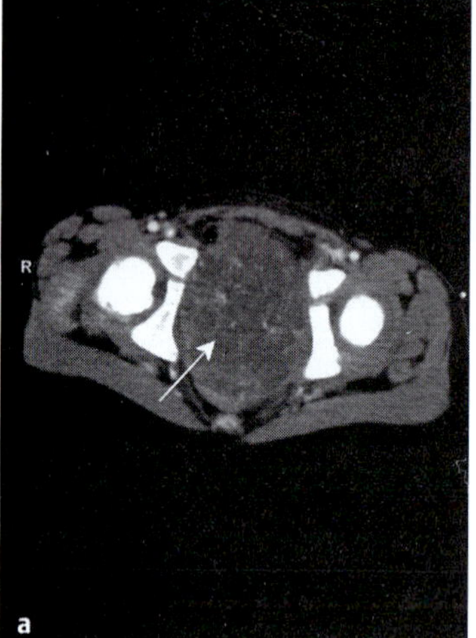

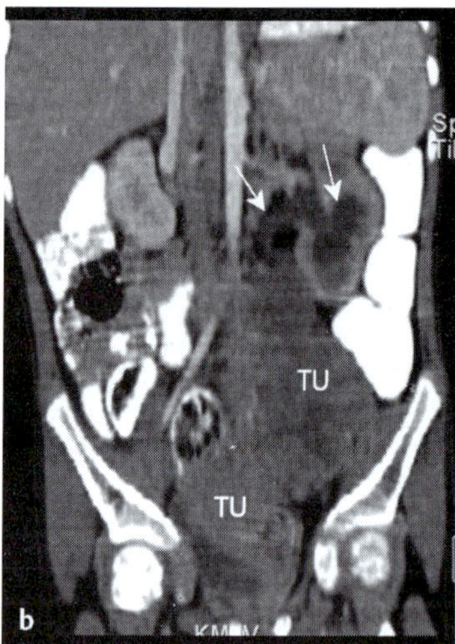

Fig. 5.22 a, b Rhabdomyosarcoma of the prostate. Axial image (**a**) and coronal multiplanar reconstruction (**b**).The large retroperitoneal tumor masses (TU) impair urinary drainage on the left, causing dilation of the renal pelvis and ureter (**b**, arrows).

Imaging Signs

- **Ultrasound findings**
  Multilobulated mass in the caudal bladder • Tumor is usually hyperechoic • Exophytic growth • Tumor is indistinguishable from the bladder wall • Tumor invasion of the ureteric orifices leads to urinary retention • Tumor may be cystic or solid • Tumor is usually large at the time of the diagnosis • Lymph node metastases • Metastases to other organs (especially the liver).
- **Color Doppler ultrasound findings**
  Tumor vascularization • Vascular compression or displacement.
- **CT findings**
  Where MRI is unavailable • Used to exclude or confirm pulmonary metastases • Heterogeneous enhancing tumor • Origin of the tumor is often difficult to determine.
- **MRI findings**
  Pelvis organs should be visualized in all three planes • T1-weighted images show intermediate tumor signal • Hyperintense on T2-weighted images • Marked enhancement • Pseudocapsule • Excellent visualization of tumor infiltration.
- **Nuclear medicine imaging**
  Nuclear medicine ^{99}Tc imaging is used to visualize bone metastases.

Clinical Aspects

- **Typical presentation**
  Dysuria • Hematuria • Tenesmus • Progressive urine retention • Palpable bladder • Visible vaginal tumor • Constipation and testicular swelling.
- **Therapeutic options**
  Primary chemotherapy • Surgical tumor resection • Radiation therapy.
- **Course and prognosis**
  Rhabdomyosarcoma of the bladder is usually already in stage III when initially diagnosed • 3-year survival rate after chemotherapy is 60–90% • The 5-year survival rate after radical surgery is 14–35%.
- **Complications**
  Tumor rupture • Metastases • Tumor invasion of adjacent pelvic structures.

Differential Diagnosis

Chronic cystitis	– Thickening of the bladder wall, especially at the trigone – Pseudodiverticulum may be present – Known causes such as indwelling catheter, neurogenic bladder, chemotherapy, hematogenous infection, bladder stones
Ovarian tumor	– Usually more pronounced cystic component – Ovarian teratomas include calcifications and fat in the tumor – Tomographic modalities visualize the organ of origin
Pelvic neuroblastoma	– Typically there are small tumor calcifications – Classic tumor growth around vascular structures – MIBG scintigraphy – Increased catecholamine production
Inflammatory pseudotumor	– Occurs in disorders such as chronic Crohn's disease – Known patient history – Typical laboratory findings – Histologic and microbiological findings
Sacrococcygeal teratoma	– Typical position – Directly adjacent to spine – Early diagnosis (usually peripartal)

Tips and Pitfalls

Initial diagnostic studies that reveal a large tumor usually do not clearly identify the organ of origin • Children with hematuria of uncertain causes should undergo ultrasound with a full bladder, as small rhabdomyosarcomas of the bladder could otherwise escape detection • A small rhabdomyosarcoma of the bladder can be misinterpreted as a chronic inflammatory reaction • MRI is indicated where the true pelvis cannot be evaluated but suspicious clinical symptoms are present.

Selected References

Ashlock R et al. Treatment modalities of bladder/prostate rhabdomyosarcoma: a review. Prostate Cancer Prostatic Dis 2003; 6: 112–120

Garel L et al. US of the pediatric female pelvis: a clinical perspective. Radiographics 2001; 21: 1393–1407

Groff DB. Pelvic neoplasms in children. J Surg Oncol 2001; 77: 65–71

Wu HY et al. Pediatric urologic oncology: bladder, prostate, testis. Urol Clin North Am 2004; 31: 619–627

Definition

- **Epidemiology**

  Incidence is 1:40 000 • Most common congenital solid tumor in newborns • Girls are affected four times as often as boys.

- **Etiology, pathophysiology, pathogenesis**

  Extragonadal germ-cell tumor • Arises from pluripotential cells • Does not necessarily contain material from all three germ layers • Usually detected and visible externally at birth • Usually a benign mature teratoma (up to 75% of all lesions) is present in newborns • Malignant teratomas are rare (7–17%) and are usually yolk sac tumors • Benign lesions can degenerate into malignant tumors • Associated with other congenital malformations—spine (5–16% of cases), urogenital anomalies such as renal dysplasia, urethral atresia, and undescended testis • 70–80% of all teratomas occur in the sacrococcygeal region • Not associated with chromosome anomalies.

Table 5.3 Variants of sacrococcygeal teratoma

Type	Location	Frequency
1	Primarily postsacral with only minimal presacral component	47%
2	Postsacral with major intrapelvic component	34%
3	Visible externally but primarily presacral and extending into the abdominal cavity	9%
4	Completely presacral without any detectable postsacral component	19%

Imaging Signs

- **Ultrasound findings**

  Primarily exophytic growth between the anal orifice and coccyx • Tumor is partially solid and partially cystic • Purely cystic tumors occur in 15% of cases • Average size at initial diagnosis (birth) is about 8 cm • Obstructed urinary drainage.

- **Color Doppler ultrasound findings**

  Tumor vascularization • Compression or displacement of pelvic vascular structures.

- **CT findings**

  Fatty tumor components are visualized (tumor is usually benign) • Hemorrhage and necrosis suggest a malignant lesion • Cystic changes • Sensitive in detecting tumor calcifications • Used for initial staging of malignant teratomas.

- **MRI findings**

  Precisely visualizes the extent of the tumor • Anterior displacement of the anus • Fatty tumor components are markedly hyperintense on T1-weighted images •

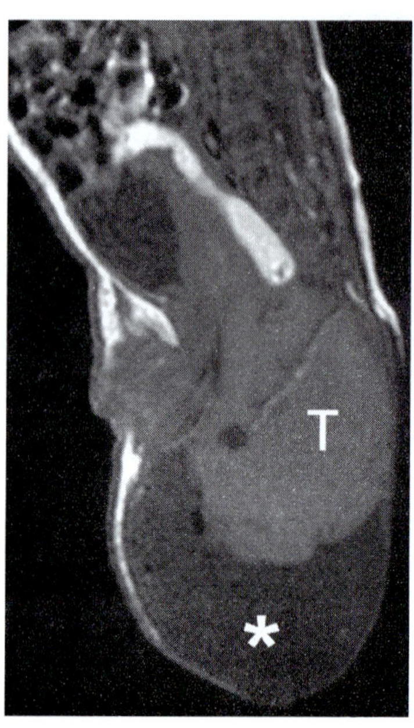

Fig. 5.23 Sacrococcygeal teratoma. MR image, sagittal T1-weighted SE sequence. Large solid tumor (T) and cystic tumor (*) components.

Chemical shift artifacts occur along fatty tissue interfaces • Associated spinal deformities may also be present • Intrapelvic tumor extensions are present in 50% of cases.

Clinical Aspects

- **Typical presentation**
  Significant deformity of the buttocks and perineal region • Diagnosis is usually made before birth • Polyhydramnios • Hydrops fetalis and heart failure occur in a hypervascularized tumor due to a steal effect and arteriovenous shunt within the tumor • Constipation • AFP is raised only in the malignant type.
- **Therapeutic options**
  Total tumor resection together with the coccyx and lower sacral vertebrae in newborns • Laparotomy is indicated only in types 3 and 4 and in primary malignant teratoma • Malignant tumors require chemotherapy and radiation therapy.
- **Course and prognosis**
  Prognosis is very good following total resection of a benign tumor • In malignant tumors, prognosis depends on the extent of the tumor, surgical treatment, and histologic type • The infant may be stillborn • In 50% of cases, there are initial metastases (peritoneal, hepatic, pulmonary, cerebral, bone) • 5-year survival rate is about 50%.

Factors that increase the risk of malignancy:
- The infant is older.
- The tumor arises early in the pregnancy.
- The tumor has a large presacral component.
- The tumor contains primarily solid components.
- The tumor was not completely resected.
- Several operations were performed on the tumor.
- The coccyx was not resected along with the tumor.

▸ **Complications**

Rate of recurrence is high without resection of the coccyx (> 30%) • The probability of malignancy increases to over 30% within several months (early resection is indicated) • Bladder and distal bowel dysfunction • Persistent constipation after surgical treatment • Massive tumor hemorrhage • Vaginal birth is rendered difficult (cesarean section may be indicated).

Differential Diagnosis

Cystic duplication anomaly of the rectum	– Relation to rectum visualized – Spine is normal – No metastases – Cystic; no solid components
Meningomyelocele	– No calcifications – Communicates directly with the spinal canal – Spinal cord and/or cauda equina fibers are displaced into the mass – Cystic components correspond to the dural sac filled with cerebrospinal fluid – Descent of the conus medullaris usually occurs
Hemangioma	– Typical hyperechoic or inhomogeneous ultrasound morphology – Hypervascular tumor – Markedly hyperintense on T2-weighted images with considerable enhancement
Lymphangioma	– Purely cystic mass – Septa between the individual cysts – Soft, compressible tumor – No solid tumor components – Color-coded Doppler ultrasound shows no vascularity – No communication with the spinal canal
Chordoma	– Midline tumor, typically in the sacrum – Can contain solid and cystic components – Bony destruction – Recurrence is common – No metastases – No associated malformations of the spine – Markedly hyperintense on T2-weighted images

Pelvic rhabdomyosarcoma	– Usually no calcifications – Arises from the urogenital tract – Spine is normal – Peak frequency between the ages of 2 and 6 years
Ependymoma	– Spinal occurrence is more common in adults than children – Predilection for the lower thoracic spinal cord, conus medullaris, and filum terminale – Tumor growth is usually not very extensive – Well demarcated – Cystic components in 50% of cases – Typically associated with syrinx – Leptomeningeal metastases
Simple skin appendage	– No solid tumor components – No presacral mass – Normal spinal findings

Tips and Pitfalls

Sacrococcygeal teratomas can grow into the spinal canal. This must not be confused with a primary spinal tumor • The diagnosis must not be based on ultrasound alone as it cannot reliably detect intraabdominal and spinal tumor components.

Selected References

Dähnert W. Sacrococcygeal teratoma. In: Dähnert W (ed.). Radiology Review Manual. Baltimore: Williams & Wilkins; 1991: 108–109

Danzer E et al. Diagnosis and characterization of fetal sacrococcygeal teratoma with prenatal MRI. AJR Am J Roentgenol 2006; 187: W350–356

Sebire NJ et al. Sacrococcygeal tumors in infancy and childhood; a retrospective histopathological review of 85 cases. Fetal Pediatr Pathol 2004; 23: 295–303

Woodward PJ et al. From the archives of the AFIP: A comprehensive review of fetal tumors with pathologic correlation. Radiographics 2005; 25: 215–242

Definition

- **Epidemiology**
  Most common gonadal germ-cell tumor in children • Incidence increases with age • Annual incidence is 0.7:100 000 • Peak frequency is at age 15–19 years.
- **Etiology, pathophysiology, pathogenesis**
  Frequency distribution of germ-cell tumors: Sacrococcygeal 45% • Gonads 35% • Head and neck 6% • Retroperitoneum 5% • Mediastinum 4% • Brain and spinal cord 4% • Other locations 1%.
  Types of teratomas: Mature cystic teratomas (dermoid cysts) • Immature teratomas • Monodermal teratomas (struma ovarii, carcinoid tumors, neurogenic tumors).
  Presumably the result of abnormal differentiation of fetal germ cells from the yolk sac • Immature teratomas occur in younger children and are usually larger than dermoid cysts (14–25 cm as opposed to 7 cm on average) • Bilateral lesions occur in 10–20% of cases • Teratomas contain tissue from all three germ layers (endoderm, ectoderm, mesoderm) and can contain fat, hair, rudimentary teeth, calcifications, and cystic components • Cystic components consist of sebum, which at body temperature is liquid • Rokitansky protuberance: Nodular area projecting into the lumen of a cyst that contains hair, bone, or rudimentary teeth • *Peritoneal gliomatosis:* Glial metastases of tumor cells in the form of small glial nodules.

Imaging Signs

- **Ultrasound findings**
  Dermoid cyst: Cystic mass with hyperechoic Rokitansky protuberances (most common form) • Diffuse or partially hyperechoic mass (sebum and hair within the cyst) • Hyperechoic bands (hair) in the cyst.
  Immature teratoma: Heterogeneous echogenicity with partially solid components • Isolated calcifications.
- **Color Doppler ultrasound**
  Differentiates perfused solid tumor components from avascular structures such as hair.
- **CT findings**
  Recommended where MRI is unavailable • Fatty components (93%) • Calcifications (56%) • Fat-fluid levels (12%) • Cyst wall has smooth margins and is 2–5 mm thick • Immature teratomas generally show a larger solid component with calcifications and fatty components.
- **MRI findings**
  Primary cross-sectional imaging modality • Used for follow-up studies especially in malignant degeneration • Visualizes the tumor origin in the ovary • Cystic components appear hypointense on T1-weighted images and hyperintense on T2-weighted images • Hair, calcific deposits, and rudimentary teeth are hypointense • Fat is hyperintense on T1-weighted images and hypointense with fat suppression.

Fig. 5.24 a, b Ovarian teratoma in an adolescent girl. Axial contrast-enhanced CT (**a**) and coronal multiplanar reconstruction (**b**). The giant immature ovarian teratoma extends into the upper abdomen. The tumor is primarily cystic but also exhibits solid components and calcifications.

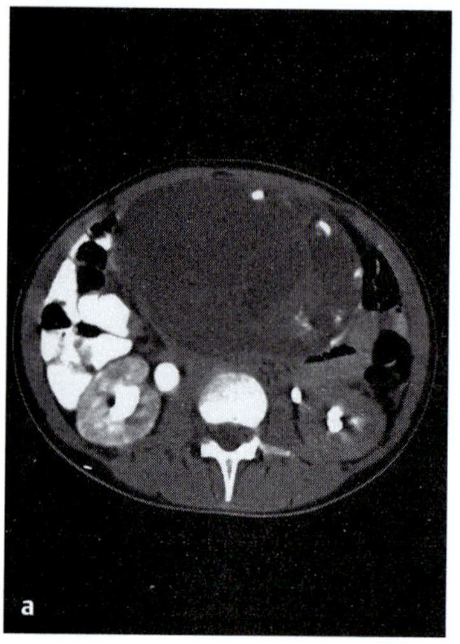

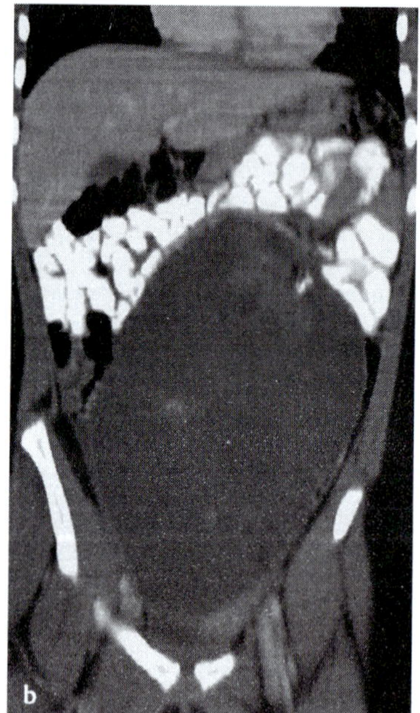

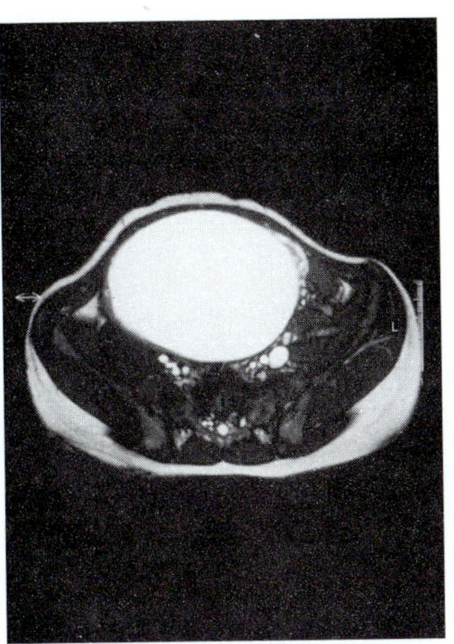

Fig. 5.25 Dermoid cyst in a 10-year-old girl. MR image, axial true FISP sequence through the pelvis. Large hyperintense dermoid cyst (8 × 15 cm) arising from the left ovary.

Clinical Aspects

- **Typical presentation**
  Abdominal pain • Increased abdominal circumference • AFP and/or β-hCG are raised in malignant lesions.
- **Therapeutic options**
  Surgical resection • Preoperative chemotherapy in malignant teratoma • Radiation therapy.
- **Course and prognosis**
  Prognosis is very good after complete resection of a benign teratoma • Prognosis is poor for malignant teratoma (5-year survival rate is less than 30%) • Prognosis for peritoneal gliomatosis is good; usually the lesions mature under chemotherapy • Large nodules are surgically resected; follow-up examinations at close intervals are indicated to monitor the remaining small lesions.
- **Complications**
  Ovarian torsion • Infection • Bleeding • Rupture • Malignant degeneration (1–2%) • Recurrence after subtotal resection • Infertility after bilateral tumor ovariectomy.

Differential Diagnosis

Ovarian cyst	– Cyst with smooth, sharp margins – Often there are small cysts on the wall within the ovarian cyst – Uncomplicated cysts are anechoic on ultrasound – Hemorrhage produces echogenic cyst contents and occasionally sedimentation – No perfusion
Ovarian torsion	– Acute pain – Enlarged hypoechoic ovary – Multiple peripheral cysts measuring 8–10 mm (fluid accumulation due to congestion in the follicles) – Free intraabdominal fluid
Cystadenoma	– Well demarcated, thin-walled cystic mass – Septa of variable thickness – Calcifications in the septa or cyst wall
Pelvic rhabdomyosarcoma	– Usually solid mass – Infiltrating – Metastases in lymph nodes and organs – Usually no calcifications

Tips and Pitfalls

Easily confused with other disorders considered in differential diagnosis • Fat suppression on MRI is useful in differentiating fatty components in teratomas and blood in ovarian cysts with hemorrhage • Contralateral ovary should also be examined as 10% of all teratomas occur bilaterally.

Selected References

Comerci JT Jr et al. Mature cystic teratoma: a clinical pathologic evaluation of 517 cases and review of the literature. Obstet Gynecol 1994; 84: 22–28

Outwater EK et al. Ovarian teratomas: tumor types and imaging characteristics. Radiographics 2001; 21: 475–490

Yamaoka T et al. Immature teratoma of the ovary: correlation of MR imaging and pathologic findings. Eur Radiol 2003; 13: 313–319

Definition

- **Epidemiology**
  Incidence is less than 1:1000 per year • Most common cause of acute scrotum in children • Rare before puberty as the disorder is often transmitted sexually.
- **Etiology, pathophysiology, pathogenesis**
  Bacterial inflammation of the epididymis • *Pathogen: E. coli* before puberty and in men over 35 years; *Chlamydia trachomatis, Neisseria gonorrhoeae* in men younger than 35 years • Secondary involvement of the testis (epididymo-orchitis) occurs in 20–40% of cases • Isolated orchitis is rare and primarily caused by viruses (mumps, echoviruses, adenoviruses, coxsackievirus).
  Associated malformations in infants: Vesicoureteral reflux • Urethral valve • Ectopic ureter • Prostatic utricle • Detrusor sphincter dyssynergia.

Imaging Signs

- **Ultrasound findings**
  Epididymis is enlarged and usually hypoechoic • Hyperechoic components are also present where hemorrhage has occurred • Inhomogeneous echo pattern • Associated hydrocele • Thickened scrotal wall.
- **Color Doppler ultrasound findings**
  Increased vascularity in the epididymis and occasionally testis as well • Increased diastolic blood flow.

Clinical Aspects

- **Typical presentation**
  Painful swelling of the testis • Scrotal edema • Abdominal pain • Lower abdominal pain • Fever • Dysuria.
- **Therapeutic options**
  Antibiotic therapy • Analgesia • Elevation of the testes • Cooling • Surgical intervention where complications occur.
- **Course and prognosis**
  Prognosis is usually good • Symptoms usually abate within a few days of treatment.
- **Complications**
  Pyocele • Abscess • Sepsis • Testicular ischemia • Testicular atrophy • Infertility in complicated bilateral lesions.

Differential Diagnosis

Testicular torsion	– Sudden pain – Enlarged testis, decreased echogenicity – Reduced or absent perfusion of the testis – Later hemorrhage, infarction, hydrocele, thickening of the scrotal wall

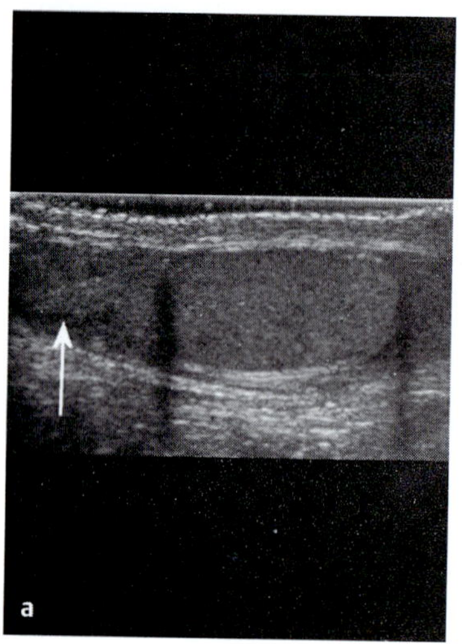

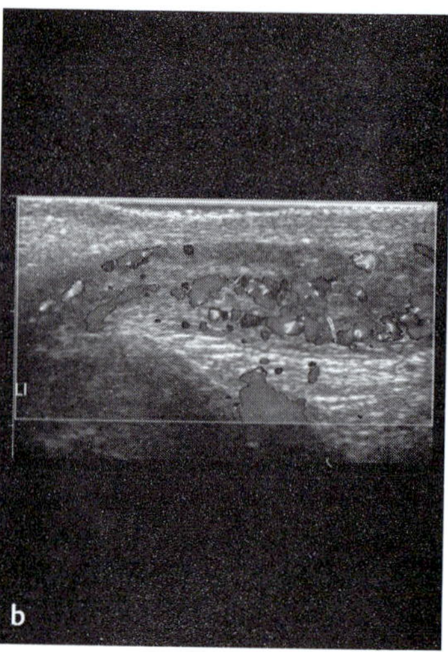

Fig. 5.26 a, b Epididymitis. Plain ultrasound (**a**) and Doppler ultrasound (**b**). Ultrasound demonstrates enlarged epididymis (arrow). Doppler ultrasound (**b**) shows increased perfusion.

Scrotal hematoma	– Extratesticular hematoma (hyperechoic) – Ruptured testis exhibits inhomogeneous echo pattern and irregular contour at the rupture site
Scrotal hernia	– Bowel in the scrotal compartment, usually with peristalsis – Normal testis and epididymis

Tips and Pitfalls

Can be confused with testicular torsion • In pediatric epididymitis, the examiner should be alert to possible associated urogenital anomalies • Elevation of the testes alleviates pain in epididymitis and exacerbates pain in testicular torsion (Prehn sign).

Selected References

Karmazyn B et al. Clinical and sonographic criteria of acute scrotum in children: a retrospective study of 172 boys. Pediatr Radiol 2005; 35: 302–310

Likitnukul S et al. Epididymitis in children and adolescents. A 20-year retrospective study. Am J Dis Child 1987; 141: 41–44

Merlini E et al. Acute epididymitis and urinary tract anomalies in children. Scand J Urol Nephrol 1998; 32: 273–275

Suzer O et al. Color Doppler imaging in the diagnosis of the acute scrotum. Eur Urol 1997; 32: 457–461

Definition

- **Epidemiology**
  Incidence is 1:4000 • Peak age is up to age 1 year and during puberty.
- **Etiology, pathophysiology, pathogenesis**
  Neonatal (extravaginal) torsion: Torsion of the spermatic cord proximal to the insertion of the tunica albuginea • *Cause:* Spermatic cord is loosely fixed in the inguinal canal • Disorder can also occur in utero with complete infarction of the affected testis • Hemorrhagic infarction with testicular necrosis • Followed by fibrosis and occasionally calcifications.
  Intravaginal torsion: Torsion of the spermatic cord within the tunica albuginea • Commonly occurs with increased testosterone levels in puberty • The "bell clapper deformity" predisposes (12% of the male population)—this involves a high insertion of the tunica albuginea on the spermatic cord with complete enveloping of the testis, epididymis, and distal spermatic cord • The left side is affected slightly more often.

Imaging Signs

- **B-mode and color Doppler ultrasound**
  Reduced or absent vascularity (sensitivity 86–88%, specificity 90–100%) • Where symptoms persist longer than 12 hours, there may be increased peritesticular blood flow.

Table 5.4 Ultrasound findings in testicular torsion

Duration of symptoms	Ultrasound and color Doppler findings
< 4 hours	Normal B-mode scan, absent or reduced testicular vascularization, spiral twisting of the spermatic cord vascular structures
4–6 hours	Swelling of the testes, decreased echogenicity, absent or reduced testicular vascularization, spiral twisting of the spermatic cord vascular structures
> 12 hours	Heterogeneous echo texture due to congestion, hemorrhaging, and infarction; associated hydrocele, thickened scrotal wall

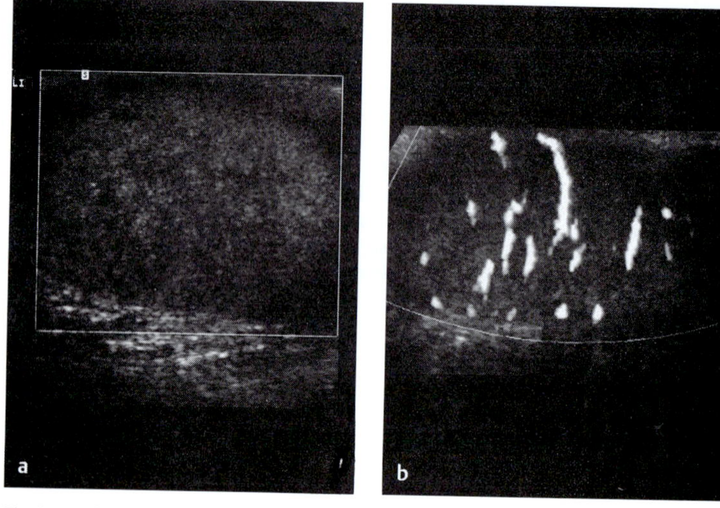

Fig. 5.27 a, b Testicular torsion. Color Doppler ultrasound. Testicular torsion (**a**) and normal contralateral testis (**b**). Enlarged, hypoechoic testis without vascularization (**a**) where pain has been present for 6 hours. Normal echogenicity and vascularization in the contralateral testis (**b**).

Clinical Aspects

- **Typical presentation**
  Sudden testicular pain • Testicular swelling • Radiating pain in the inguinal canal and lower abdomen • Nausea • Vomiting • Absent cremasteric reflex • Fever • Protracted clinical course in half of cases.
- **Therapeutic options**
  Surgical exploration • Detorsion of the testis • Resection of a necrotic testis • Orchidopexy of the contralateral side.
- **Course and prognosis**
  Preservation of the testis depends on the duration of symptoms:
  - Shorter than 6 hours: 85–97%.
  - Longer than 12 hours: less than 20%.
- **Complications**
  Infarction with loss of the testis.

Differential Diagnosis

Epididymo-orchitis	– Enlarged epididymis – Inhomogeneous echo pattern – Increased perfusion of the epididymis and of the testis where orchitis is also present – Associated hydrocele – Scrotal wall is thickened
Torsion of the testicular appendages	– Acute scrotum – Cremasteric reflex intact – Small hardened nodule on the upper margin of the testis – Normal perfusion of both testes – Enlarged testicular appendage (> 6 mm) with increased peripheral perfusion – Reactive hydrocele
Testicular tumor	– Intratesticular mass – Inhomogeneous echo pattern – Abnormal tumor perfusion
Hernia	– Bowel structures in the scrotal compartment, usually with peristalsis – Normal testis and epididymis
Testicular trauma	– Inhomogeneous echo pattern and irregular contour of the testis in testicular rupture – Enlarged testis – Hyperechoic extratesticular hematoma

Tips and Pitfalls

Findings on B-mode ultrasound can be completely normal in the initial stage • In incomplete torsion, color Doppler ultrasound can show normal vascularity.

Selected References

Eaton SH et al. Intermittent testicular torsion: diagnostic features and management outcomes. J Urol 2005; 174: 1532–1535

Hörmann M et al. Imaging of the scrotum in children. Eur Radiol 2004; 14: 974–983

Kravchick S. Color Doppler sonography: its real role in the evaluation of children with highly suspected testicular torsion. Eur Radiol 2001; 11: 1000–1005

Livne PM et al. Testicular torsion in the pediatric age group: diagnosis and treatment. Pediatr Endocrinol Rev 2003; 1: 128–133

Definition

- **Epidemiology**
  Peak age: 4–18 months.
- **Etiology, pathophysiology, pathogenesis**
  Defective mineralization with loss of physiologic organization in the growth plates • In contrast, osteomalacia involves decreased calcification of osteoid tissue • Both occur in children, but only osteomalacia occurs in adults.
  Calcium-deficiency rickets: Raised parathormone level.
  - Vitamin D deficiency rickets (most common form): Insufficient intake of exogenous calcium • Gastrointestinal malabsorption as in sprue or cystic fibrosis • Insufficient exposure to sunlight • Antiepileptic therapy (phenobarbital or phenytoin can interfere with intestinal absorption of calcium).
  - Vitamin D dependent rickets: Autosomal recessive disorder involving impaired synthesis of 1,25-dihydroxy vitamin D (type I) or defective vitamin D receptor (type II).
  - Renal osteopathy: Chronic renal insufficiency • Chronically depressed 1,25-dihydroxy vitamin D synthesis • Signs of rickets with bony changes accompanied by secondary hyperparathyroidism.

  Phosphate deficiency rickets: Normal parathormone level.
  - Vitamin D resistant rickets (most common form, accounting for 80% of all cases). Phosphate diabetes • Usually x-linked dominant • Hypophosphatemia • Hyperphosphaturia • Normal serum levels of calcium and vitamin D.
  - Tumor-induced rickets: Usually benign mesenchymal tumors • Fibroblast growth factor impairs phosphate resorption in the renal tubules • Secondary hypophosphatemia • Occurs later than early childhood.
  - Phosphate deficiency in premature infants: Premature birth • Furosemide.

Imaging Signs

- **Radiographic findings**
  Typical location: Distal radius and ulna, knee • Deficient mineralization of the center of the growth plates with delayed appearance of ossification centers • Irregularly widened growth plates • Splaying and cupping of the metaphyses • Costochondral beading (rachitic rosary) • Cortical thinning • Periosteal reaction • Bowing of long bones • Looser's zones (pseudofractures in osteomalacia) • Rib fractures in premature infants • Greenstick fractures • Coarse trabeculation of the bone.

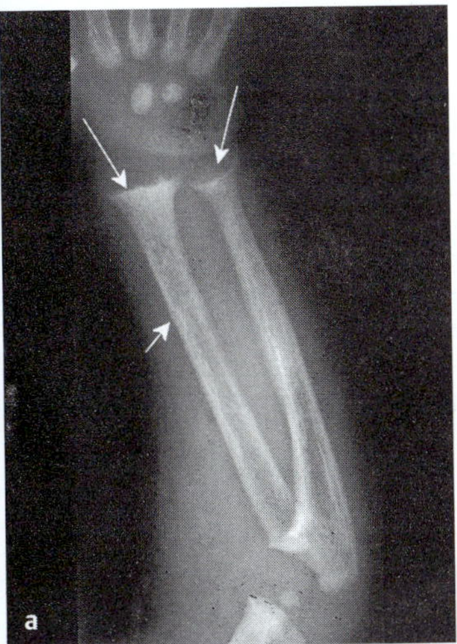

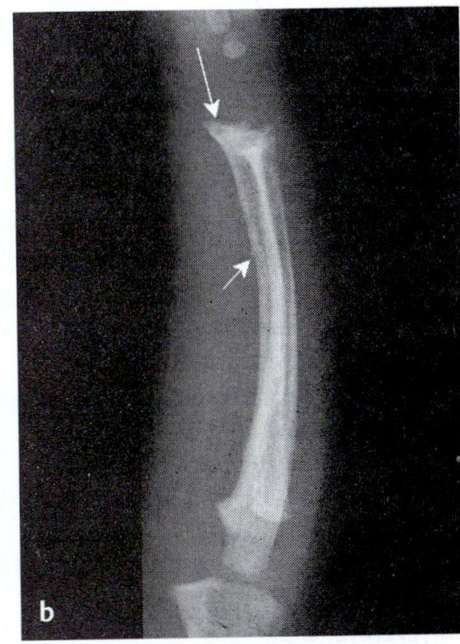

Fig. 6.1 a, b Rickets. Forearm in two planes. Typical changes in rickets with widening and cupping of metaphyses of the distal forearm bones (large arrows). Mid-shaft green-stick radial fracture of the mid-shaft radius (small arrow).

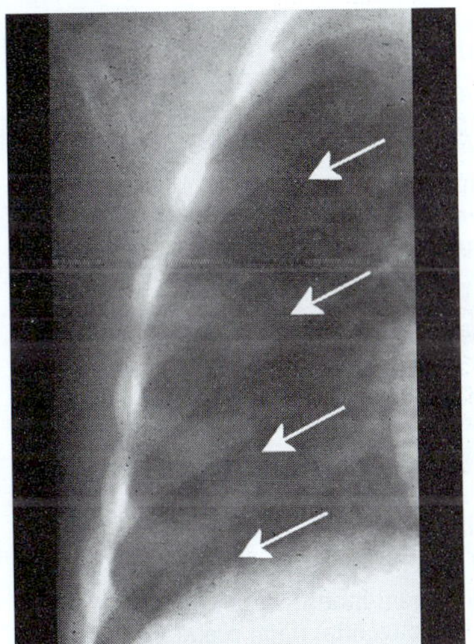

Fig. 6.2 "Rachitic rosary" with typical costochondral beading (arrows).

Clinical Aspects

- **Typical presentation**
  Bone pain • Craniotabes • Rachitic rosary • Bowlegs • Disproportionately small stature • Decreased muscle tone • Delayed closure of the fontanelles • Delayed tooth eruption • Tooth enamel defects.
  - *Vitamin D deficiency rickets:* Alkaline phosphatase and parathormone are elevated • 1,25-dihydroxy vitamin D is normal to raised.
  - *Phosphate deficiency rickets:* Alkaline phosphatase is raised • Parathormone and 1,25-dihydroxy vitamin D are normal.
- **Therapeutic options**
  Vitamin D prophylaxis in infants • Phosphate substitution and calcitriol in phosphate diabetes.
- **Course and prognosis**
  This depends on the underlying disorder and when the disorder is diagnosed.
- **Complications**
  Fractures • Bony deformities • Small stature.

Differential Diagnosis

Blount disease	– Aseptic osteonecrosis of the medial tibial metaphysis – Depression of the medial tibial plateau leading to secondary bilateral genu varum deformities – Above age 6 years – More common in black children; girls are affected more often than boys
Osteogenesis imperfecta	– Cortical thinning – Reduced diaphyseal diameter – “Corner sign” is rare – Diaphyseal fracture is common – Family history (autosomal dominant inheritance) – Blue sclera may be present
Congenital deformity	– Presumably due to abnormal fetal position
Renal tubular acidosis	– Demineralization due to buffer effect of bone on H^+ ions. – Radiographically indistinguishable from vitamin D deficiency rickets
Fanconi syndrome	– Generalized defect of the proximal renal tubules – Glucosuria – Hyperphosphaturia – Aminoaciduria
Neurofibromatosis type I	– Autosomal dominant inheritance – Deformity with congenital tibial pseudarthrosis – Known CNS manifestations in neurofibromatosis type I (brainstem gliomas, optic gliomas) and type II (bilateral acoustic neurinomas, predisposition for meningiomas and ependymomas)

Tips and Pitfalls

Bowlegs are physiologic until age 2 years and should not be confused with a bowing deformity • The cause of rickets cannot be inferred from the radiologic appearances • Rickets should not be confused with osteomalacia.

Selected References

Cheema JI et al. Radiographic characteristics of lower-extremity bowing in children. Radiographics 2003; 23: 871–880

Gissel T et al. Adverse effects of antiepileptic drugs on bone mineral density in children. Expert Opin Drug Saf 2007; 6: 267–278

Leonard MB. Assessment of bone mass following renal transplantation in children. Pediatr Nephrol 2005; 20: 360–367

Nield LS et al. Rickets: not a disease of the past. Am Fam Physician 2006; 74: 619–626

Definition

- **Epidemiology**
  Affects 3% of all children and adolescents • Most commonly occurs between the ages of 5 and 7 years • Can occur up to age 13 years • Two to three times more common in boys than girls.
- **Etiology, pathophysiology, pathogenesis**
  Etiology is unknown • Often there is a history of previous respiratory tract infection (40–50%) • Not a bacterial or viral hip infection • Legg–Calvé–Perthes disease can be induced by effusion and compression of the intraarticular epiphyseal vessels.

Imaging Signs

- **Ultrasound findings**
  Usually an anechoic joint effusion is present with widening of the medial joint space and balloonlike expansion of the capsule • In chronic cases the capsule is often thickened, a sign of synovitis.
- **Radiographic findings**
  Useful in excluding other bone disorders such as Legg–Calvé–Perthes disease • Joint space is widened due to effusion (in 25% of cases) • Effusion may also cause lateral displacement of the femoral head • Regional osteoporosis is present in 30% of cases.
- **MRI findings**
  Useful in excluding early-stage Legg–Calvé–Perthes disease or osteomyelitis • Fat-suppressed T2-weighted images show a hyperechoic joint effusion • Normal bone marrow signal • T1-weighted images show synovial enhancement after contrast administration, consistent with synovitis.

Clinical Aspects

- **Typical presentation**
  Sudden hip or knee pain • Compensatory limp • Patient avoids weight bearing with the affected leg • Reduced mobility • Affected leg is usually slightly flexed, abducted, and externally rotated (positive figure of four test) • Range of motion testing is painful.
- **Therapeutic options**
  - *Slight pain:* Bed rest for 2–3 days • Anti-inflammatory agents • Analgesics.
  - *Marked pain:* Aspiration of the effusion and/or traction therapy where indicated.
- **Course and prognosis**
  Prognosis is very good • Resolves completely • Children usually recover within a few days or within 1–2 weeks at the latest.

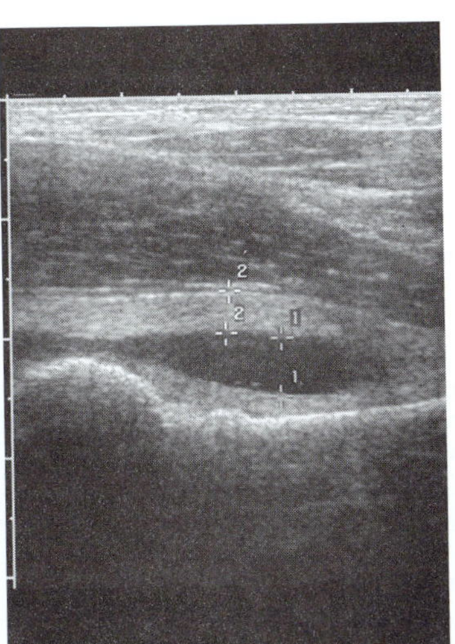

Fig. 6.3 Transient synovitis of the hip. Hip ultrasound. Anechoic joint effusion (1) and capsular thickening (2).

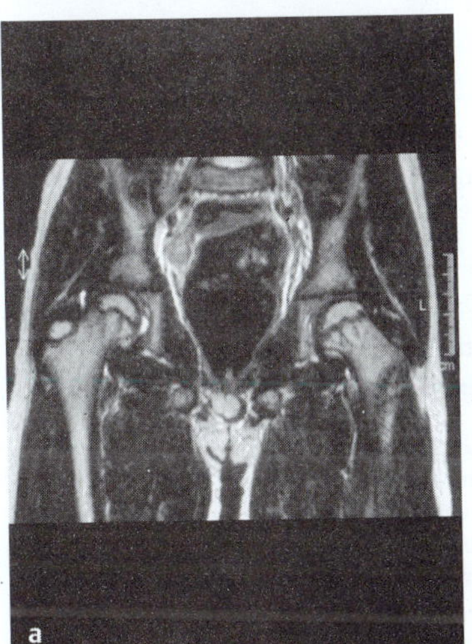

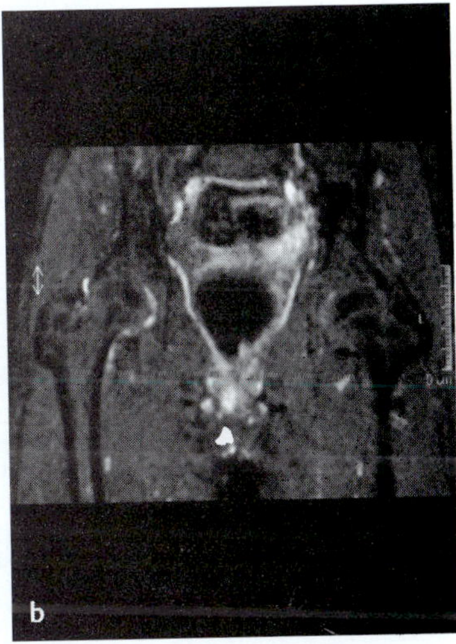

Fig. 6.4 a, b School-age child with transient synovitis of the right hip. MR image of the hip. The T2-weighted TSE image (**a**) shows a hyperintense joint effusion with normal bone marrow signal in the femoral heads. After intravenous contrast administration, the T1-weighted image (subtraction, **b**) shows synovial enhancement in the right hip (synovitis). Femoral head perfusion is unimpaired.

▸ **Complications**

Administration of analgesics and lack of immobilization can lead to protracted clinical course • Condition can recur • Suppurative effusion secondary to joint aspiration.

Differential Diagnosis

Septic arthritis	– Severely ill child – Hip pain and decreased range of motion are considerably more severe; abnormal blood count – Radiographs show joint space widening to over 2 mm
Legg–Calvé–Perthes disease	– Symptoms do not resolve within a few days – Early stages detectable on MRI – Joint effusion, altered signal in the epiphysis
Slipped capital femoral epiphysis	– At age 12–15 years – Ultrasound shows step off in the growth plate – Lauenstein view shows posteromedial displacement of the growth plate relative to the metaphysis
Rheumatoid arthritis	– Rare in the hip – Symptoms are progressive – Synovitis, pannus

Tips and Pitfalls

Antibiotic treatment has recently been an issue as it can mask symptoms of septic arthritis • Consider, that cildren up to the age of 4 years often project hip pain in the knee • The diagnosis of transient synovitis of the hip is only certain when symptoms resolve within a week.

Selected References

Bosch R et al. Value of ultrasound in differential diagnosis of pediatric hip joint effusion (Perthes disease, C. fugax, epiphysiolysis capitis femoris). Z Orthop Ihre Grenzgeb 1998; 136: 409–412

Jung ST et al. Significance of laboratory and radiologic findings for differentiating between septic arthritis and transient synovitis of the hip. J Pediatr Orthop 2003; 23: 368–372

Lee SK et al. Septic arthritis versus transient synovitis al MR imaging preliminary assessment with signal intensity alterations in bone marrow. Radiology 1999; 211: 459–465

Yang WJ et al. MR imaging of transient synovitis: differentiation from septic arthritis. Pediatr Radiol 2006; 36: 1154–1158

Zamzam MM. The role of ultrasound in differentiating septic arthritis from transient synovitis of the hip in children. J Pediatr Orthop B 2006; 15: 418–422

Definition

- **Epidemiology**
  Acute osteomyelitis primarily affects children • Half of all patients are younger than 5 years old.
- **Etiology, pathophysiology, pathogenesis**
  Inflammation of bone marrow, cancellous bone, cortex, and periosteum • Route of infection is hematogenous or exogenous (traumatic or iatrogenic) • Pathogens in newborns include *Staphylococcus aureus*, group B streptococci, and *Escherichia coli*; in children, *Staphylococcus aureus* • No pathogen can be identified in primary chronic osteomyelitis • Occurs most often in the lower extremity (75% of cases) and less often in the spine (53%), especially in the lumbar spine.
  - *Acute hematogenous osteomyelitis:* Manifestation reflects physiologic age-related changes in the vascular supply to the metaphysis and epiphysis.
  - *Chronic osteomyelitis:* Occurs secondary to acute osteomyelitis or as a primary chronic disorder with sequestration and/or external fistula.
  - *Brodie abscess:* Extensive granulation tissue surrounds the abscess • This prevents further expansion • Typically occurs in the tibial metaphysis.
  - *Plasma cell osteomyelitis:* Chronic recurrent multifocal osteomyelitis (CRMO) • Mucoid exudate is surrounded by plasma cell granulation tissue in a bony cavity • Not induced by bacterial infection • Clavicle is often affected • A special case is SAPHO syndrome (synovitis, acne, pustulosis palmaris et plantaris, hyperostosis, osteitis).
  - *Sclerosing, nonsuppurative Garré osteomyelitis:* Occurs primarily in the tibia and mandible • Chronic form does not involve liquefaction • Periosteal apposition.

  Acute hematogenous osteomyelitis in infants: Infantile type • Occurs before the age of 18 months • Inflammation spreads from the metaphysis to the epiphysis through the common vascular supply present at this age (septic arthritis).
  Acute hematogenous osteomyelitis in children: Juvenile type • Occurs prior to closure of the growth plates • As the metaphysis and epiphysis have separate vascular supplies at this age, the disorder shows a predilection for the metaphysis of the long bones • Large cortical sequestra • Subperiosteal abscesses.
  Acute hematogenous osteomyelitis in adolescents and adults: Adolescent type • Occurs after closure of the growth plates • Epiphysis and metaphysis again share a common vascular supply • Septic arthritis • Suppurative inflammation of the diaphyseal medulla • Progresses to chronic stage • Fistulas.

Imaging Signs

- **Radiographic findings**
  Acute hematogenous osteomyelitis: Early phase (up to 10 days after onset of symptoms) usually shows normal findings • Metaphyseal soft tissue swelling with blurred fat planes • Osteopenia • Bone destruction • Lamellar and spiculated areas of periosteal reaction • Bone sequestra • Joint space widening in septic arthritis.

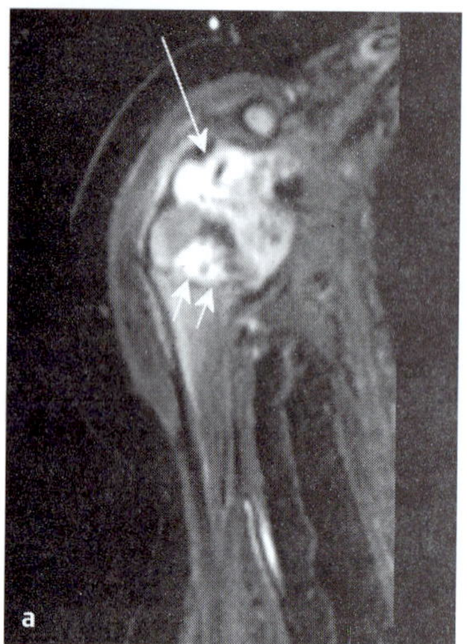

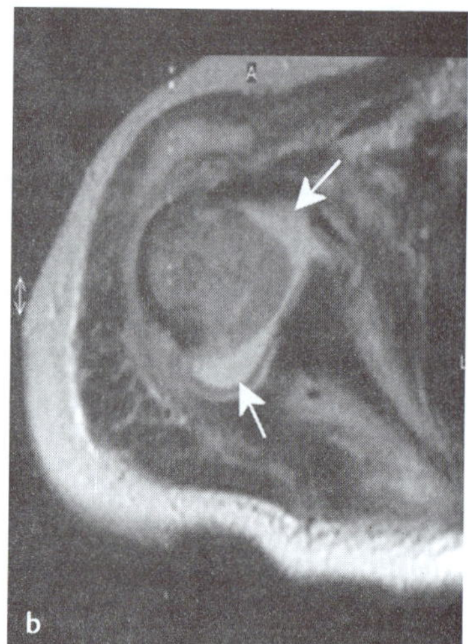

Fig. 6.5 a–c Septic arthritis in a 6-week-old infant. MR image of the right shoulder. Coronal STIR (**a**), axial T2-weighted TSE (**b**), and axial T1-weighted SE images after contrast administration (**c**): Suppurative arthritis (**a**, large arrow; **b**, arrows) with associated synovitis (**c**, arrows), and metaepiphyseal osteomyelitis (**a**, small arrows).

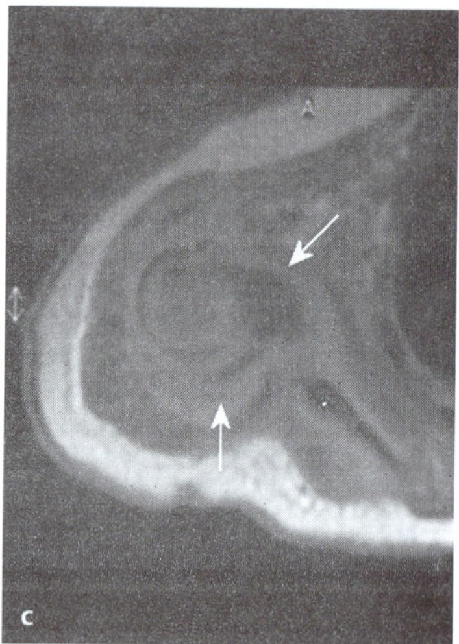

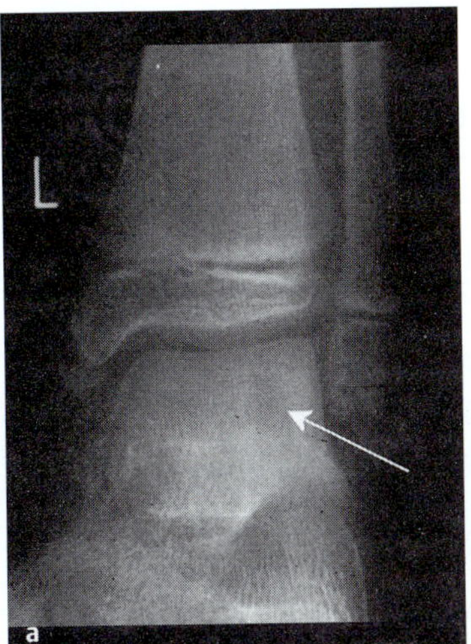

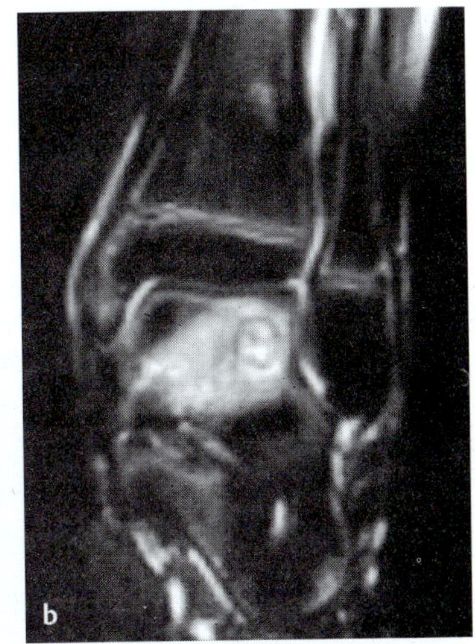

Fig. 6.6 a, b Brodie abscess. A-P radiograph of the ankle (**a**) and MR image (**b**). The radiograph shows a Brodie abscess of the lateral talus (**a**, arrow), recognizable by the sharply demarcated oval radiolucency with a discrete sclerotic margin. The MRI fat-suppressed T2-weighted image (**b**) shows the abscess cavity with a fine hypointense sclerotic margin and a perifocal talar edema.

Chronic osteomyelitis: Irregular bone sclerosis with areas of increased transparency • Periosteal separation • Increased bone volume.
Sclerosing nonsuppurative Garré osteomyelitis: Cortical thickening • Bone sclerosis • No subperiosteal abscesses.
Brodie abscess: Circumscribed, sharply demarcated area of osteolysis • Marginal sclerosis of the defect • No periosteal reaction.

▸ **Ultrasound findings**
Hyperechoic inhomogeneous extraosseous soft tissue component • Joint effusion, occasionally with hyperechoic contents (pus) • Subperiosteal abscess.

▸ **MRI findings**
The extent of the inflammatory intramedullary lesion is well visualized on the fat-suppressed T2-weighted images • Abscesses are clearly visualized as nonenhancing areas on post-contrast images • Excludes or confirms joint involvement • Shows fistulas and sequestration • Soft tissue inflammation.

▸ **Bone scan**
High sensitivity (three-phase nuclear medicine skeletal imaging, nuclear medicine leukocyte imaging) • Multiple lesions are readily detected.

Clinical Aspects

► **Typical presentation**

Fever (septic temperature) • Diminished general health • Pain • Erythema and swelling • Compensatory posture • Laboratory inflammation parameters are raised • Only discrete symptoms are present in chronic form.

► **Therapeutic options**

Conservative: Intravenous antibiotics for more than 3 weeks • Followed by oral antibiotic treatment • Immobilization.

Surgical: Decompression • Removal of sequestra and abscesses • Cancellous graft where indicated • Fistula excision • Joint involvement requires aspiration and irrigation.

► **Course and prognosis**

Chronic osteomyelitis usually exhibits a long and complicated clinical course • Prognosis is good for the acute form with no joint involvement when treatment is adequate.

► **Complications**

Accelerated growth due to inflammatory hyperemia • Soft tissue abscess • Fistula • Pathologic fracture • Septic arthritis • Bony deformation with premature closure of the growth plate • Joint destruction in septic arthritis • Pyomyositis.

Differential Diagnosis

Osteosarcoma or Ewing sarcoma	– Usually no signs of inflammation – Often indistinguishable from other disorders considered in differential diagnosis (biopsy indicated) – No subperiosteal abscesses – Bone marrow edema usually more sharply demarcated – Metastases
Metastases	– Known underlying disorder often present – Multiple bone lesions – Inflammation parameters not raised
Langerhans cell histiocytosis	– See relevant section
Lymphoma	– Lymph node involvement – Extraosseous manifestation – Circumscribed lesions – Inflammation parameters not elevated

Tips and Pitfalls

The greatest difficulty in differential diagnosis is distinguishing osteomyelitis from osteogenic sarcoma or Ewing sarcoma • Where osteomyelitis is suspected but there is no detectable lesion, three-phase nuclear medicine is indicated as the initial study, followed by additional specific diagnostic studies • Immediate MRI is indicated to evaluate any clearly abnormal local findings • Normal plain radiographs do not exclude osteomyelitis. Therefore, immediate MRI is indicated to confirm or exclude a purely clinical suspicion • Osteomyelitis in infants inevitably leads to joint destruction from septic arthritis unless adequate treatment is promptly initiated.

Selected References

Blickman JG et al. Current imaging concepts in pediatric osteomyelitis. Eur Radiol 2004; 14 Suppl 4: L55–64

Dähnert W. Osteomyelitis. In: Dähnert W (ed.). Radiology Review Manual. Baltimore: Williams & Wilkins; 1991: 66–67

Earwaker JW et al. SAPHO: syndrome or concept? Imaging findings. Skeletal Radiol 2003; 32: 311–327

Jurik AG. Chronic recurrent multifocal osteomyelitis. Semin Musculoskelet Radiol 2004; 8: 243–253

Offiah AC. Acute osteomyelitis, septic arthritis and discitis: differences between neonates and older children. Eur J Radiol 2006; 60: 221–232

Robben SG. Ultrasonography of musculoskeletal infections in children. Eur Radiol 2004; 14 Suppl 4: L65–77

Definition

▸ **Epidemiology**

Incidence is 30% in children and adolescents • Boys are affected twice as often as girls • Peak age is 7–8 years • Usually occurs prior to closure of the growth plates • Fibrous cortical defect and nonossifying fibroma are the most common bone lesions.

▸ **Etiology, pathophysiology, pathogenesis**

Periosteum penetrates the cortex • Predilection for long bones • In a cortical defect, the lesion is limited to the cortex • Nonossifying fibroma extends into the medullary cavity • *Histology:* Spindle cells and histiocytes, multinucleated giant cells resembling osteoclasts, lymphocytes, plasma cells • Predilection for the distal medial femur, proximal tibia and femur, and proximal humerus.

Imaging Signs

▸ **Radiographic findings**

Cystic bone lesion • Typically occurs in an eccentric metaphyseal location • Slight marginal sclerosis, occasionally resembling a seashell • Elliptical shape • Longitudinal axis of the tumor is parallel to the longitudinal axis of the bone • Cortical thinning • Initially occurs in close proximity to the growth plate • Typical signs of malignancy are absent • Physiologic bone growth increases the distance between the lesion and the growth plate, and the lesion becomes increasingly sclerotic (ossifying fibroma).

▸ **Ultrasound findings**

Well-demarcated bone defect • Filled with hypoechoic material • Doppler mode shows prominent vascularization within the lesion • The echogenicity of the lesion increases and its size decreases over time.

▸ **MRI findings**

Not required to confirm the diagnosis • Usually an incidental finding • Appears isointense to muscle on T1-weighted images • Hyperintense on T2-weighted images • T1-weighted and T2-weighted images show a hypointense halo of marginal sclerosis • Slight contrast enhancement, especially at the margin • No periosteal reaction.

Clinical Aspects

▸ **Typical presentation**

Asymptomatic • Usually an incidental finding • Large lesions can lead to pathologic fractures.

▸ **Therapeutic options**

Curettage and cancellous grafting are indicated when the lesion covers more than 50% of the cross-section of the medullary cavity.

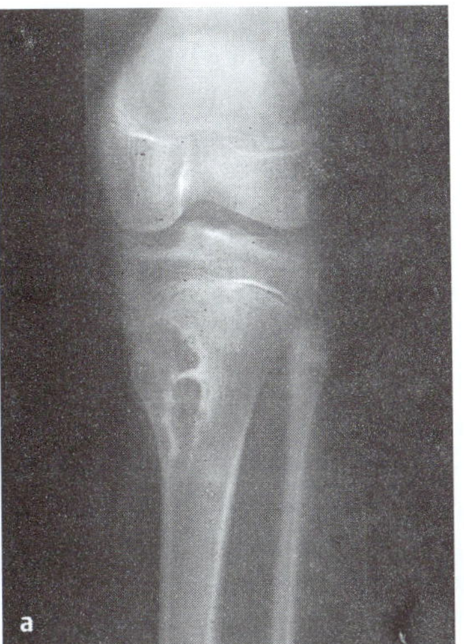

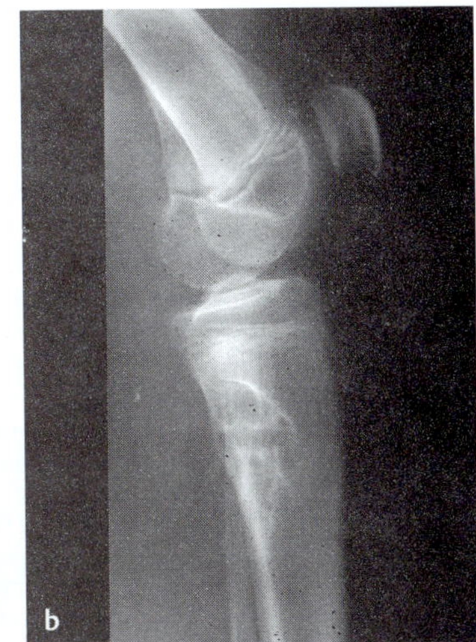

Fig. 6.7 a, b Nonossifying fibroma. Radiographs of the knee in two planes. Classic radiographic appearance of a nonossifying fibroma in the proximal posteromedial tibial metaphysis.

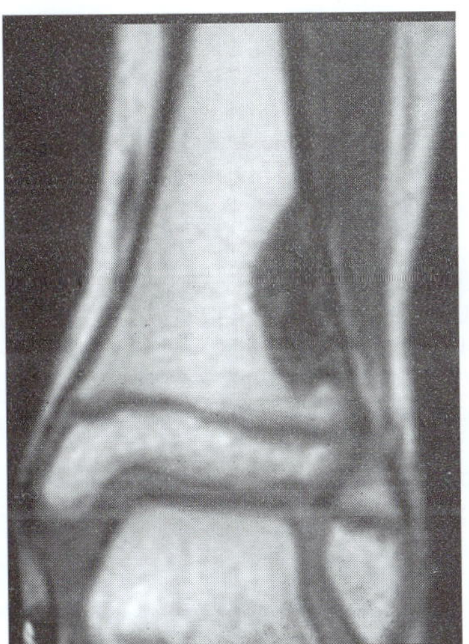

Fig. 6.8 MR image, unenhanced T1-weighted image. Nonossifying fibroma of the distal lateral tibial metaphysis.

- **Course and prognosis**
  Most lesions heal spontaneously by ossification within 2–4 years • Further growth can occur • Lesions do not recur after surgery.
- **Complications**
  Pathologic fracture.

Differential Diagnosis

Benign fibrous histiocytoma	– Usually occurs before age 25 years – Can cause pain – Can recur after curettage – Radiologically indistinguishable
Periosteal desmoid	– Primarily occurs between the ages of 12 and 20 years – Predilection for posterior aspect of medial femoral condyle – Resembles fibrous cortical defect – May exhibit characteristics of malignancy – Usually remits spontaneously – Biopsy is contraindicated
Fibrous dysplasia	– Monostotic or polyostotic – Predilection for femur, tibia, and ribs – Arises in the center of the bone – Vesicular form – Occurs in disorders such as McCune–Albright syndrome

Tips and Pitfalls

A healing nonossifying fibroma must not be confused with osteosclerotic bone malignancies • MRI and CT are not indicated for evaluation of a fibrous cortical defect • Biopsy of fibrous cortical defects is contraindicated.

Selected References

Araki Y et al. MRI of fibrous cortical defect of the femur. Radiat Med 1994; 12: 93–98

Dähnert W. Fibrous cortical defect. In: Dähnert W (ed.). Radiology Review Manual. Baltimore: Williams & Wilkins; 1991: 36

Huzjan R et al. The value of ultrasound in diagnosis and follow-up of fibrous cortical defect. Ultraschall Med 2005; 26: 420–423

Yanagawa T et al. The natural history of disappearing bone tumours and tumour-like conditions. Clin Radiol 2001; 56: 877–886

Definition

- **Epidemiology**
Occurs primarily in children • 90% of all patients are younger than 20 years • Accounts for 7% of all benign bone tumors • No sex predilection.
- **Etiology, pathophysiology, pathogenesis**
Aneurysmal bone cysts occur de novo as primary lesions in 65–99% of cases. Usually they are posttraumatic • Secondary aneurysmal bone cysts account for 1–35% of all lesions and develop in existing, usually cystic lesions such as fibrous dysplasia, giant cell tumor, chondroblastoma, nonossifying fibroma, solitary bone cyst, and osteosarcoma • Half of all lesions occur in the diaphyseal-metaphyseal junction of long bones • Less common locations include the diaphysis of long bones, flat bones such as the scapula and pelvis, and spine (12–30%) • Aneurysmal bone cysts may be intraosseous or extraosseous (usually posttraumatic). *Histology:* Multiple blood-filled sinusoidal spaces and isolated solid segments of fibrous, highly vascularized tissue • The walls of the sinusoids may contain both osteoid and mature bone • Rarely multinucleated giant cells are present.

Imaging Signs

- **Radiographic findings**
Multicystic, eccentric, expansive vesicular lesion • Usually occurs in the center of the bones of the distal extremities • Large extraosseous tumor components, especially in the ribs and pelvis, with "eggshell" periosteal ossification • Occasionally there is a sclerotic margin • Lesion contains trabeculae and septa (bony ridges due to irregular bone resorption); these occur less often in the spine • Lesion never crosses the growth plate • Slight periosteal reaction may occur, usually after a fracture • Pronounced expansion of the vertebral appendages.
- **CT findings**
Extent and proximity to the spinal canal • Cortical thinning • No cortical destruction visualized • No periosteal reaction typical of malignancy • Fluid level is present in hemorrhage (10–35% of cases) • Used for guiding percutaneous biopsy.
- **MRI findings**
Extent and proximity to the spinal canal • Multicystic tumor • Cysts exhibit variable signal intensities depending on the age of the hemorrhage • Typical cystic hemorrhages with sedimentation signs • Hypointense halo (sclerotic zone, such as in periosteal thickening).
- **Angiographic findings**
Marked vascularization particularly pronounced on the periphery • Allows selective embolization of the aneurysmal bone cyst.

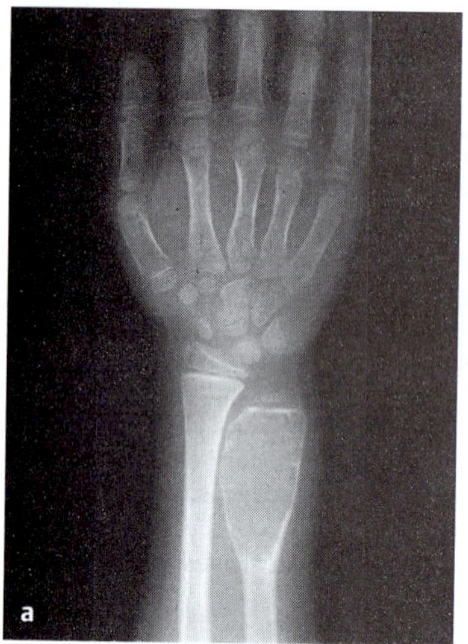

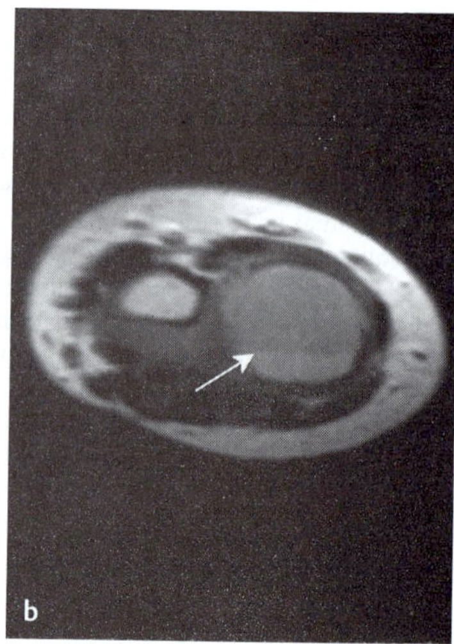

Fig. 6.9 a, b Aneurysmal bone cyst. Radiograph (**a**) and MR image (**b**). The conventional radiograph shows a large aneurysmal bone cyst in the metaphysis and diaphysis of the distal ulna. On the T1-weighted MR image, the cystic tumor exhibits hyperintense sedimentation (**b**, arrow) secondary to hemorrhage.

Clinical Aspects

- **Typical presentation**
  Pain • Swelling • Limited range of motion • Neurologic symptoms in spinal involvement due to compression of the spinal cord and/or spinal nerves • Often an incidental finding in a pathologic fracture.
- **Therapeutic options**
  Curettage is performed and defect filled with cancellous graft or cement, using phenol or liquid nitrogen where indicated • Selective arterial embolization in the spine • Supplementary radiation therapy where indicated.
- **Course and prognosis**
  May increase in size slowly or cause rapid bone destruction.
- **Complications**
  Pathologic fracture (5% of cases) • Hemorrhage • Recurrence (10–15% of all lesions, with incomplete curettage) • Large spinal tumors can lead to paraplegia.

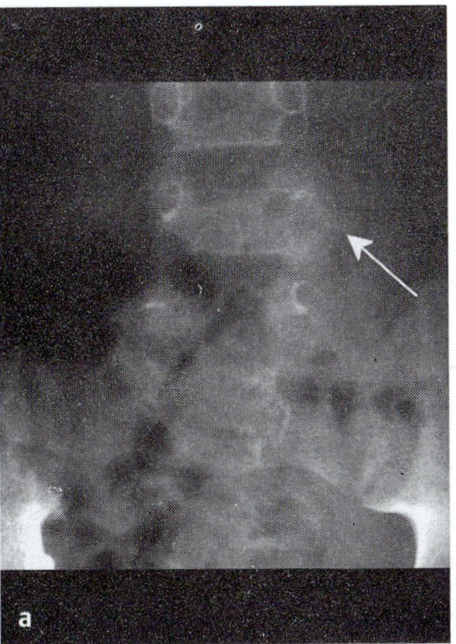

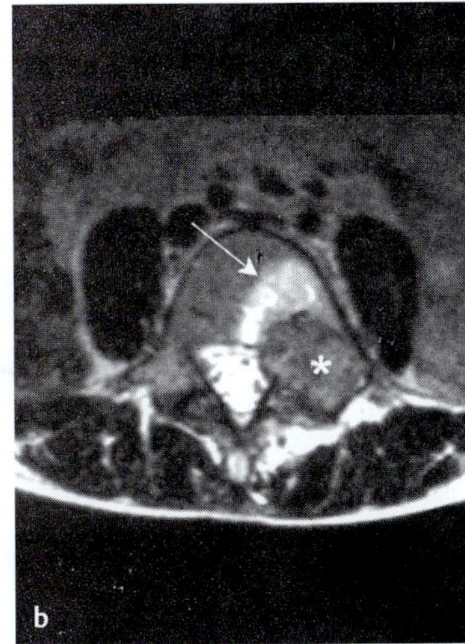

Fig. 6.10 a, b Aneurysmal bone cyst in the left vertebral arch of vertebra L4. Radiograph (**a**) and MR T2-weighted TSE image (**b**). The conventional radiograph only shows cortical expansion of the vertebral arch (**a**, arrow); the left pedicle is not clearly visualized. The MR image (**b**) not only visualizes the tumor (*), which extends into the spinal canal, but also demonstrates bone marrow edema in the vertebral body (arrow).

Differential Diagnosis

Giant cell tumor (osteoclastoma)	– Predilection for metaphysis and epiphysis in long bones – Less pronounced trabeculation – No matrix calcification – Small extraosseous tumor component – Older patients
Juvenile bone cyst	– Central position – Minimal expansion – Considerable marginal sclerosis, no central trabeculation – Pathologic fracture may occur
Enchondroma	– Typical focal or stranded calcifications – Usually lies in a central location – Oval shape with cortical thinning and cortical expansion
Telangiectatic osteosarcoma	– Histologic examination often required for differential diagnosis – Fluid level in hemorrhage

Fibrous dysplasia	– Ground-glass bone structure – Finely nodular or coarse calcifications – Honeycomb cystic appearance – Cortical expansion and bending deformity
Osteoblastoma	– Also affects the spine – Smaller soft tissue component than aneurysmal bone cyst – Often focal calcifications in the center – Solid tumor components are common – Usually solitary lesion
Pseudotumor in hemophilia	– Known coagulation disorder

Tips and Pitfalls

Where findings include an aneurysmal bone cyst, one must be careful to exclude an underlying bone tumor • Fluid levels in the cyst are not pathognomonic as they also occur in lesions such as osteosarcomas.

Selected References

Cottalorda J et al. Aneurysmal bone cysts of the pelvis in children: a multicenter study and literature review. J Pediatr Orthop 2005; 25: 471–475

Keenan S et al. Musculoskeletal lesions with fluid-fluid level: a pictorial essay. J Comput Assist Tomogr 2006; 30: 517–524

Mankin HJ et al. Aneurysmal bone cyst: a review of 150 patients. J Clin Oncol 2005; 23: 6756–6762

Woertler K. Benign bone tumors and tumor-like lesions: value of cross-sectional imaging. Eur Radiol 2003; 13: 1820–1835

Definition

- **Epidemiology**
  Usually diagnosed in early childhood • There is no known increased familial incidence or involvement of hereditary factors • No sex predilection.
- **Etiology, pathophysiology, pathogenesis**
  Disorder shows predilection for one half of the body • Strictly unilateral involvement may occur (Ollier disease) • Affects only those skeletal structures initially present as cartilaginous primordia • Etiology is not fully understood • Nests of ectopic cartilage develop in the growth plates and migrate to the metaphysis, where they proliferate • The cartilage cells and growth plate fail to mature • This leads to limb shortening • Histologic findings are indistinguishable from solitary endochondroma (may be slightly more hypercellular).
  Common sites: Proximal humerus • Distal forearm • Metacarpals and phalanges • Pelvis and proximal femur • Knee (distal femur, proximal tibia) • Distal tibia.

Imaging Signs

- **Radiographic findings**
  Well-demarcated, round radiolucencies • Column-like highly radiolucent strips extend from the growth plate into the diaphysis • Fan-shaped lesions on the iliac crest • Cortical expansion in the metaphysis and adjacent diaphysis leads to skeletal deformities • Typical limb shortening • Growth plates in older children are irregular, and epiphyseal involvement is present • Focal, popcorn-like, or ring-shaped patterns of calcification occur with increasing age • Madelung deformity.
- **MRI**
  Not required for diagnosis • May be useful for visualizing individual enchondromas (hyperintense on T2-weighted images, hypointense on T1-weighted images).

Clinical Aspects

- **Typical presentation**
  Growth disturbances with shortening of the arm or leg • The initial symptom usually only is a limp due to slight leg shortening • Hand and foot deformities.
- **Therapeutic options**
  Surgery to correct functional impairment (lengthening osteotomy, Ilizarov fixator) or treat malignant degeneration.
- **Course and prognosis**
  This depends on the severity of the disorder and resulting skeletal deformity.

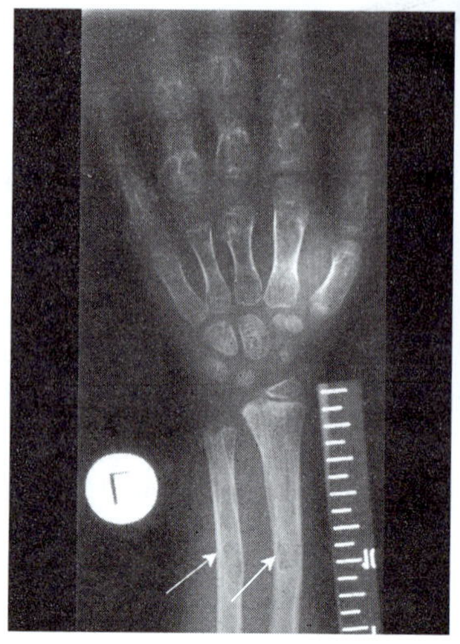

Fig. 6.11 Enchondromatosis. A-P radiograph of the left hand showing involvement of the metacarpals, phalanges, and distal forearm bones (arrows).

▸ **Complications**

Associated with juvenile granulosa cell ovarian tumor.

Sarcomatous degeneration occurs in 25–30% of cases.

- Osteosarcoma occurs in young adults.
- Chondrosarcoma (including lesions in the bones of the distal extremities) or fibrosarcoma occurs in older patients.

Differential Diagnosis

Maffucci syndrome	– Congenital, not hereditary – Enchondromatosis and soft tissue hemangiomatosis – Multiple calcified phleboliths in the soft tissue – Identical distribution of bone lesions as in Ollier disease – Ultrasound search for intraabdominal hemangiomas
Simple solitary enchondroma	– Mature hyaline cartilage – Central or juxtacortical location – Usually occurs between ages 10 and 40 years – No sex predilection – Most often in the bones of the distal extremities – Usually asymptomatic unless pathologic fracture occurs

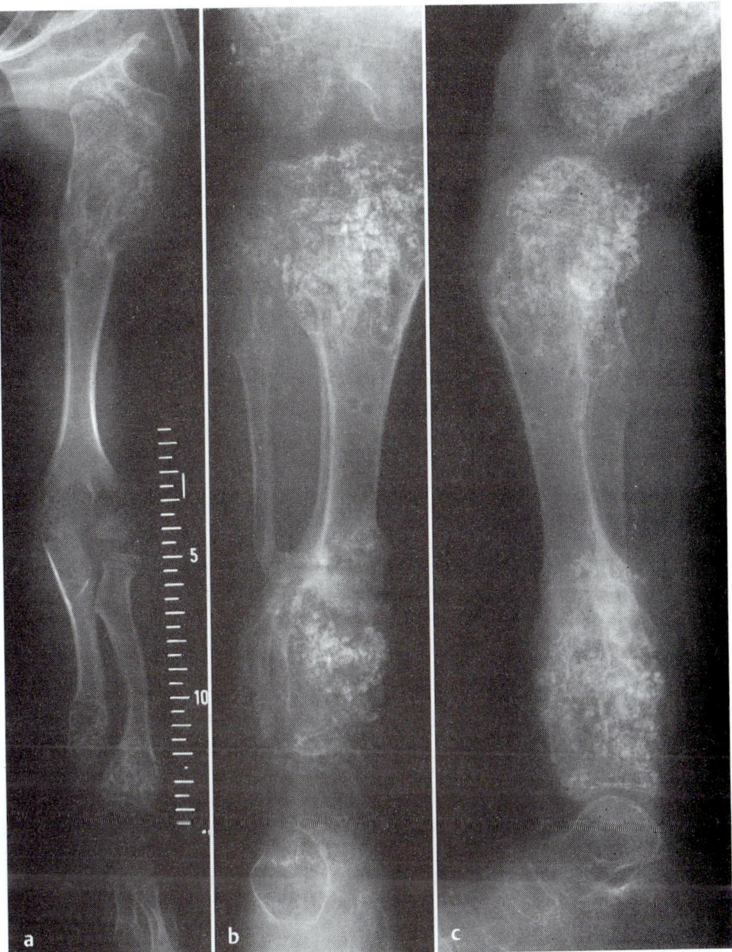

Fig. 6.12 a–c Multiple large enchondromas in the upper (**a**) and lower extremity (**b, c**) with typical shortening, deformation, and cortical expansion of the bone. The enchondromas show typical calcifications.

Osteochondroma	– Autosomal dominant inheritance – Typical morphology with bony outgrowth arising from the surface of the bone – Cartilage cap – Exhibits its own growth plate – Growth ceases with skeletal maturity – Usually occurs in the metaphysis of the long bones, usually in the knee and proximal humerus
Fibrous dysplasia (polyostotic form)	– Usually also shows a predilection for one side – Ground-glass bone structure due to loss of trabeculation – No epiphyseal involvement – Significant bone deformities – Cortical thinning with "seashell" configuration of the inner cortex – Pathologic fracture may be present ("shepherd's crook" deformity of the proximal femur) – Bone scan visualizes all lesions
McCune–Albright syndrome	– Fibrous dysplasia (polyostotic form) – Café-au-lait spots – Precocious puberty
Metaphyseal dysplasia	– Autosomal recessive inheritance – Abnormal metaphyseal ossification – Short stature of varying severity with limb shortening – Joint deformity

Tips and Pitfalls

Can be confused with other disorders considered in the differential diagnosis.

Selected References

Bukte Y et al. A case of multiple chondrosarcomas secondary to severe multiple symmetrical enchondromatosis (Ollier's disease) at an early age. Clin Radiol 2005; 60: 1306–1310

Dähnert W. Radiology Review Manual. Baltimore: Williams & Wilkins; 2003: 71

Flemming DJ et al. Enchondroma and chondrosarcoma. Semin Musculoskelet Radiol 2000; 4: 59–71

Kolodziej L et al. The use of the Ilizarov technique in the treatment of upper limb deformity in patients with Ollier's disease. J Pediatr Orthop 2005; 25: 202–205

Noel G et al. Chondrosarcomas of the base of the skull in Ollier's disease or Maffucci's syndrome–three case reports and review of the literature. Acta Oncol 2004; 43: 705–710

Definition

▸ **Epidemiology**

Solitary osteochondroma: Most common benign tumor of bone (35% of cases) • Accounts for 9% of all bone tumors • No sex predilection.

Multiple osteochondromas: Autosomal dominant inheritance • Only occurs after age 30 years • Males are affected three times as often as females.

▸ **Etiology, pathophysiology, pathogenesis**

Cartilage capped bony exostosis arising on the external surface of the bone containing a marrow cavity that is continuous with that of the underlying bone (World Health Organization definition) • Presumably ectopic enchondral ossification centers from the physeal region • Occurs in the vicinity of the growth plate • Histologic structure is typical of a growth plate (proliferative cartilage, columnar cartilage, calcification zone, and ossification zone) • Cartilage cap is usually only a few millimeters thick in active osteochondromas • Growth terminates with closure of the growth plates.

Typically occurs in the metaphysis of long bones—distal femur (25% of all lesions), proximal tibia (14%), and proximal humerus (17%) • Other locations are the scapula, pelvis, vertebral arches, spinous processes, ribs, and phalanges.

Imaging Signs

▸ **Radiographic findings**

Forms: Pedunculated, mushroom-shaped, broad-based (sessile) • Half of all solitary osteochondromas are pedunculated • Up to 80% of multiple osteochondromas are sessile • Cancellous bone of the bone of origin is continuous with the cancellous bone of the exostosis • Arciform, ring-shaped, popcorn-shaped, and clustered matrix ossifications occur.

▸ **Ultrasound findings**

Visualizes noncalcified cartilage cap • Findings may include bursitis.

▸ **MRI findings**

Useful in anatomic regions such as the pelvis, spine, and scapula where overlapping structures obscure the region of interest • The cartilage cap is hyperintense on T2-weighted images • A cartilage cap thicker than 2 cm suggests malignancy.

Clinical Aspects

▸ **Typical presentation**

Often an incidental finding • Palpable mass or protrusion • Impingement of capsular insertions, nerves, vascular structures, or muscles causes pain, as does traumatic avulsion • Growth disturbances occur, especially in multiple hereditary cartilaginous exostoses • Where accessory bursae develop, signs of irritation and inflammation (bursitis) may occur • In malignant degeneration, additional growth and pain will often occur after puberty.

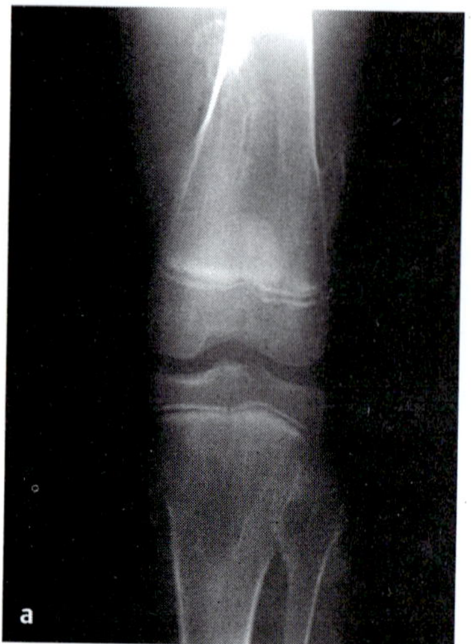

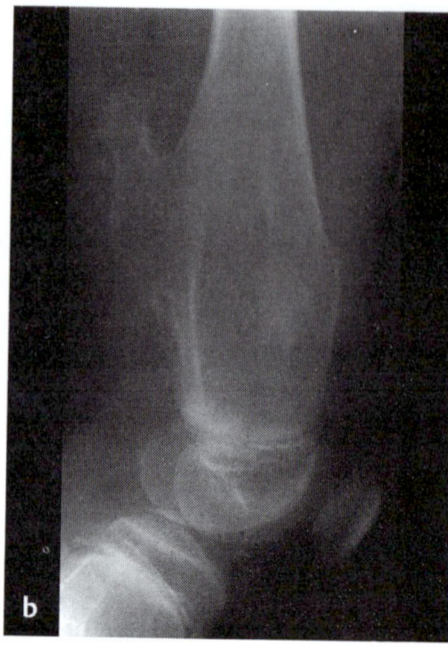

Fig. 6.13 a, b Osteochondroma. Radiographs of the knee in two planes. Multiple, primarily sessile metaphyseal osteochondromas. Metaphyses are widened and thickened.

- **Therapeutic options**

  Observation • Symptomatic osteochondromas require surgical excision.

- **Course and prognosis**

  Solitary osteochondromas become malignant (chondrosarcoma) in less than 1% of cases • In multiple hereditary cartilaginous exostoses, malignant degeneration occurs in 5–10% of cases • Risk of malignant degeneration is highest in osteochondromas in the shoulder or pelvis.

- **Complications**

  Impingement of capsular insertions, nerves, vascular structures, and muscles • Traumatic avulsion • Recurrence after resection, growth disturbances, or fracture of the host bone may occur • Malignant degeneration.

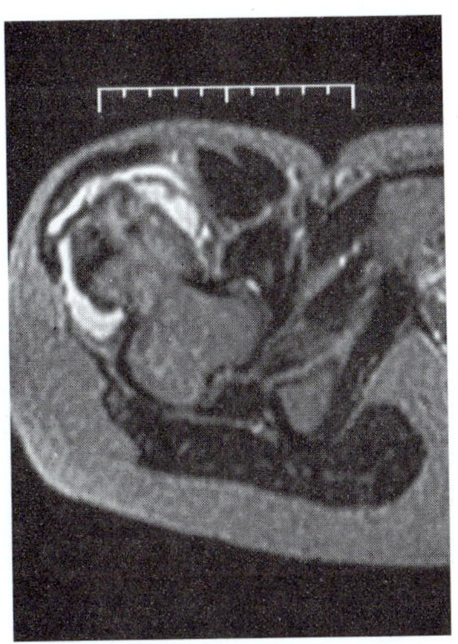

Fig. 6.14 MR axial T2-weighted TSE image through the right femoral neck. Large, broad-based osteochondroma extending anteriorly from the bone. Hyperintense cartilage cap.

Differential Diagnosis

Normal variant as in a supracondylar process	– Hook-shaped, resembling an exostosis – On the flexor aspect of the diaphysis and metaphysis – Base arises directly from the cortex
Bizarre parosteal osteochondromatous proliferation	– 25% of cases occur in long bones – Ossifications arising directly from the cortex – Cartilage cap
Juxtacortical periosteal chondroma	– Metaphysis – Eroding lesion of the outer cortex – Sharply defined border – Key-shaped defect – Overhanging bony margins along the proximal and distal borders – Tumor matrix calcifications
Parosteal osteosarcoma	– Cortical thickening – Parosteal tumor component – Dense matrix ossification – Spicules
Chondrosarcoma adjacent to exostosis	– Growth continues puberty – Fine, diffuse, amorphous calcifications remote from the base of the tumor – Cartilage cap thicker than 2 cm

Tips and Pitfalls

Osteochondromas can also be induced by radiation therapy in children, especially in the spine and pelvis • Cartilage caps thicker than 2 cm and irregular calcifications remote from the base of the tumor suggest a secondary chondrosarcoma • Even dynamic contrast-enhanced MRI often cannot distinguish between benign and malignant lesions.

Selected References

Lee KC et al. Imaging the complications of osteochondromas. Clin Radiol 2002; 57: 18–28

Malghem J et al. Benign osteochondromas and exostotic chondrosarcomas: evaluation of cartilage cap thickness by ultrasound. Skeletal Radiol 1992; 21: 33–37

Murphey MD et al. Imaging of osteochondroma: variants and complications with radiologic-pathologic correlation. Radiographics 2000; 20: 1407–1434

Oviedo A et al. Bizarre parosteal osteochondromatous proliferation: case report and review of the literature. Pediatr Dev Pathol 2001; 4: 496–500

Woertler K et al. Osteochondroma: MR imaging of tumor-related complications. Eur Radiol 2000; 10: 832–840

Definition

- **Epidemiology**
  Usually occurs between the ages of 10 and 30 years • Predilection for the long bones, especially femur and tibia.
- **Etiology, pathophysiology, pathogenesis**
  Etiology is unknown, possibly neoplastic or inflammatory • Benign bone-forming neoplasm • Central nidus is characteristic • Nidus is usually smaller than 1 cm • Reactive new bone formation is seen around the lesion • Usually in the metaphyseal region, especially in the femur • Lesions in the spine (thoracolumbar junction) usually involve the posterior elements (pedicle, spinous process, and vertebral arch) • Multicentric or multifocal osteoid osteomas exhibit more than one nidus • *Forms:* Cortical, intramedullary, subperiosteal, periarticular (intracapsular) • Composed of osteoid or mineralized immature bone • Osteoid island (nidus) surrounded by highly vascularized connective tissue • Dense bone of varying maturity surrounds the nidus.

Imaging Signs

- **Radiographic findings**
  Usually there is cortical thickening with a central radiolucent nidus with or without central calcification • Conventional tomography may be helpful in visualizing the nidus.
- **CT**
  For precisely localizing the nidus and determining its size • May be useful in planning interventional therapy.
- **MRI findings**
  On T2-weighted images, the nidus appears hyperintense with extensive perifocal bone marrow edema • Pronounced, early contrast enhancement of the viable nidus • Essential study for evaluating the success of interventional ablation of the nidus as it can detect a residual nidus.
- **Bone scan**
  Highly sensitive in demonstrating even small osteoid osteomas.

Clinical Aspects

- **Typical presentation**
  Pain increases at night and improves with administration of acetylsalicylic acid (in up to 75% of cases) • Prostaglandin E_2 is elevated within the nidus.
- **Therapeutic options**
  Total en bloc resection • Interventional procedures such as CT-guided radiofrequency ablation are increasingly used.
- **Course and prognosis**
  Complete removal of the nidus is curative • No growth tendency • Spontaneous regression is rare.

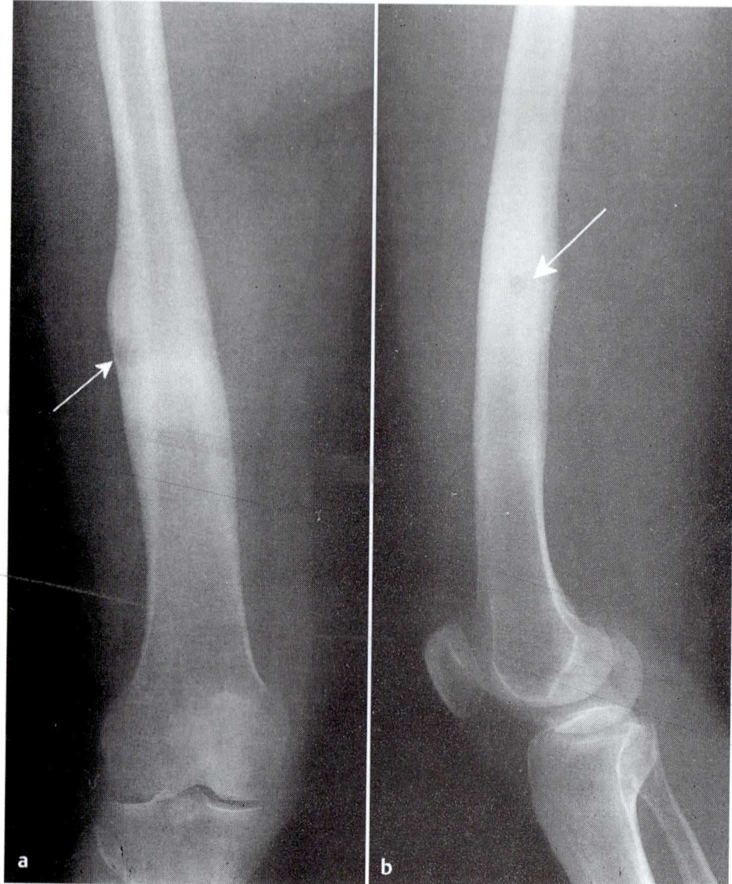

Fig. 6.15 a, b Osteoid osteoma. Radiographs of the femur in two planes. Typical appearance of an osteoid osteoma in the lateral femoral cortex. The radiolucent nidus (arrow) is surrounded by a broad margin of sclerotic bone. There is marked cortical thickening.

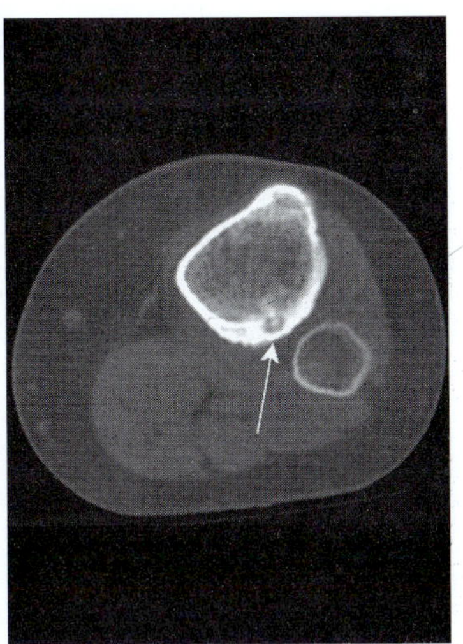

Fig. 6.16 CT, bone window. Slightly calcified nidus (arrow) in the center of the posterior tibia.

▸ **Complications**

Accelerated bone growth where the lesion lies adjacent to the growth plate • Compensatory scoliosis due to pain where the spine is affected • Early osteoarthritis with an intracapsular osteoid osteoma.

Differential Diagnosis

Bone abscess (Brodie's abscess)	– Fistula (usually extending to the nearest growth plate) – Constant pain that does not increase at night – Laboratory values indicative of inflammation
Osteoma (cortical island)	– Asymptomatic incidental finding – Normal nuclear medicine imaging findings – Multiple lesions in osteopoikilosis
Stress fracture	– Radiolucent line in bone coursing perpendicular (not parallel) to the cortex – Cortical thickening – Callus formation – Typical location, for example, in metatarsals – Radiographic signs appear about 10 days after fracture
Osteoblastoma	– Resembles osteoid osteoma (> 1.5–2 cm) – Usually occurs in the spine – May also occur in long bones – Patients may not have any symptoms; much weaker response to salicylates

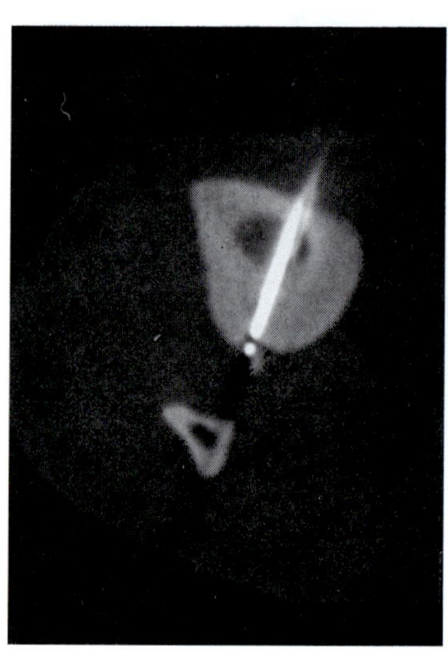

Fig. 6.17 CT. Radiofrequency ablation of an osteoid osteoma of the tibia with a bipolar probe.

Tips and Pitfalls

It is often impossible to distinguish an osteoid osteoma or osteoblastoma from an aneurysmal bone cyst, especially in the spine • A bone scan is indicated where typical clinical symptoms are present in the absence of a proven osteoid osteoma • The viable nidus often can only be clearly visualized in the early contrast phase and may escape detection in the later contrast phase, especially on MRI • Complete removal of the nidus should be verified on an MRI follow-up study after every interventional procedure • Intracapsular osteoid osteomas usually escape detection on plain radiographs.

Selected References

Allen SD et al. Imaging of intra-articular osteoid osteoma. Clin Radiol 2003; 58: 845–852

Assoun J et al. Osteoid osteoma: MR imaging versus CT. Radiology 1994; 191: 217–223

Cantwell CP et al. Current trends in treatment of osteoid osteoma with an emphasis on radiofrequency ablation. Eur Radiol 2004; 14: 607–617

Gaeta M et al. Magnetic resonance imaging findings of osteoid osteoma of the proximal femur. Eur Radiol 2004; 14: 1582–1589

Definition

▸ **Epidemiology**
Second most common bone tumor in children and adolescents • Boys are affected more often than girls (3:2) • Most common in boys between the ages of 10 and 15 years.

▸ **Etiology, pathophysiology, pathogenesis**
Small-cell and round-cell tumor • Presumably arises from postganglionic cholinergic neurons • Occurs most often in the diaphysis (60% of cases) of the long bones (25% in the femur, also in the tibia, humerus, fibula, and ribs) • Occurs less often in flat bones (pelvis and scapula) • Periosteal Ewing sarcomas are rare • Extraosseous occurrence is extremely rare • Most often metastasizes to other bones and the lungs.

Imaging Signs

▸ **Radiographic findings**
Tumor with very aggressive appearance • Poorly demarcated • Usually has a soft tissue component (displaces the intramuscular fat planes) • Often infiltrates adjacent soft tissue • Permeative or moth-eaten osteolysis • *Periosteal reaction:* Lamellar, onion-skin appearance, spicules, Codman triangle • Mixed osteolytic and sclerotic forms occur • Purely sclerotic lesions often occur in the pelvis • *Extraosseous form:* Massive parosteal tumor component, erosion, and periosteal reaction in the adjacent bone.

▸ **Ultrasound findings**
Interrupted cortical reflections • Hyperemic soft tissue tumor with convex margin.

▸ **CT**
Helpful in visualizing bone destruction • Chest CT is indicated to exclude metastases.

▸ **Contrast MRI findings**
Modality of choice for visualizing local extent of tumor for planning biopsy, and follow-up during treatment • Differentiates tumor from peritumoral edema • Changes in the contrast dynamics of the tumor under treatment are a prognostic criterion • Hyperintense to skeletal muscle on T2-weighted images • Hypointense to normal bone marrow or intermediate signal on T1-weighted images • Inhomogeneous contrast enhancement on T1-weighted images.

▸ **Bone scan**
For identifying bone metastases.

▸ **PET**
FDG-PET for follow-up under therapy • For identifying metastases • Useful in differentiating recurrence from postoperative changes.

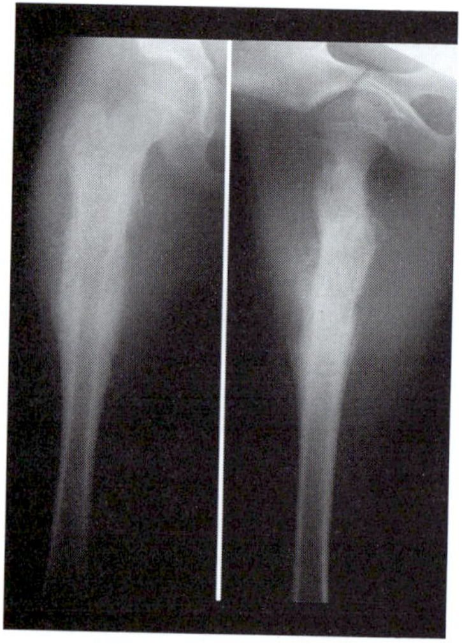

Fig. 6.18 Ewing sarcoma. Radiographs in two planes. Moth-eaten areas of osteolysis and extensive periosteal reaction in the proximal femur, lamellar and spiculated appearance, Codman triangle, large soft tissue tumor displacing the fat planes.

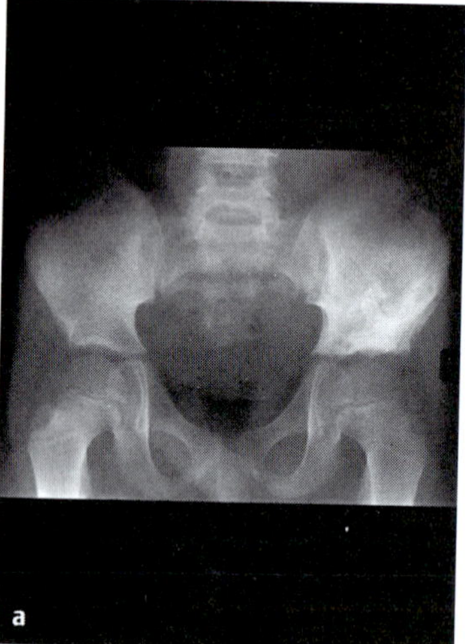

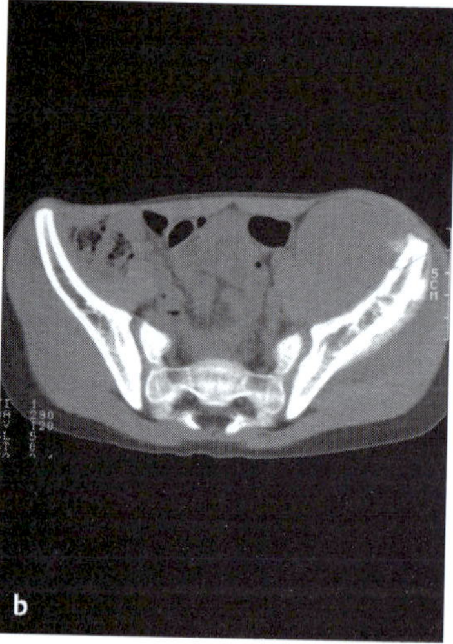

Fig. 6.19 a, b Ewing sarcoma in the left iliac wing in a 6-year-old boy. The pelvis radiograph (**a**) shows primarily sclerotic changes in the left ileum. The CT image (**b**) also shows a primarily spiculated area of periosteal reaction and a large soft tissue tumor on the inner aspect of the ileum.

Clinical Aspects

- **Typical presentation**
  Pain and swelling in the region of the tumor • Malaise • Weight loss • Fever • Abnormal blood count (leukocytosis, anemia, raised erythrocyte sedimentation rate) • Spinal involvement can lead to pathologic fracture and gibbus • Neurologic symptoms can occur with expansion into the spinal canal.
- **Therapeutic options**
  Polychemotherapy (vincristine, doxorubicin, cyclophosphamide or ifosfamide, actinomycin D, and possibly etoposide) • This is followed by local treatment (surgery and radiation therapy where indicated) • Then additional chemotherapy for up to one year.
- **Course and prognosis**
  Five-year survival rate depends on the tumor stage at the time of the diagnosis • Probability of survival is higher in patients with tumors in long bones (65% of cases) than in those with flat bones (54%) • Prognosis is unfavorable in cases with a large tumor volume and metastases at the time of the diagnosis.
- **Complications**
  Pathologic fracture • Infiltration of neurovascular bundles • Recurrence • Postoperative granulomas and scarring may occur • Sequelae of radiation therapy.

Differential Diagnosis

Osteomyelitis	– More common in children under age 5 years – More rapid worsening of symptoms – Metaphyseal location – Uninterrupted normal periosteal formation of new bone (lamellar) – No tumor matrix on MRI
Osteosarcoma	– Tumor sclerosis occurs more frequently – Moth-eaten destruction
Eosinophilic granuloma	– Not always distinguishable – Often diaphyseal location – Relatively sharply demarcated osteolysis, although moth-eaten osteolysis may also occur – Lamellar periosteal reaction may occur
Neuroblastoma metastasis	– More common in children under age 3 years – Moth-eaten destruction with or without sclerosis – Ill-defined, usually interrupted periosteal reaction
Embryonal rhabdomyosarcoma with bone infiltration	– Radiologically identical to a Ewing sarcoma – Histologic differentiation is often difficult as well

Tips and Pitfalls

A Ewing sarcoma can easily be confused with osteomyelitis on the basis of similar radiographic findings, clinical presentation, and changes in laboratory values • FDG-PET can be helpful in distinguishing recurrence of the lesion from therapy-induced changes • Lamellar, onion-skin periosteal reactions only occur in about 25% of all Ewing sarcomas and are not pathognomonic as they also occur in osteomyelitis and eosinophilic granuloma.

Selected References

Eggli KD et al. Ewing's sarcoma. Radiol Clin North Am 1993; 31: 325–337

Kutluk MT et al. Treatment results and prognostic factors in Ewing sarcoma. Pediatr Hematol Oncol 2004; 21: 597–610

Rodriguez-Galindo C et al. Analysis of prognostic factors in ewing sarcoma family of tumors: review of St. Jude Children's Research Hospital studies. Cancer 2007; 110: 375–384

Shapeero LG et al. Periosteal Ewing sarcoma. Radiology 1994; 191: 825–831

Spunt SL et al. Ewing sarcoma-family tumors that arise after treatment of primary childhood cancer. Cancer 2006; 107: 201–206

Definition

- **Epidemiology**

  Medullary osteosarcomas are the most common primary malignant bone tumors • Peak frequency is between ages 10 and 20 years • Boys are affected more often than girls by a ratio of 1.5:1 • Accounts for 60% of malignant bone tumors in children.

- **Etiology, pathophysiology, pathogenesis**

  Etiology is unclear • A genetic disposition with increased familial incidence has been shown • The tumor can form osteoid and calcified bone • Occurs in the metaphysis of long bones • 58% of all lesions occur in the distal femur or proximal tibia • Grows into the epiphysis in 75% of cases • Flat bones and spine are affected in 20% of cases • Usually unicentral • Multicentric bone involvement with skip lesions is rare.

Table 6.1 WHO classification of osteogenic sarcomas

Primary osteosarcoma
Central (medullary) osteosarcoma: • Classic osteosarcoma • Telangiectatic osteosarcoma (highest malignancy, less common in children, males > females) • Well differentiated (low grade) osteosarcoma • Small-cell (mesenchymal) osteosarcoma
Superficial (juxtacortical) osteosarcoma: • Parosteal osteosarcoma (very rare, more common metadiaphyseal) • Periosteal osteosarcoma (age 20–50) • High-grade osteosarcoma (conventional osteosarcoma)
Secondary osteosarcoma • Secondary to irradiation • Secondary to Paget disease

Imaging Signs

- **Radiographic findings**

  Classic osteosarcoma: Ill-defined areas of osteolysis with cortical destruction • Permeative growth • New bone formation occurs even in the adjacent soft tissue tumor • Malignant periosteal reactions such as Codman triangle and spicules • Onion-skin periosteal reaction is rare.

  Telangiectatic osteosarcoma: Large osteolytic areas • Osteosclerotic reactions are almost completely absent.

  Parosteal osteosarcoma: Very dense due to its high calcium content • Tumor envelops the shaft of the bone • Fine radiolucencies are formed by periosteum lying between the tumor and the underlying cortex.

  Periosteal osteosarcoma: Broad-based lesion on the surface of the bone • Tumor exhibits inhomogeneous density • Cortical thickening.

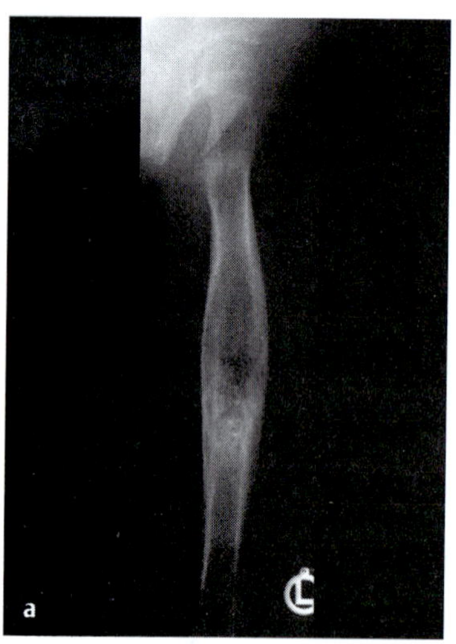

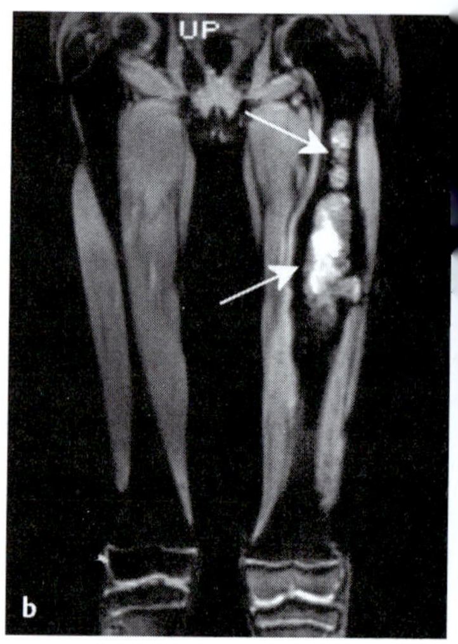

Fig. 6.20 a, b Telangiectatic osteosarcoma of the left femur in an 8-year-old girl. Radiograph (**a**) and MRI (**b**). The radiograph shows primarily osteolytic bone lesions. Isolated osteosclerotic changes are visualized in the lower part of the tumor. The coronal STIR image (**b**) demonstrates the full extent of the tumor (arrows).

- **CT findings**
  Optimally visualizes bony destruction and new bone formation • Soft tissue processes are not ideally detected • Primarily suitable for excluding or confirming pulmonary metastases.
- **MRI findings**
  Modality of choice for visualizing the entire extent of the tumor including soft tissue involvement and possible skip lesions • Tumor volume • Relationship to adjacent neurovascular structures • Particularly suitable for follow-up examinations • Demonstrates hemorrhages and possible fluid levels in telangiectatic osteosarcoma.
- **DSA findings**
  Demonstrates abnormal tumor vascularization • Allows preoperative tumor embolization.
- **Ultrasound**
  For screening local and regional lymph nodes • Excluding abdominal metastases.
- **Bone scan**
  Used for visualizing bone metastases • Not used as a primary diagnostic study.

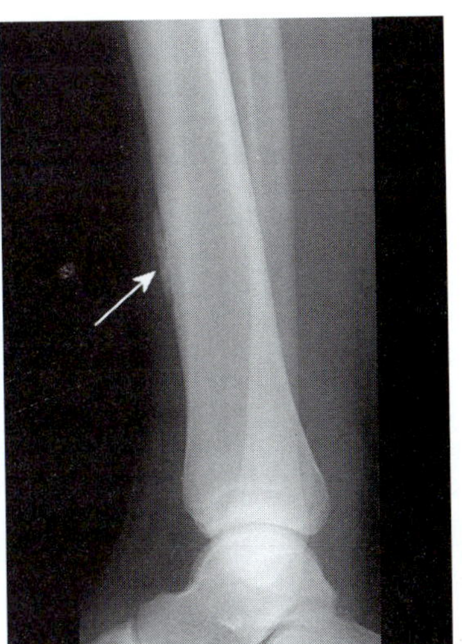

Fig. 6.21 Parosteal osteosarcoma. Radiograph of the tibia. Anterior to the bone there is a shell-like lesion with a narrow space between the tumor and the adjacent bone.

Clinical Aspects

- **Typical presentation**
  Pain of uncertain origin • Local swelling • Enlarged lymph nodes • Signs of inflammation (erythema, swelling, hyperthermia) • Unintentional weight loss, including cachexia • Poor general condition • Pathologic fracture • B-type symptoms • Laboratory findings include raised alkaline phosphatase level.
- **Therapeutic options**
  Neoadjuvant chemotherapy • Surgical resection of the tumor is indicated; curative surgery is not possible in the presence of extrapulmonary metastases.
- **Course and prognosis**
  In 20% of cases, a distant metastasis is present at the time of the diagnosis • Left untreated, tumor progression is fatal • Survival rate for local osteosarcoma with adequate treatment is over 70% • Surgical removal of the pulmonary focal lesions greatly improves the survival rate for pulmonary metastases (30–50%).
- **Complications**
  Early hematogenous metastases (to lung and bone).

Differential Diagnosis

Ewing sarcoma	– Typically diaphyseal – Often onion-skin periosteal reaction – Follow-up includes monitoring of neuron-specific enolase levels
Chondrosarcoma	– Calcified cartilage matrix – Most common location: pelvis, femur, humerus – Malignant degeneration of an enchondroma or osteochondroma close to the trunk
Chronic osteomyelitis	– History and laboratory values – No extensive soft tissue process – Abscesses may be present – Can mimic any bone tumor
Myositis ossificans	– Typical zones around an active germinal center – Sharply demarcated against the bone – Often history of trauma or immobilization
Bone metastases	– Usually multiple – Known underlying disorder often present, if not differential diagnosis should consider cancer of unknown primary – Osteolytic or osteosclerotic – Tumor markers – Periosteal reactions are less common
Aneurysmal bone cyst	– Cystic lesion with intralesional hemorrhage and fluid levels as in telangiectatic osteosarcoma

Tips and Pitfalls

Where a malignant solid bone tumor is suspected, closed biopsy procedures should only be performed after consultation with the surgeon. The approach to the biopsy site must lie within the surgical approach so that any malignant cells displaced into the aspiration canal can be resected • Cross-sectional modalities should not be used without first obtaining conventional radiographs.

Selected References

Hoffer FA. Primary skeletal neoplasms: osteosarcoma and Ewing sarcoma. Top Magn Reson Imaging 2002; 13: 231–239

Kim SJ et al. Imaging findings of extrapulmonary metastases of osteosarcoma. Clin Imaging 2004; 28: 291–300

Murphey MD et al. The many faces of osteosarcoma. Radiographics 1997; 17: 1205–1231

Murphey MD et al. Telangiectatic osteosarcoma: radiologic-pathologic comparison. Radiology 2003; 229: 545–553

Murphey MD et al. Imaging of periosteal osteosarcoma: radiologic-pathologic comparison. Radiology 2004; 233: 129–138

Schajowicz F. Tumors and Tumorlike Lesions of Bone. Berlin: Springer; 1994

Definition

- **Epidemiology**
  Overall incidence is about 0.4:100 000 children below the age of 15 years • Over 75% of cases occur before age 10 years.
- **Etiology, pathophysiology, pathogenesis**
  Earlier classification of Langerhans cell histiocytosis:
  Eosinophilic granuloma: Primarily involves bone • At least 10% of patients later develop multifocal or extraosseous lesions • Peak incidence is between the ages of 5 and 10 years • Predilection for male sex • Accounts for 60–80% of cases of Langerhans cell histiocytosis.
  Letterer–Siwe disease: Acute disseminated fulminant form of histiocytosis X • Usually affects children younger than 12 months • Hepatosplenomegaly • Lymphadenopathy • Lung involvement • Accounts for 10% of cases of Langerhans cell histiocytosis.
  Hand–Schüller–Christian disease: Chronic disseminated fulminant form of histiocytosis X • Peak age 3–6 years • Hepatosplenomegaly • Exophthalmos • Diabetes insipidus occurs with CNS involvement • Skin involvement • Calvarial osteolytic lesions of the skull.
  Etiology is unclear • Various manifestations • Reactive proliferation and/or accumulation of dendritic cells • Presumably a defect in intercellular communication with cytokine imbalance • The skeleton is most often affected when the disease involves only one organ system (eosinophilic granuloma) • The skeleton is the second most often affected organ system where the disease involves more than one system • The skull is involved particularly often.

Table 6.2 Classification according to the Histiocytic Society

Classification
Involvement of a single organ system
Localized disease
• Monostotic bone involvement
• Solitary skin lesion
• Involvement of a solitary lymph node
• Solitary lung lesion
• Solitary CNS lesion
Multiple lesions
• Involvement of multiple bones
• Involvement of multiple lymph nodes
Multisystemic disease
• Involvement of two or more organs or organ systems
• With or without organ dysfunction

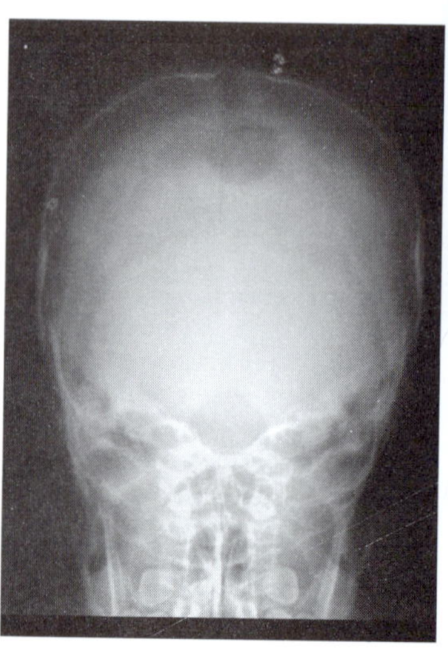

Fig. 6.22 Eosinophilic granuloma. Skull radiograph. In the high occipital region there is a sharply demarcated osteolytic lesion.

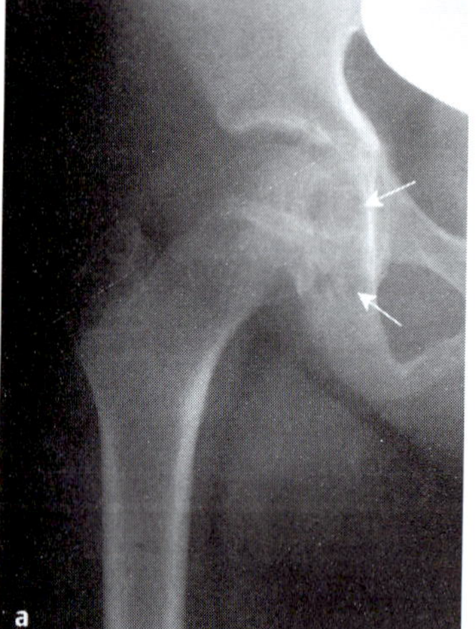

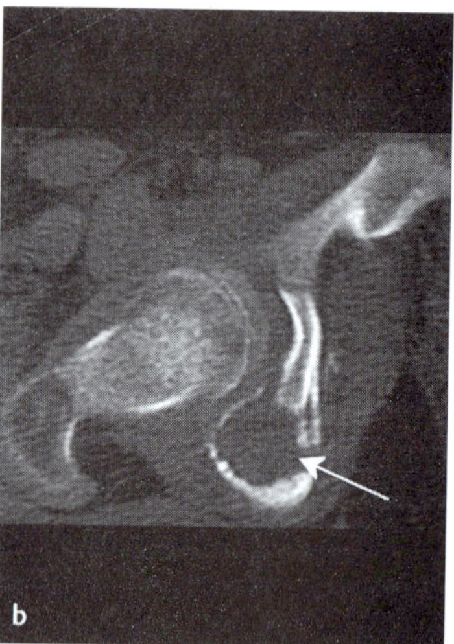

Fig. 6.23 a, b A 9-year-old girl with pelvic involvement in Langerhans cell histiocytosis. Radiograph (**a**) and CT (**b**). The radiograph shows vesicular, inhomogeneous bone structure in the acetabulum and along the posterior column (**a**, arrows). The CT image better demonstrates the extensive bone destruction (**b**, arrow).

Imaging Signs

- **Radiographic findings**
  Solitary (50–75% of cases) or multiple • Locations include the skull (50%), mandible, spine, ribs, long bones, and pelvis.
  Skull: Osteolytic lesions appear to be punched out • Occasionally their margins may also be ill-defined, especially in the acute phase • Marginal sclerosis is present in the healing phase (50% of all lesions) • Central "button" bone sequestra may occur • The cranium may exhibit a "raindrop" pattern • Extensive involvement produces a maplike appearance • Destruction of the sella, mastoid (with chronic otitis media), orbits, and petrous bone • "Floating" teeth in the upper jaw and mandible • Vertebra plana.
  Long bones and pelvis: Destructive osteolysis • Lamellar periosteal reaction • Cortical destruction • Later focal sclerotic lesions increasingly appear • Large oval bands of destruction are present.
- **Chest radiograph findings**
  Cystic structures • Bullae develop with risk of spontaneous pneumothorax (25% of cases) • Bilateral disseminated reticulonodular pathology • Later progresses to fibrosis and honeycomb lung.
- **Ultrasound findings**
  Hepatosplenomegaly with granulomas • Lymphadenopathy • Soft tissue nodules are present over the bony lesions.
- **CT findings**
  High-resolution CT of the chest: Symmetric nodular lesions (up to 10 mm in size) and cystic lesions in the lung • Predilection for upper and middle lung segments • Bullae (usually < 2 cm) • Lung fibrosis • Honeycomb lung • Hilar lymphadenopathy is rare.
  Bone CT: Precisely visualizes the extent of bony lesions • Soft tissue involvement may be better visualized with other modalities.
- **MRI findings**
  Cerebral involvement: Granulomatous lesions with the same signal characteristics as other inflammatory granulomas • Meninges and/or brain parenchyma (primarily hypothalamus, cerebellum, temporal and occipital lobes, and spinal cord) are involved • Most often the hypothalamus–pituitary axis is affected • Granulomatous thickening of the pituitary stalk • The posterior pituitary is not hyperintense on unenhanced T1-weighted images.
  Bone involvement: Bone marrow edema • Diffuse contrast enhancement • Soft tissue nodules may be present immediately adjacent to the bone • In skull involvement, the outer and inner tables exhibit a typical funnel-shaped configuration • Low signal intensity on T1-weighted images • High signal intensity on T2-weighted images.
- **Nuclear medicine imaging**
  Disseminated bone involvement • One-third of all inactive lesions do not show up on nuclear medicine imaging.

Clinical Aspects

▸ **Typical presentation**

Symptoms are highly variable • Asymptomatic until there is disseminated organ involvement • Most common initial symptoms include bone pain, swelling, and skin lesions • "Typical" symptoms such as exophthalmos, chronic otitis media in involvement of the mastoid bone, and premature loss of teeth are only present in 1–2% of all initial occurrences • *Typical skin involvement:* Brown to red papules with blistering, ulceration, crusting, and hemorrhages • These occur primarily on the trunk and scalp • Isolated nodular lesions may be present • Anemia • Pancytopenia • Mucosal ulceration • Neurologic symptoms in CNS involvement • Diabetes insipidus • Coughing and dyspnea in pulmonary involvement.

▸ **Therapeutic options**

Surgical excision is indicated for solitary skeletal and localized skin lesions • Local cortisone therapy • Extensive skin involvement is treated with photochemotherapy • Involvement of multiple organ systems and multiple bone lesions require systemic therapy with corticosteroids, cytostatic agents, and immunosuppressive agents • Radiation therapy is only used as a last resort.

▸ **Course and prognosis**

Prognosis is good for involvement of a single organ system, regardless of the treatment • Unfavorable prognostic factors in multiple organ system involvement include age less than 2 years, multiple organ involvement, and organ dysfunction (liver, lung, and/or bone marrow) • The most important prognostic factors include involvement of one or more "risk organs" at the time of diagnosis (liver, spleen, lung, and hemopoietic tissue) and the response to therapy during the first 6–12 weeks • Five-year survival rate is 80% • Lesions recur in 45% of these cases (usually bone, skin, and pituitary) • Chronic recurrent course is rare • Mortality in multiple organ system involvement is 20%.

▸ **Complications**

Late sequelae may occur depending on organ involvement • Scoliosis in vertebra plana • Loss of teeth • Pulmonary fibrosis • Cirrhosis of the liver • Pituitary insufficiency (oligomenorrhea, hypothyroidism, short stature, diabetes insipidus).

Differential Diagnosis

▸ **Bone involvement**

Osteomyelitis	– Varied pattern with osteolytic and sclerotic changes – Periosteal reactions – Signs of inflammation – Vertebra plana also occurs in chronic recurrent multifocal osteomyelitis
Ewing sarcoma	– Rarely multifocal – Vertebra plana may also occur – Soft tissue involvement – Typically diaphyseal – Onion-skin periosteal reaction

Osteosarcoma	– Typically metaphyseal – Often associated with new bone formation (osteosclerotic form) – Malignant periosteal reactions – Occasionally with large soft tissue component (calcifications) – Biphasic age distribution
Plasmacytoma	– Ill-defined osteolytic areas – Soft tissue tumor component – Peak age much later – Laboratory values include typical protein electrophoresis findings (Bence Jones proteinuria may be present)
Lymphoma	– Ill-defined osteolytic areas – Periosteal reactions – Soft tissue component without calcifications – Extraosseous involvement
Fibrous dysplasia	– Osteolytic vesicular lesion – Signs of benign lesion with sharply defined marginal sclerosis – Bending deformities in bone – Polyostotic and monostotic
Bone cysts	– Usually a solitary lesion and incidental finding (pathologic fracture may occur) – Sharply demarcated marginal sclerosis – Usually occurs in the proximal shaft of the humerus and femur

▸ **Lung involvement**

Idiopathic fibrosing lung disease	– Such as Hamman–Rich disease – Restrictive impairment of ventilation and diffusion – Typical decline in PO_2 with exercise – Diffuse reticular or nodular densities, usually symmetric
Atypical pneumonia	– Chronologic course is typical – Laboratory and clinical signs of inflammation – Interstitial changes with ill-defined margins – Usually no bullae (differential diagnosis should consider an abscess)
Sarcoidosis	– Bilateral hilar lymphadenopathy – Later involves interstitial pulmonary changes – Irreversible pulmonary fibrosis occurs only in the late stage – Bronchial lavage and laboratory diagnostic tests (elevated ACE) confirm the diagnosis – Findings improve rapidly with corticoid treatment

Tips and Pitfalls

The heterogeneity of the disorder often leads to late diagnosis • Langerhans cell histiocytosis should be considered wherever bone lesions are accompanied by chronic skin or mucosal pathology and/or treatment-resistant otitis media or mastoiditis or diabetes insipidus • Histologic examination is indicated as the disease is difficult to distinguish from other disorders considered in differential diagnosis.

Selected References

Favara BE et al. A contemporary classification of histiocytic disorders. The WHO committee on histiocytic/reticulum cell proliferations. Reclassification Working Group of the Histiocytic Society. Med Ped Oncol 1997; 29: 157–166

Gadner H et al. A randomised trial of treatment for multisystem Langerhans' cell histiocytosis. J Pediatr 2001; 138: 728–734

Ghirardello S et al. The diagnosis of children with central diabetes insipidus. J Pediatr Endocrinol Metab 2007; 20: 359–375

Isaacs H Jr. Fetal and neonatal histiocytoses. Pediatr Blood Cancer 2006; 47: 123–129

Ladisch S et al. LCH-I: A randomized trial of etoposide versus vinblastine in disseminated langerhans cell histiocytosis. Med Pediatr Oncol 1994; 23: 107–110

Lahey E. Histiocytosis X: an analysis of prognostic factors. J Pediatr 1975; 87: 184–189

Minkov M et al. Response to initial treatment of multisystem Langerhans cell histiocytosis: an important prognostic indicator. Med Pediatr Oncol 2002; 39: 581–585

Willman CL et al. Langerhans cell histiocytosis (histiocytosis X): a clonal proliferative disease. NEJM 1994; 331: 154–160

Definition

- **Epidemiology**
  Most common malignant disorder in children • Accounts for 27% of all malignant disorders • Peak age is between 2 and 6 years • Boys are affected more often than girls by a ratio of 1.2:1.
- **Etiology, pathophysiology, pathogenesis**
  Malignant disease of hemopoietic stem cells • Normal hemopoietic bone marrow is diffusely infiltrated or displaced by immature or minimally differentiated lymphoblasts • Hyperemic and hemorrhagic bone marrow • Destruction of bone trabeculae • The cytomorphologic subclassification of the French, American, and British (FAB) study group identifies groups L1–L3 • Cytochemical differentiation (peroxidase, esterase, and acid phosphatase) is helpful in distinguishing acute lymphatic leukemia from acute myeloid leukemia • *Immunologic differentiation:* c-ALL, T-ALL, pre-B ALL, B-ALL • Incidence is higher in children with Down syndrome or genetic translocations.

Imaging Signs

- **Radiographic findings**
  Can be normal initially • Diffuse osteopenia in the vertebrae and long bones with trabecular rarefaction; collapse of the superior and inferior vertebral endplates • Compression fractures of the vertebral body • Vertebra plana may be present.
  Metaphyseal radiolucent bands ("leukemic bands"): These are due to reduced enchondral ossification • Horizontal radiolucent bands in the metaphyses of the long bones • Often appear as linear densities after treatment.
  Focal bone lesions: Sharply demarcated circumscribed bone lesions • Moth-eaten or permeative appearance • Coarsening or widening of the diploe of the skull • Disseminated confluent areas of osteolysis.
  Periostitis in the long bones: Onion-skin or lamellar periosteal changes • Subperiosteal infiltration by leukemia cells • Subperiosteal hemorrhage • Pathologic fractures, often in the metaphysis.
- **CT findings**
  Only required where large areas of bone destruction are present • May be helpful in spinal involvement.
- **MRI findings**
  Modality of choice for visualizing medullary expansion • Useful where it is difficult to make a diagnosis • Useful in the presence of complications under therapy • Whole-body MRI (with fat suppression) is not yet established as a routine staging method • Focal or diffuse bone marrow infiltration exhibits slight to intermediate signal intensity on T1-weighted images (indistinguishable from hemopoietic marrow in younger children) • T1 relaxation time of the infiltrated marrow is prolonged • Hyperintense to normal bone marrow on T2-weighted images.
- **Bone scan**
  Increased tracer uptake • Can lead to underestimation of the extent of bone marrow involvement.

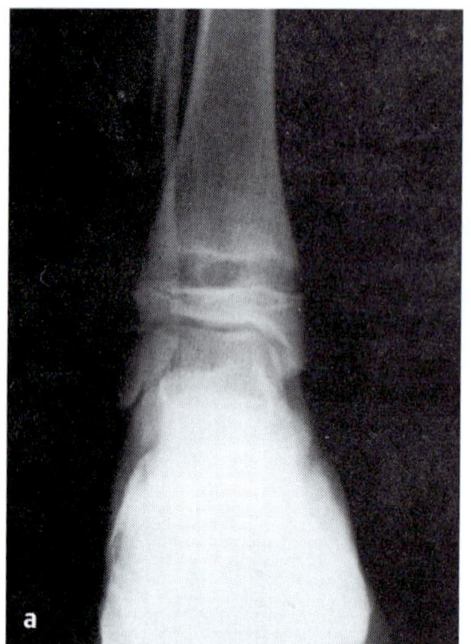

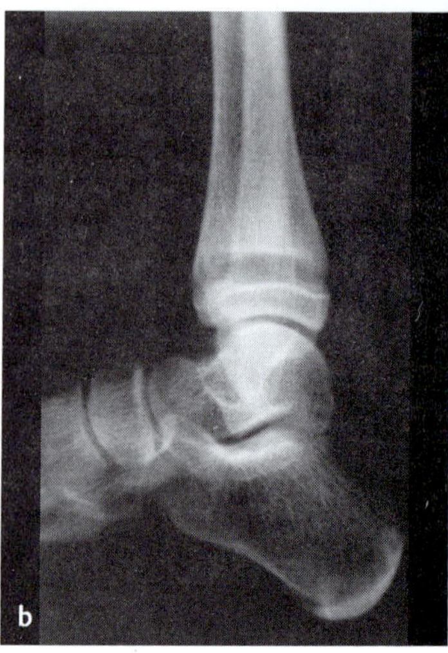

Fig. 6.24 a, b Acute lymphatic leukemia in a 12-year-old boy. Radiograph of the ankle in two planes. Metaphyseal radiolucent bands in the distal tibia and fibula.

▸ **PET**

Extramedullary involvement • Evaluation of the success of therapy.

Clinical Aspects

▸ **Typical presentation**

Often there are uncharacteristic symptoms • Protracted clinical course • Pallor • Fatigue • Loss of appetite • Weight loss • Fever • Patients tend to develop recurrent persistent infections • Hematomas and/or petechial skin and mucosal hemorrhages • Bone and joint pain is often present • Joint effusion • Headache, nausea, and vomiting occur in CNS involvement • Lymph nodes are moderately enlarged • Splenomegaly and/or hepatomegaly • Mikulicz syndrome (leukemic infiltration in the lacrimal and salivary glands) occurs in rare cases.

▸ **Therapeutic options**

Polychemotherapy: Induction therapy • CNS prophylaxis • Reinduction therapy with or without prophylactic irradiation of the cranium • Long-term therapy.
Supportive therapy: Prophylaxis against infections.

▸ **Course and prognosis**

Prognosis depends on the absolute lymphoblast count in peripheral blood • Liver and spleen size determine whether the patient belongs to a risk group.

- *Unfavorable prognostic factors:* Poor response to the preliminary prednisone phase of therapy • Persistence of lymphoblasts after 1 month of chemotherapy • Recurrence within 18 months of the diagnosis.

- *Favorable prognostic factors:* Long initial remission phase • 80% probability of survival without recurrence.

▸ **Complications**

Pathologic fractures • Osteonecrosis during treatment • Joint effusion • Bleeding • Bacterial infections • Fungal infections during chemotherapy • Carcinomatous meningitis in CNS involvement.

Differential Diagnosis

Neuroblastoma metastases	– More common in children under age 3 years – Moth-eaten destruction with or without sclerosis – Ill-defined, usually interrupted periosteal reaction
Eosinophilic granuloma	– Osteolytic lesions that appear punched out – Lamellar periosteal reaction – Cortical destruction
Osteomyelitis	– Bony destruction can mimic leukemic infiltration – Periosteal reactions – Signs of inflammation
Lymphoma	– Usually a solitary lesion, occasionally multifocal – Ill-defined osteolytic bone lesions are common – Pathologic fractures – Parosteal soft tissue component
Ewing sarcoma	– Typically diaphyseal – No metaphyseal radiolucent lines – Aggressive periosteal reaction (lamellar, spicules, Codman triangle) – Bone destruction (permeative, moth-eaten) – Large soft tissue component

Tips and Pitfalls

When joint pain, joint effusion, and accelerated erythrocyte sedimentation rate are present, the disorder can easily be confused with rheumatic fever, rheumatoid arthritis, and osteomyelitis • Metaphyseal radiolucent bands also occur in healing rickets, hypervitaminosis D, congenital syphilis, rubella, cytomegalovirus infection, toxoplasmosis, and scurvy.

Selected References

Benz G et al. Radiological aspects of leukaemia in childhood: an analysis of 89 children. Pediatr Radiol 1976; 20; 4: 201–213

Gallager DJ et al. Orthopedic manifestations of acute pediatric leukemia. Orthop Clin North Am 1996; 27: 635–644

Goncalves M et al. Diagnosis of malignancies in children with musculoskeletal complaints. Sao Paolo Med J 2005; 123: 21–23

Müller HL et al. Acute lymphoblastic leukaemia with severe skeletal involvement: a subset of childhood leukaemia with a good prognosis. Pediatr Hematol Oncol 1998; 15: 121–133

Definition

- **Epidemiology**
  Incidence is approximately 3% of all newborns • Eight times more common in girls than boys • Unilateral dislocation affects the left hip twice as often as the right hip • Over 25% of affected infants have bilateral dislocation.
- **Etiology, pathophysiology, pathogenesis**
  Etiology is unknown • Several risk factors have been postulated—familial history (especially maternal), breech presentation, foot deformities, oligohydramnios • Late or deficient hip development • Malposition of the femur to the acetabulum • Abnormal development of the roof of the acetabulum and the acetabular cavity itself • Loose joint capsule due to maternal hormones exacerbates joint instability • Incongruity of the articular surfaces can lead to interposition of connective tissue or joint capsule.
  Sequelae of joint deformity:
  - Shallow acetabulum with a steep angle of the acetabular roof.
  - Deformed femoral head.
  - Steep angle of the femoral neck.

Imaging Signs

- **Ultrasound findings**
  Patient is examined in the lateral position with the hip slightly flexed and internally rotated and the knee flexed (5–7.5 MHz) • Dynamic examination with compression and traction applied to the thigh.
  Landmarks for the standard imaging plane: The inferior margin of the ilium is clearly visualized • The anterior margin of the ilium forms a straight line • The bony acetabular convexity is well visualized • The acetabular labrum is clearly demarcated.
  Reference lines and angles:
  - *Base line:* Caudal tangent along the ilium.
  - *Line of the acetabular roof:* Tangent along the inferior margin of the acetabular roof.
  - *Line of the cartilaginous roof:* From the bony convexity through the acetabular labrum.
  - *Acetabular inclination angle (α):* Between the base line and the line of the acetabular roof.
  - *Cartilage roof angle (β):* Between the line of the acetabular roof and the line of the cartilaginous roof.

  Qualitative evaluation: Shape of the acetabulum • Position of the femoral head • Shape of the bony and cartilaginous rim • Reflection of the cartilaginous acetabular convexity • Position of the acetabular labrum.
  Quantitative evaluation: Acetabular inclination angle (α) • Cartilage roof angle (β).
- **Color Doppler ultrasound**
  Not yet a standard diagnostic procedure • Allows evaluation of femoral head perfusion.

Table 6.3 Ultrasound stages according to Graf

Type	Characteristics	Bony modeling	Bony rim	Cartilage roof triangle
Ia (every age)	• Mature hip • $\alpha \geq 60°$ • $\beta < 55°$	Good	Angular	Good coverage
Ib (every age)	• Mature hip • $\alpha \geq 60°$ • $\beta > 55°$	Good	Blunt	Good coverage
II a+ (normal age-related aturation deficit)	• Physiologically immature • $\alpha = 50–59°$ (normal age-related reading) • $\beta > 55°$	Sufficient	Round	Good coverage
II a– (maturation deficient until 3 months old)	• Physiologically immature • $\alpha = 50–59°$ (reading shows maturation deficit) • $\beta > 55°$	Deficient	Round	Good coverage
II b (maturation deficient after 3 months old)	• Delayed ossification • $\alpha = 50–59°$ • $\beta > 55°$	Deficient	Round	Good coverage
II c (every age)	• Hazard range • $\alpha = 43–49°$ • $\beta < 77°$	Highly deficient	Round to flat	Satisfactory coverage
II d	• Beginning eccentricity • $\alpha = 43–49°$ • $\beta > 77°$	Highly deficient	Round to flat	Displaced
III a	• Eccentric joint • $\alpha < 43°$ • $\beta > 77°$	Poor	Flat	Cranially displaced without structural alteration
III b	• Eccentric joint • $\alpha < 43°$ • $\beta > 77°$	Poor	Flat	Cranially displaced with structural alteration
IV	• Eccentric joint • $\beta > 77°$	Poor	Flat	Medially and caudally displaced

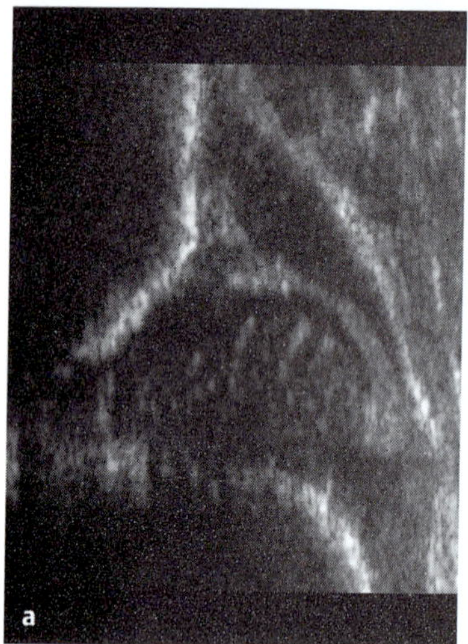

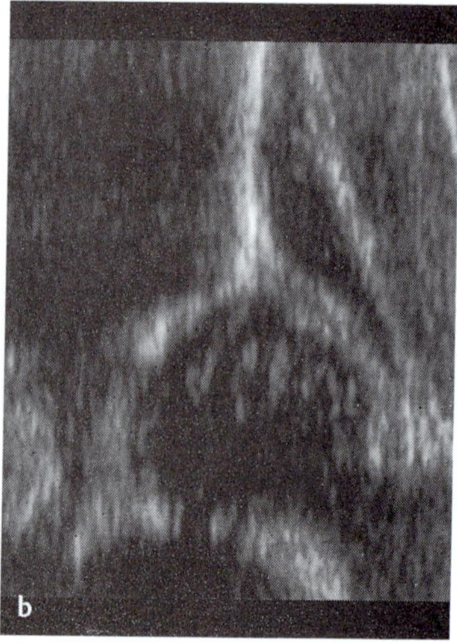

Fig. 6.25 a, b Developmental dysplasia of the left hip. Ultrasound scans of the affected side (**a**) and normal contralateral side (**b**). Eccentric left hip with poor bony modeling. The bony rim is flat and the cartilaginous labrum is cranially displaced without structural alteration (α: 40°, β: 80°, hip type III a according to Graf classification).

Fig. 6.26 Infant with an irreducible dislocation of the dysplastic left hip. MRI (T2-weighted TSE image) of both hips. The epiphyseal center of the left femoral head is smaller than the contralateral side. Hip dislocation and cartilage hypertrophy in the left acetabulum.

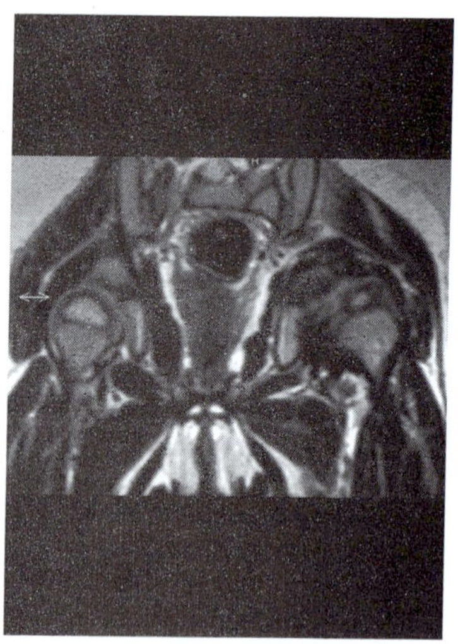

- **Plain pelvis radiograph**
  Useful primarily after the onset of epiphyseal ossification • Demonstrates the extent of defective acetabular ossification • Demonstrates the severity of subluxation or dislocation of the femoral head.
  Common measurements include:
  - *Hilgenreiner or Y line:* Passes through the superior margin of the triradiate cartilage bilaterally • Shows the relationship between femoral head and acetabulum • Provides the basis for other indicators.
  - *Acetabular index:* Angle between the tangent along the acetabular roof and the Hilgenreiner line • Normal value = 25–29°.
  - *Perkins–Ombrédanne line:* Vertical line from the farthest corner of the ossified acetabular cartilage to the Hilgenreiner line • The epiphysis of the femoral head should lie in the inner lower quadrants of the crosshair figure created by the intersection of the lines.
  - *Shenton's line:* Arc from the medial aspect of the femoral neck to the superior margin of the obturator foramen • Interrupted in dislocation.
  - *Andre von Rosen line:* Defines the position of the longitudinal axis of the femoral shaft relative to the acetabulum • Image is obtained with the hip abducted 45° and internally rotated • In a normal hip, the line intersects the pelvis at the margin of the acetabulum.
- **Arthrography**
  Useful where there are impediments to reduction.
- **CT**
  Sometimes used preoperatively to obtain a three-dimensional representation of the extent of subluxation or dislocation • Occasionally used postoperatively to verify proper hip position.
- **MRI**
  Used only in difficult cases • For postoperative follow-up.

Clinical Aspects

- **Typical presentation**
  Abduction is limited with the hip flexed • Inguinal fold is deepened or asymmetric • Leg appears shortened • Ortolani sign is present • Limited range of motion • Positive Allis or Galeazzi sign • Positive Trendelenburg test • Waddling gait in older children.
- **Therapeutic options**
  Pavlik harness to maintain hip abduction, flexion and external rotation is indicated for stage II c or greater according to Graf • Duration of therapy depends on the age and severity of dysplasia • Regular follow-up is indicated • Surgical hip reduction and use of a splint or cast may be necessary • Pelvic osteotomy (Salter or triple osteotomy) may be required to improve coverage of the femoral head.
- **Course and prognosis**
  With early diagnosis and treatment, the disorder usually resolves without complication • Left untreated, the disorder increases the risk of early osteoarthritis of the hip • Surgery can improve the prognosis in cases that are diagnosed late.

▸ **Complications**

Where treatment is performed late, residual acetabular dysplasia, coxa valga with anteversion, or a combination of both may persist • Dysplasia with degenerative joint disease • Avascular necrosis of the femoral head (rare).

Differential Diagnosis

Poliomyelitis, neuromuscular disorders	– Increased muscle tone leads to deformities – Capsular ligaments are tight – No bony deformities
Suppurative arthritis	– Clinical signs of infection – Hip effusion – Synovitis – Aspirated purulent synovial fluid
Proximal femoral focal deficiency	– Shortened femur with deformed or absent head and neck – Enlarged obturator foramen – Horizontal or dysplastic acetabulum – Hypertrophy of the sartorius leads to flexion, abduction, and external rotation in the hip.

Tips and Pitfalls

Precise patient positioning is required for the plain pelvis radiograph to prevent inaccurate measurements due to improper rotation • Delayed ossification of the epiphysis (delayed maturation) can be a sign of developmental dysplasia of the hip • Where typical ultrasound visualization of the hip is not possible, a pelvis radiograph is indicated to determine the cause (for example, skeletal dysplasia).

Selected References

Cady RB. Developmental dysplasia of the hip: definition, recognition and prevention of late sequelae. Pediatr Ann 2006; 35: 92–101

Harcke HT. Screening newborns for developmental dysplasia of the hip: the role of sonography. Am J Roentgenol 1994; 162: 395–397

Jaramillo D et al. Gadolinium-enhanced MR imaging of pediatric patients after reduction of dysplastic hips: assessment of femoral head position, factors impeding reduction, and femoral head ischemia. AJR Am J Roentgenol 1998; 170: 1633–1637

Rosendahl K et al. Ultrasound in the diagnosis of developmental dysplasia of the hip in newborns. The European approach. A review of methods, accuracy and clinical validity. Eur Radiol 2007; 17: 1960–7

von Kries R et al. Effect of ultrasound screening on the rate of first operative procedures for developmental hip dysplasia in Germany. Lancet 2003; 362: 1883–1887

US Preventive Services Task Force. Screening for developmental dysplasia of the hip: recommendation statement. Pediatrics 2006; 117: 898–902

Definition

▸ **Epidemiology**
Incidence is 1:10 000 • Peak age in girls is 8–15 years, in boys 10–17 years • Boys are affected three times as often as girls • Bilateral in 2–40% of cases • Contralateral slipped capital femoral epiphysis often occurs within a year of the initial manifestation.

▸ **Etiology, pathophysiology, pathogenesis**
In children the femoral head and neck are connected by the growth plate • Body weight can produce a fracture (Salter–Harris type I) in areas with hypertrophic chondrocytes • The epiphysis slides off the metaphysis.
Predisposing factors: Obesity • Acute growth spurt • Primary hypothyroidism • Growth hormone deficiency • Developmental dysplasia of the hip • Down syndrome.

Imaging Signs

▸ **Ultrasound findings**
Examination performed with hip in various degrees of rotational positions • Joint effusion • Synovial thickening.

▸ **Radiographic findings**
Anteroposterior and lateral frog-leg views are indicated • Loss of the Capener triangle sign (triangular shadow due to the medial aspect of the femoral neck overlapping the posterior wall of the acetabulum). The Klein tangent (along the outer cortex of the femoral neck) no longer intersects the epiphysis • Periarticular osteoporosis • Later there is asymmetric widening and loss of definition in the growth plate • Apparent reduction in the height of the epiphysis • Posteromedial and caudal displacement of the epiphysis • Ill-defined margin or sclerosis of the metaphysis • In chronic cases, the femoral neck comes to resemble a pistol grip • Severity is graded according to the displacement of the slipped capital femoral epiphysis
Lateral head/shaft angle: This slip angle is measured on the frog-leg lateral radiograph and describes the difference between the femoral shaft and a perpendicular of the femoral epiphysis (< 10° is normal).
Classification:
- *Grade I:* Mild form, < 30°
- *Grade II:* Moderate form, 30–50°
- *Grade III:* Severe form, > 50°

Postoperative evaluation of implant position and union in the growth plate.

▸ **CT findings**
May be used to evaluate the extent of displacement when conventional radiographs do not provide sufficient information • Findings include widened growth plates.

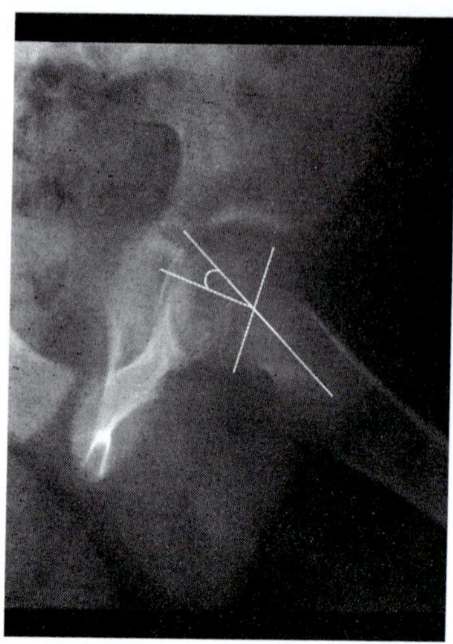

Fig. 6.27 Slipped capital femoral epiphysis. Frog-leg lateral view of the left hip. Posteromedial and cranial epiphyseal displacement. The slip angle is 20°, representing the mild (grade I) slipped capital femoral epiphysis.

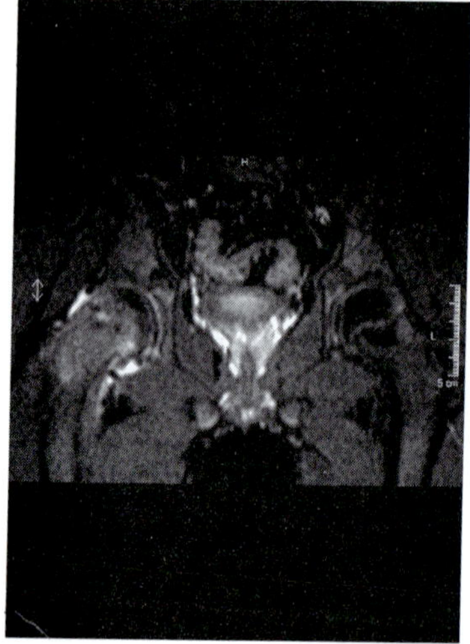

Fig. 6.28 Acute moderate right slipped capital femoral epiphysis. MR STIR image. Joint effusion, widened hyperintense physis (growth plate), and metaphyseal and epiphyseal bone marrow edema. Left side appears normal.

- **MRI findings**
  Widening of the physis (growth plate) is detectable sooner than on conventional radiographs • The growth plate is hyperintense on T2-weighted (STIR) images • Morphologic distortion of the growth plate • Bone marrow edema in the metaphysis and epiphysis • Joint effusion • Contrast-enhanced dynamic MRI may be used to evaluate perfusion of the femoral head before and after surgery (internal fixation with titanium pins or screws).
- **Bone scan**
  Tracer uptake in the hip is increased in synovitis • Tracer uptake in the growth plate is decreased in avascular necrosis.

Clinical Aspects

- **Typical presentation**
  Classification according to severity and duration of clinical symptoms:
  - *Acute:* Acute pain in the groin or the knee and limited motion • Children are suddenly unable to walk • Leg moves into compensatory abduction and external rotation when the hip is flexed (positive Drehmann sign).
  - *Chronic:* Symptoms for more than 3 weeks • Fatigue after weight bearing • Limp • Often dismissed as harmless • Limited motion and external rotation deformity.
  - *Acute-on-chronic:* Acute symptoms in the setting of chronic slipped capital femoral epiphysis • Acute worsening of the epiphyseal slippage angle as displacement of the epiphysis increases.
  - *Preslip:* Mild clinical symptoms with a widened and irregular growth plate • No detectable slippage of the epiphysis on conventional radiographs.

  A further distinction is made between stable and unstable slipped capital femoral epiphysis, which reflects whether the patient is able to walk or not.
- **Therapeutic options**
  Emergency • Immediate bed rest with no weight bearing • Brief traction treatment may be considered • Transepiphyseal pinning or screw fixation is usually carried out without any attempt at reduction.
- **Course and prognosis**
  Prognosis is good for cases diagnosed early and treated surgically by epiphysiodesis • Unstable lesions have a less favorable prognosis • Chances of healing are directly proportional to the severity of the lesion.
- **Complications**
  Chondrolysis occurs in about 30–35% of cases • Early osteoarthritis of the hip (25–30%) • Joint space narrowing • Pain • Limited range of motion • Associated synovitis may also occur.
  Avascular necrosis of the femoral head: Frequency: 25% • Also occurs as a postoperative complication • Pain • Limited range of motion • Displacement of implants.

Differential Diagnosis

Acute transient synovitis of the hip	– Hip effusion – Normal growth plate – No slipped capital femoral epiphysis
Legg–Calvé–Perthes disease	– Children are younger (age 5–8 years) – Fragmentation of the femoral head, flattening of the growth plate, and subsequent coxa magna – Bone marrow edema in the femoral head with impaired perfusion on contrast-enhanced MRI – Joint effusion, synovitis
Traumatic slipped capital femoral epiphysis	– Clear history of trauma – Rarely, occurs in newborns as birth trauma

Tips and Pitfalls

Normal findings on conventional radiographs do not exclude slipped capital femoral epiphysis • Be alert to the possibility of bilateral slipped capital femoral epiphyses when comparing the affected hip with the contralateral hip.

Selected References

Bhatia NM et al. Body mass index in patients with slipped capital femoral epiphysis. J Pediatr Orthop 2006; 26: 197–199

Billing L et al. Slipped capital femoral epiphysis. The mechanical function of the periosteum: new aspects and theory including bilaterality. Acta Radiol Suppl 2004; 432: 1–27

Katz DA. Slipped capital femoral epiphysis: The importance of early diagnosis. Pediatr Ann 2006; 35: 102–111

Kennedy JG et al: Osteonecrosis of the femoral head associated with slipped capital femoral epiphysis. J Pediatr Orthop 2001; 21: 189–193

Loder RT et al. Slipped capital femoral epiphysis. J Bone Joint Surg 2000; 82: 1170–1188

Staatz G et al. Evaluation of femoral head vascularization in slipped capital femoral epiphysis before and after cannulated-screw fixation with use of contrast-enhanced MRI: initial results. Eur Radiol 2007; 17: 163–168

Definition

- **Epidemiology**

  Incidence is 1:1000–5000 • Occurs between 3 and 12 years • Peak age is about 5–6 years • Bilateral involvement occurs in 10–20% of cases • Boys are affected four times as often as girls.

- **Etiology, pathophysiology, pathogenesis**

  Aseptic necrosis • Etiology is unclear • Suggested possible causes include idiopathic osteonecrosis, impaired blood supply to the epiphyseal center of the femoral head, bone infarction due to repeated microtrauma • Initially, epiphyseal blood supply is impaired • This leads to bone necrosis • A growth disturbance then occurs in the femoral head with hypertrophy of the epiphyseal cartilage • During the fragmentation stage, the necrotic bone is resorbed • Cartilage-containing cysts or pseudocysts occurs in the metaphysis • The articular surface of the femoral head collapses over necrotic zones (subchondral fracture) • Loss of bony support in the lateral column leads to lateral displacement and subluxation of the femoral head • Rapid subsidence of the epiphysis leads to incongruity of the articular surfaces (hinge abduction: impingement of the superolateral portion of the femoral head on the lateral lip of the acetabulum) • In the repair stage, bone cells recolonize and rebuild the femoral head.

  Classification according to Catterall (reflects the extent of epiphyseal changes):

  - *Stage 1:* Less than 25% of the epiphysis (anteromedial portion) is involved • There is no subchondral collapse • No fragmentation of the femoral head.
  - *Stage 2:* Less than half of the epiphysis is affected • Collapse of the involved segment • The medial and lateral segments are still well preserved • Minor cystic changes in the metaphysis.
  - *Stage 3:* Almost the entire epiphysis is affected • Epiphysis appears dense with a “head-within-a-head appearance” • Diffuse metaphyseal involvement • Femoral neck is widened.
  - *Stage 4:* Entire epiphysis shows collapse and sequestration • Femoral head is flattened.

  Catterall supplemented this classification with risk factors (head at risk):

  - Lateral subluxation of the femoral head.
  - Horizontal growth plate.
  - Calcifications lateral to the epiphysis
  - Radiolucent V-shaped segment in the outer portion of the femoral head (Gage sign).
  - Extensive metaphyseal involvement.

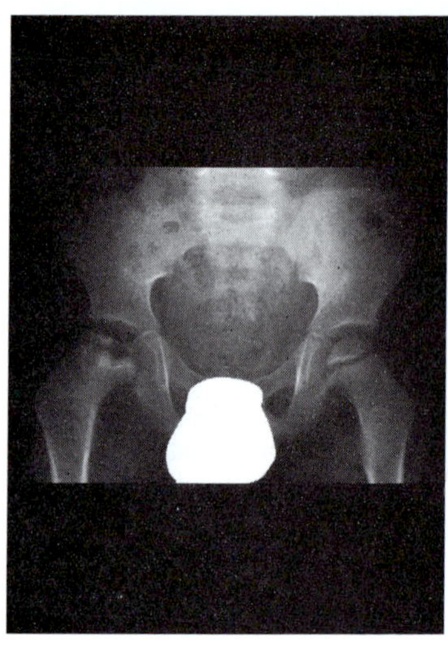

Fig. 6.29 Fragmentation stage of Legg–Calvé–Perthes disease in the right pelvis of a 5-year-old boy. Pelvic radiograph. Severe collapse of the right capital femoral epiphysis (stage IV according to Caterall). Large cystic lesions in the metaphysis, joint space widening, and beginning shortening and widening of the femoral neck.

Imaging Signs

- **Radiographic findings (plain pelvis radiograph, frog-leg view)**
  Stages according to Waldenström:
  - *Initial stage:* Widened joint space • Laterally displaced femoral head.
  - *Condensation stage:* Increased density of the femoral head • Subchondral fracture (superior and anterolateral) • Widened joint space • Laterally displaced femoral head.
  - *Fragmentation and reabsorption stage:* Fragmentation and collapse of the epiphysis • Metaphyseal cysts and pseudocysts.
  - *Reossification stage:* Reossification of the epiphysis • Enlargement and deformation of the femoral head (coxa magna) • Shortening and widening of the femoral neck • Cranial displacement of the greater trochanter.
  - *Healing stage:* Articular surfaces exhibit physiologic or pathologic congruity or incongruity (mushroom-shaped coxa magna, coxa vara with cranially displaced greater trochanter).
- **Ultrasound findings**
  Joint effusion • Flattening of the epiphysis • Epiphyseal contour is irregular • Occasionally fragmentation will be detectable.
- **MRI**
  Morphologic changes are visualized • Joint effusion • Cartilage hypertrophy • Subluxation of the femoral head • Coxa magna • Signal changes vary with the specific stage of the disorder:
  - The signal characteristics of the femoral head are initially unchanged • The contrast-enhanced images show reduced perfusion.

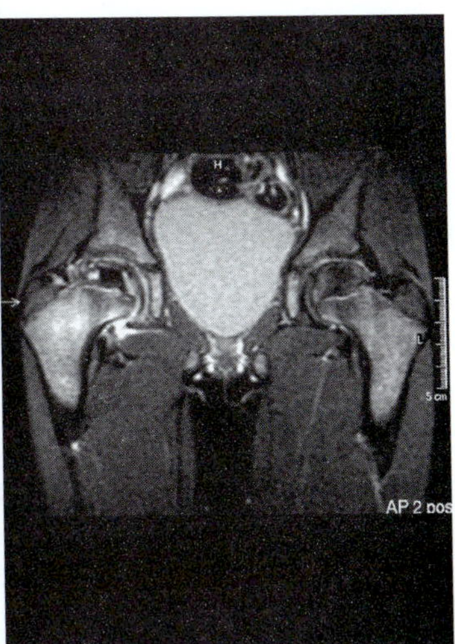

Fig. 6.30 Fragmentation stage of Legg–Calvé–Perthes disease in the right hip. MR STIR image. The medial and lateral fragments of the femoral head exhibit a bone marrow edema consistent with viable bone. The central fragment is nonviable and shows a signal void.

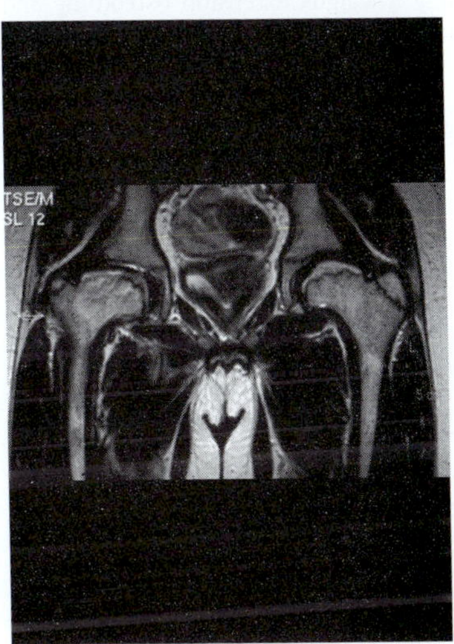

Fig. 6.31 Reossification stage of Legg–Calvé–Perthes disease. MR T2-weighted TSE image. Bilaterally enlarged femoral heads with mushroom deformity, shortened and widened femoral necks. No joint effusion, and the capital femoral epiphyses exhibit normal signal behavior indicative of reparative processes.

- Fragmentation stage: Viable fragments show bone marrow edema (hyperintense on T2-weighted images) and contrast enhancement • Nonviable fragments are hypointense or show signal-void (STIR, T2-weighted images) and do not enhance • Metaphyseal involvement is visualized as round lesions that appear hyperintense on T2-weighted images.
- Reossification stage: Bone marrow edema regresses • Perfusion of the femoral head returns to normal • Coxa magna.

► **Bone scan**
Tracer uptake in the early stage is reduced due to ischemia • Uptake is increased in the late stage due to revascularization and reparative processes.

Clinical Aspects

► **Typical presentation**
Limp due to pain in the hip, thigh, and knee • Range of motion is limited (internal rotation, abduction) • Adduction • No history of trauma.

► **Therapeutic options**
Up to 50% of cases resolve spontaneously • *Conservative treatment:* Suspension in a Thomas splint • *Surgical treatment:* Intertrochanteric varus osteotomy, Salter pelvic osteotomy, or triple osteotomy • Valgus extension osteotomy and Chiari pelvic osteotomy are used to treat late findings where the hip can no longer be reduced.

► **Course and prognosis**
Prognosis is better in young children • Prognosis is worse in children older than 8 years • Unfavorable prognostic factors include female sex, calcifications lateral to the epiphysis, metaphyseal radiolucencies, and involvement of more than 50% of the epiphysis.

► **Complications**
Leg length difference • Arthritis • Hip dislocation (may occur with a large deformed femoral head) • Coxa magna • Coxa plana • Osteoarthritis of the hip.

Differential Diagnosis

Meyer dysplasia	– Bilateral – Epiphyseal dysplasia of the femoral heads – Most common at 2–5 years – Asymptomatic – MRI does not show any impaired perfusion or bone marrow changes
Transient synovitis of the hip	– Acute, self-limiting disorder (3–10 days) – Common in boys younger than 4 years – Synovitis and joint effusion – No bony changes
Juvenile osteonecrosis	– Avascular necrosis in the presence of a known underlying disorder such as sickle cell anemia, thalassemia, or a coagulation disorder

Septic arthritis	– Acute malaise; hip flexed, abducted, and externally rotated – Signs of inflammation – Severe joint effusion, synovitis – Bone marrow edema on MRI
Juvenile rheumatoid arthritis	– Fever, positive antinuclear antibodies, rash, atrophy of the thigh muscles – Synovitis – Signs of ischemia in the femoral head in chronic disease
Slipped capital femoral epiphysis	– Caudal and posteromedial displacement of the femoral capital epiphysis – Metaphyseal and diaphyseal bone marrow edema – Widening and distortion of the physis (growth plate)

Tips and Pitfalls

It is important to recognize the early clinical signs as the radiographic findings and manifest disease only occur later • Hip symptoms that persist longer than a week suggest Legg–Calvé–Perthes disease • Radiographs are indicated and MRI should be considered in patients presenting with inexplicable hip symptoms.

Selected References

Crofton PM et al. Children with acute Perthes'disease have asymmetrical lower leg growth and abnormal collagen turnover. Acta Orthop 2005; 76: 841–847

Dezateux C et al. The puzzles of Perthes' disease: definitive studies of causal factors are needed. J Bone Joint Surg [Br] 2005; 87: 1463–1464

Lamer S et al. Femoral head vascularisation in Legg–Calve–Perthes disease: comparison of dynamic gadolinium-enhanced subtraction MRI with bone scintigraphy. Pediatr Radiol 2002; 32: 580–585

Mahnken et al. MR signal intensity characteristics in Legg–Calve–Perthes disease. Value of fat-suppressed (STIR) images and contrast-enhanced T1-weighted images. Acta Radiol 2002; 43: 329–335

van Campenhout A et al. Serial bone scintigraphy in Legg-Calve-Perthes disease: correlation with the Catterall and Herring classification. J Pediatr Orthop 2006; 15: 6–10

Definition

- **Epidemiology**

  Hemangioma: Most common mass in children • Affects 2% of all children • Higher incidence (15%) in premature infants • Girls are affected three times as often as boys.

  Arteriovenous malformation: Vascular malformations are the most common congenital abnormalities • No sex predilection.

- **Etiology, pathophysiology, pathogenesis**

  Hemangioma: A genuine neoplasm of proliferative endothelial cells • 60% of hemangiomas occur in the head and neck, 25% in the trunk, and 15% in the extremities • Lesions may be solitary (80%), multiple (20%), or diffuse • In 60% of cases, lesions are not present at birth or are very small • Size increases rapidly during the first few weeks of life • Spontaneous involution often occurs over a period of years • Residual lesions are present in up to 50% of cases • *Types:* Capillary (common, present at birth), cavernous (less common, occurring in infants) and arteriovenous hemangiomas.

  Arteriovenous malformation: Not a genuine neoplasm, rather a congenital vascular malformation • Dysplastic arteries and veins • Malformation arises due to defective differentiation of the embryonal vascular plexus in a capillary network • Arteriovenous shunts persist • Vascular convolutions without a soft tissue component • Lesions may suddenly expand under stress, with trauma, or with hormonal changes • Proliferative growth does not occur • Lesions grow proportionately with the child • Involution does not occur • These are "high-flow" lesions.

Imaging Signs

- **Ultrasound findings**

  Hemangioma: Lobulated, well demarcated lesion • Mixed echogenicity • Often located in the subcutaneous tissue • Increased flow on color Doppler and power Doppler studies • Increased vascular density.

  Arteriovenous malformation: Heterogeneous echogenicity • Vascular convolution • No soft tissue component • Color Doppler shows high vascularity, many tortuous vessels, and an arterial feeder and draining veins • Power Doppler demonstrates systolic bruit, arteriovenous shunt, and pulsatile venous flow.

- **Radiographic findings**

  Hemangioma: Soft tissue proliferation • Phleboliths may be present.

  Arteriovenous malformation: Lesions occasionally contain fatty tissue and can mimic soft tissue proliferation • Bone involvement is rare; findings include bone destruction or hypertrophy.

- **Contrast CT findings**

  Hemangioma: CT is used for lesions in the mediastinum, head, or neck • Circumscribed lobulated lesion with large draining vein showing diffuse contrast enhancement.

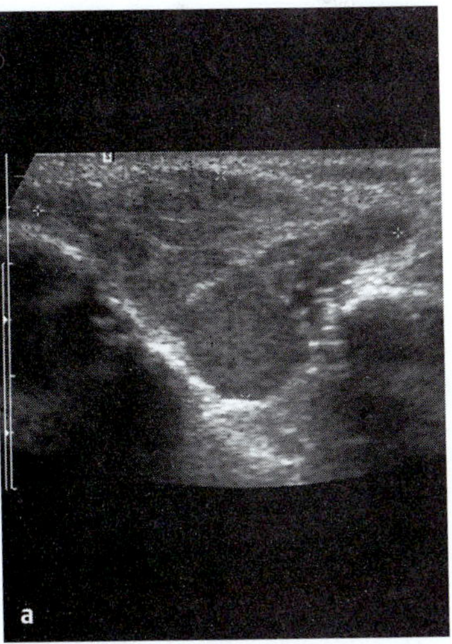

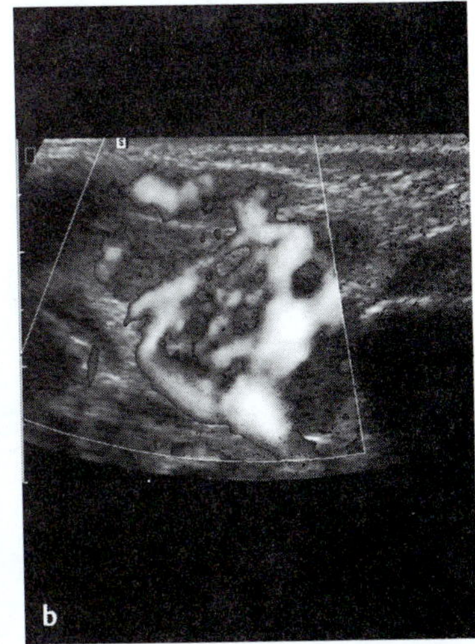

Fig. 6.32 a, b Soft tissue hemangioma. Ultrasound (**a**) and power Doppler (**b**). Well demarcated, primarily hyperechoic lesion. Power Doppler demonstrates hyperperfusion (high-flow hemangioma).

Arteriovenous malformation: CT is only used where lesions are poorly accessible to ultrasound and MRI is contraindicated.

▸ **Contrast MRI findings**

Hemangioma: Circumscribed lobulated lesion • Hyperintense on T2-weighted images with fat suppression • Isointense to muscle on T1-weighted images • Draining vein is detectable as a flow artifact or as a high-flow vessel on GRE images • Diffuse contrast enhancement • Can contain fat in the involution stage.

Arteriovenous malformation:

- T1-weighted images: Vascular convolution with multiple flow artifacts.
- T2-weighted images: Flow artifacts in multiple vessels • No soft tissue component • In edema, the surrounding tissue is occasionally hyperintense.
- T2*-weighted GE images: Hyperintense where blood flow is fast.
- T1-weighted images with contrast: Marked enhancement in the vascular structures.
- MR angiography: Helpful in preoperative planning • Vascular convolution with arterial feeder and draining vein (much larger than the artery).

▸ **Angiography**

Hemangioma: When complications are present • When embolization is planned • In a circumscribed lesion.

Arteriovenous malformation: When planning and carrying out embolization • To exclude an anastomosis with intracranial vessels in lesions located in the head • Visualization of often multiple afferent vascular structures.

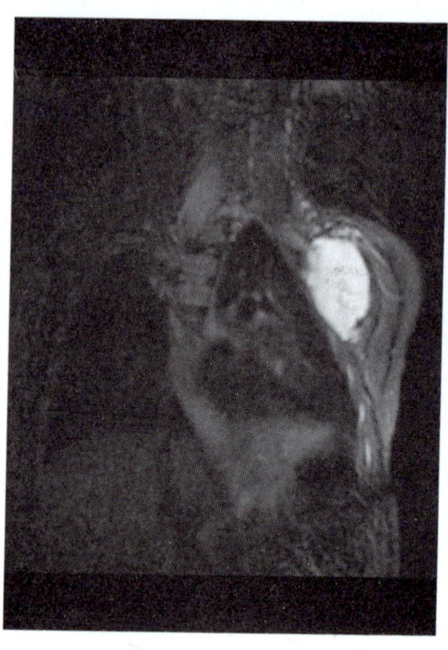

Fig. 6.33 Hemangioma in the chest wall of an infant. MR coronal STIR image. Well demarcated, markedly hyperintense mass in the soft tissue of the left anterolateral chest wall. No intrathoracic component.

Clinical Aspects

- **Typical presentation**

  Hemangioma: Bright red lesion where skin is involved • Subcutaneous lesions have a bluish appearance • Venous hum, pulsation, and a sensation of warmth during the proliferation phase • Fissures • Ulcerations • Bleeding.
  Arteriovenous malformation: Pulsatile structure • Venous hum • Warming • Skin changes • Pain • Bleeding where ulceration occurs • Heart failure • Steal syndrome.

- **Therapeutic options**

  Hemangioma: This depends on the child's age and the position, depth, and size of the hemangioma.
  - Less than 2 mm in depth and less than 1.5 cm in diameter: Cryotherapy.
  - Less than 2 mm in depth and more than 1.5 cm in diameter: Pulsed-dye laser.
  - More than 2 mm in depth in the face: Nd:Yag laser.
  - More than 2 mm in depth in the eyelid or hair-covered areas: Surgery.
  - In the face: Cryotherapy • Laser • Secondary surgery may be indicated.
  - Eyelid and hair-covered scalp: Cryotherapy • Surgery.
  - Trunk and extremities: Often no treatment is required.
  - With complications and in rapidly growing hemangiomas: Systemic cortisone • Interferon.

  Arteriovenous malformation: Embolization with coils, gel particles, or ethanol • Surgery (after embolization).

- **Course and prognosis**
  Hemangioma: 90% of all lesions involute spontaneously by age 9 years • A residual lesion remains in 40–50% of cases (telangiectasia, pigmentation, scarring, fibrotic fatty tissue).
  Arteriovenous malformation: These lesions do not resolve spontaneously • Most cases require treatment.
- **Complications**
  Hemangioma: Ulceration and bleeding • Compression of vital structures • Kasabach–Merritt syndrome (disseminated intravascular coagulation) • Psychologic distress • Heart failure.
  Arteriovenous malformation: Ulceration • Bleeding • Steal syndrome • Heart failure • Bone involvement may lead to length difference in the extremities.

Differential Diagnosis

Venous malformation	– Congenital, does not involute spontaneously – Multiple tortuous vascular structures, hyperintense on T2-weighted images – Hypointense on GRE images
Lymphatic malformation	– Congenital – Cystic septated lesion, occasionally with hemorrhage – Hyperintense on T2-weighted images – Contrast enhancement of the septa – No flow sign
Soft tissue sarcoma	– Soft tissue component – Pseudocapsule

Tips and Pitfalls

A convolution of high-flow vessels without a soft tissue component suggests an arteriovenous malformation • A lesion with a soft tissue component is more likely a hemangioma or vascular tumor • In multiple hemangiomas (hemangiomatosis), visceral hemangiomas should be excluded.

Selected References

Abernethy LJ. Classification and imaging of vascular malformations in children. Eur Radiol 2003; 13: 2483–2497

Gorincour G et al. Imaging characteristics of two subtypes of congenital hemangiomas: rapidly involuting congenital hemangiomas and non-involuting congenital hemangiomas. Pediatr Radiol 2005; 5: 1178–1185

Konez O et al. Magnetic resonance of vascular anomalies. Magn Reson Imaging Clin North Am 2002; 10: 363–388

Lee BB et al. Management of arteriovenous malformations: a multidisciplinary approach. J Vasc Surg 2004, 39: 590–600

Steven M et al. Haemangiomas and vascular malformations of the limb in children. Pediatr Surg Int 2007; 23: 565–569

Definition

- **Epidemiology**
  Incidence is 1:6000 • In 50% of cases, a lesion can be demonstrated immediately after birth • In 90%, a lesion occurs by age 2 years.
- **Etiology, pathophysiology, pathogenesis**
  Cysts lined by epithelium • Contents are serous and milky • Macrocystic and microcystic forms occur • Disorder is associated with Turner syndrome; trisomy 21, 18, and 13; fetal alcohol syndrome; and Noonan syndrome • Common sites include the neck (75% of lesions), mediastinum (3–10% of which half are continuous with neck lesions), axilla (20%), and chest wall (14%) • Mesenteric occurrence is less common • Can occur secondary to congenitally impaired lymph drainage (lack of communication between the jugular lymphatic chain and the jugular vein, Virchow node).

Imaging Signs

- **Ultrasound findings**
  Fluid-filled mass with thin septa • Usually a very extensive process • Hyperechoic when hemorrhages are present • Compressible with the transducer • The microcystic variant can appear primarily solid.
- **Color Doppler ultrasound findings**
  Septa are at most slightly vascularized • Lesion compresses adjacent vascular structures.
- **CT findings**
  Extensive cystic mass with peripheral contrast enhancement • Density values vary with protein content and hemorrhages • Adjacent structures are displaced • Vascular compression.
- **MRI findings**
  Fluid-filled spaces are particularly well visualized on T2-weighted images • The signal intensity on T1-weighted images depends on protein content and hemorrhages • There may be fluid levels within the cysts (hemorrhage) • No detectable flow • Moderate contrast enhancement in the septa • Mass effect is recognizable.

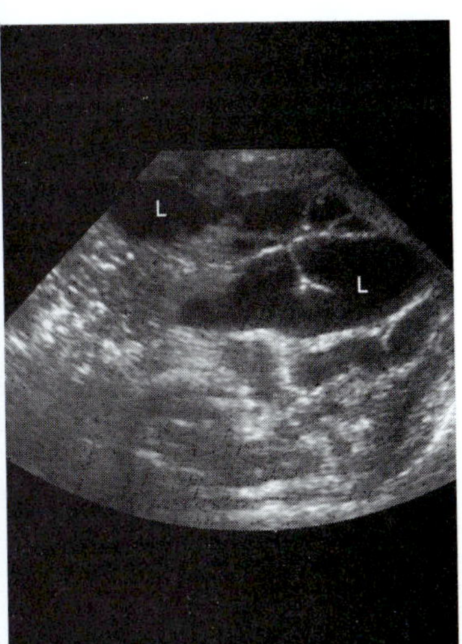

Fig. 6.34 Lymphangioma in a newborn. Ultrasound. Large cystic right cervical lymphangioma (L). Typical ultrasound morphology: Multicystic multiseptated mass that exhibits no flow signal on color Doppler ultrasound.

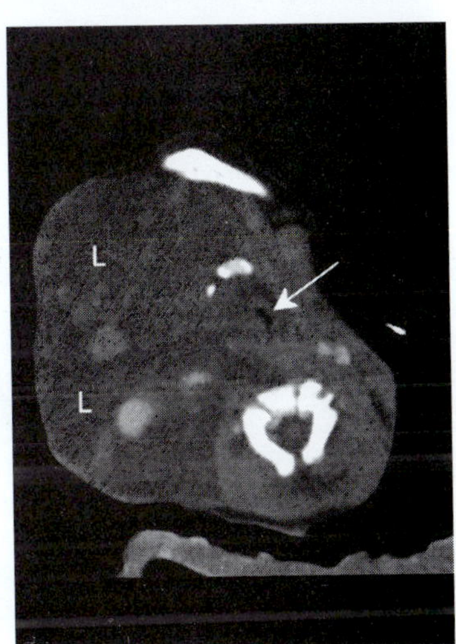

Fig. 6.35 Contrast-enhanced CT. The extent of the lymphangioma (L) is better visualized and hemorrhages are demonstrated. The tumor also extends into the parapharyngeal and retropharyngeal regions, displacing and compressing the upper respiratory tract (arrow).

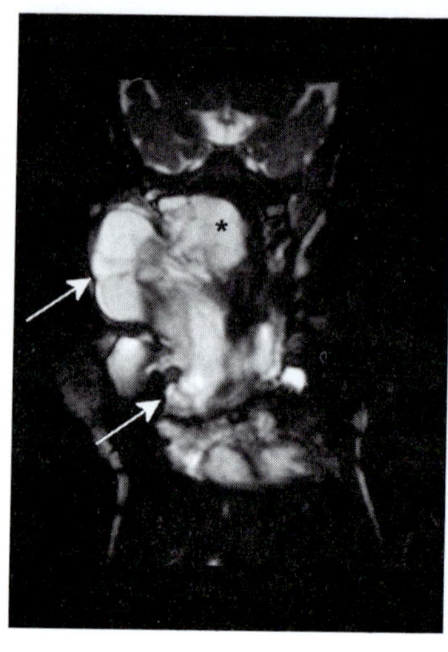

Fig. 6.36 MR fluid-sensitive sequence. Lymphangioma (arrows) appears hyperintense. The parapharyngeal component of the tumor (*) displaces and compresses the lumen of the pharynx.

Clinical Aspects

- **Typical presentation**
  Nonimmune-related hydrops • Peripheral edema • Fetal ascites • Depending on the location of the lesion, adjacent structures may show signs of involvement (e.g., dyspnea, upper inflow tract congestion) • Lesion is soft on palpation.
- **Therapeutic options**
  Surgical resection • Interferon • Percutaneous sclerotherapy • Tracheotomy is indicated in respiratory tract compression.
- **Course and prognosis**
  Slow or rapidly progressive growth • Intrauterine death (33% of cases) • Mortality in hydrops is 100% • Lesion may recur after resection, especially when there was infiltrative growth.
- **Complications**
  Airway compression • Superinfection • Hemorrhage.

Differential Diagnosis

Cervical meningocele or encephalocele	– Spinal origin – Nonseptate mass
Cystic teratoma	– Findings may include calcification – Findings may include fat – Usually also includes more solid components
Thymus cyst	– Caudal to the hyoid bone immediately adjacent to the vascular structures – Can extend into the mediastinum
Cervical cysts	– Median or lateral cystic structure – Much smaller – Septa are rare
Soft tissue sarcoma	– Pseudocapsule – Usually not extensively cystic – Viable tumor components showing marked enhancement
Vascular malformation	– Blood flow detectable on color Doppler ultrasound – Arteriovenous shunts – Flow murmur may be present – Vascular contrast enhancement on CT and MRI
Mesenteric duplication or mesenteric cyst	– Usually nonseptate – Less readily compressible – Does not enhance – Typical position

Tips and Pitfalls

A lymphangioma with hemorrhage must not be confused with a solid process • Cross-sectional imaging is always indicated in large cervical lymphangiomas to visualize the extent into thorax or mediastinum.

Selected References

Dähnert W. Lymphangioma. In: Dähnert W. (ed.) Radiology Review Manual. Baltimore: Williams & Wilkins; 1991: 497

Fliegelman LJ et al. Lymphatic malformation: predictive factors for recurrence. Otolaryngol Head Neck Surg 2000; 123: 706–710

Orvidas LJ et al. Pediatric lymphangiomas of the head and neck. Ann Otol Rhinol Laryngol 2000; 109: 411–421

Won JH et al. Percutaneous sclerotherapy of lymphangiomas with acetic acid. J Vasc Interv Radiol 2004; 15: 595–600

Definition

- **Epidemiology**

  The incidence in central Europe is 21–25 fractures/1000 children per year • The risk of a fracture before end of puberty is estimated at 5–45% • Far more common in boys than girls (13:1).
- **Etiology, pathophysiology, pathogenesis**

  The upper extremity is involved in 74% of cases, the lower extremity in 26% • 65% of fractures are metaphyseal, 25% diaphyseal, and 10% epiphyseal • Forearm fractures are the most common injuries in all age groups.

  Incomplete fractures: Impacted and greenstick fractures • Caused by axial forces acting on the bone • Bones in children are more elastic than in adults • Force is absorbed over a longer portion of the bone • This leads to plastic deformation.
  - Impacted fracture/buckle fracture: Metaphyseal fracture • Cancellous bone and cortex are impacted • Occurs most often in the humerus, radius, and ulna.
  - Greenstick fracture: Bending fracture • The cortex on one aspect of the bone is incompletely fractured whereas the opposite cortex is completely fractured • Most often occurs in the forearm.

  Salter–Harris fractures: Fractures involving the growth plate • These occur because the capsular ligaments are stronger than the physis • With the exception of the femoral head and radial head, the epiphysis and metaphysis have separate vascular supply • Epiphyseal fractures do not impair the blood supply to either structure in cases other than the two exceptions mentioned • Injury is caused by shear, traction, or compression forces acting on the bone • Most common sites include the radius, phalanges, and distal tibia.

Table 6.4 Salter–Harris classification of epiphyseal fractures

Type	Definition
I	Fracture through the growth plate (physis)
II	Fracture through the growth plate and metaphysis (most common)
III	Fracture through the growth plate and epiphysis, intraarticular
IV	Fracture through the metaphysis, growth plate and epiphysis, intraarticular
V	Crush fracture of the growth plate

Supracondylar fracture: Typical fracture of the distal humerus • Mechanism of injury is either extension trauma (95%, fall on the outstretched arm) or flexion trauma (fall on the elbow) • Can be associated with injuries to the olecranon, medial epicondyle, distal radius, brachial artery, ulnar nerve, and median nerve.

Toddler fractures: Common in children learning to walk • The fracture occurs because the bone is not yet adapted to the new loads • Causes include compression, torsion, and bending forces • Common sites include the tibia, fibula, calcaneus, talus, tarsals, and metatarsals.

Transitional fractures of late adolescence: These occur in older adolescents in whom physiologic closure of the growth plates has begun • *Forms:* These include

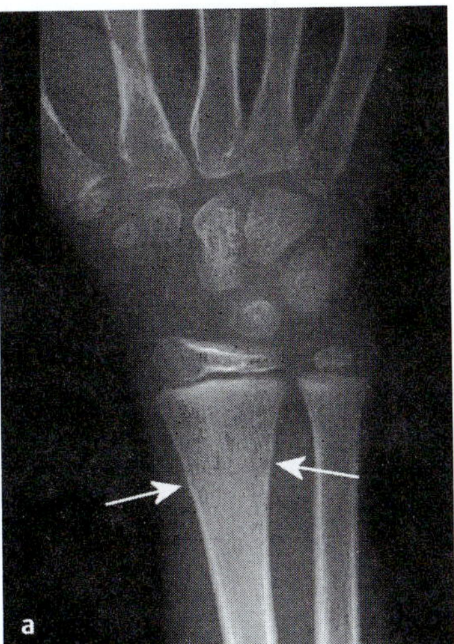

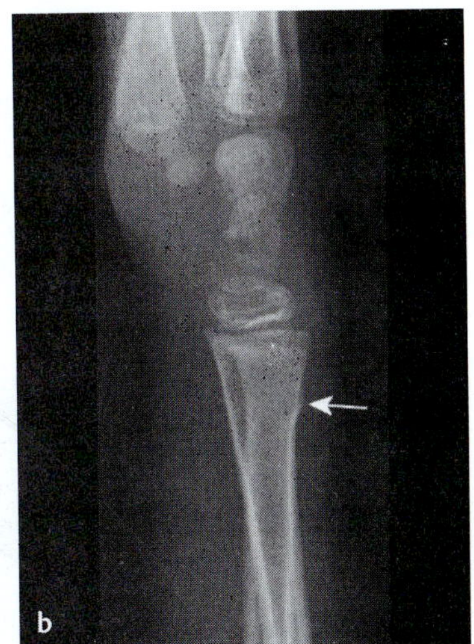

Fig. 6.37 a, b Buckle fracture of the distal radius. Radiographs in two planes. Metaphyseal cortical expansion due to impaction (arrows) is only moderate on the A-P film (**a**) but is clearly visualized on the lateral film (**b**).

two-plane fractures involving a purely epiphyseal fracture and triplane I and II fractures with an additional metaphyseal bending wedge.

Imaging Signs

- **Radiographic findings**

Impacted fracture buckle fracture: Deformation or protrusion of the cortex due to compressive forces • There may be slight angulation of the distal fragment.

Greenstick fracture: Diaphyseal bending fracture with fracture of the convex cortex • Opposite cortex is incompletely fractured • Periosteum is intact.

Salter–Harris fracture: Partial or complete widening of the growth plate • Radiolucent line in the epiphysis and/or metaphysis.

Supracondylar fracture: Positive "fat pad" sign • In extension trauma, the fracture line will extend from a proximal posterior point to a distal volar point • In flexion trauma, the line extends a proximal volar point to a distal posterior point • In up to 25% of cases, there is no visible fracture line • A tangent along the anterior cortex of the humerus intersects the anterior third of the capitellum of the humerus (Rogers line) • Malrotation can be detected by observing the volar bone spur on the lateral film.

Toddler fracture: In the tibia, there will be a hairline spiral fracture (visible as a radiolucent or radiodense line) or protrusion of the anterior cortex and an oblique fracture of the posterior cortex • Other bones exhibit plastic deforma-

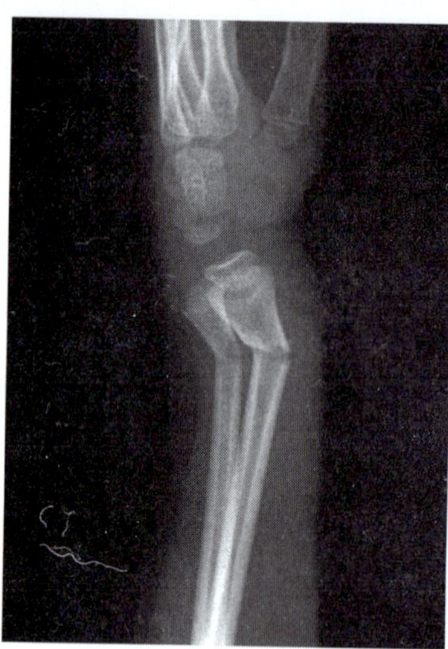

Fig. 6.38 Greenstick fracture of the forearm. Lateral radiograph. Bending fracture with complete disruption of the anterior cortex and partial fracture of the posterior cortex of the radius and ulna.

tion, impacted fracture, compression fracture, or a vertical or horizontal subcortical radiodense line.

Transitional fracture:

- Two-plane fracture: Epiphyseal fracture with avulsed lateral fragment.
- Triplane I fracture: Additional metaphyseal bending wedge; the metaphyseal fracture ends at the growth plate.
- Triplane II fracture: Additional metaphyseal bending wedge; the metaphyseal fracture continues into the growth plate (posterior Volkmann fracture).

► **CT**

Rarely, used in incomplete fractures when the conventional radiograph cannot exclude epiphyseal involvement • Rarely used in epiphyseal fractures and supracondylar fractures for preoperative evaluation of the extent of the fracture and degree of displacement.

► **MRI**

Used in pediatric fractures of the thoracic spine • For detecting occult fractures (bone marrow edema on T2-weighted images) • Preoperatively in premature closure of the growth plate.

Clinical Aspects

► **Typical presentation**

Pain • Swelling • Compensatory posture • Limited range of motion.

► **Therapeutic options**

Immobilization in a plaster cast • Open reduction and internal fixation is indicated in higher grade Salter–Harris fractures or supracondylar fractures.

- **Course and prognosis**

  Pediatric fractures usually heal without sequelae • The prognosis is usually very good • Prognosis is good for Salter–Harris type I and type II fractures and worse for types III–V.
- **Complications**

  Malrotation deformities • Involvement of neurovascular structures • Premature closure of the growth plate with premature cessation of growth in the limb • Joint involvement may lead to incongruity of the articular surfaces with early osteoarthritis.

Differential Diagnosis

Child abuse	– Multiple fractures of varying ages – Avulsed metaphyseal fragments – Posterior rib fractures – Subperiosteal hemorrhages
Osteogenesis imperfecta	– Family history (autosomal dominant inheritance) – Cortical thinning – Reduced diaphyseal diameter – Diaphyseal fractures are common – Rarely there are avulsed metaphyseal fragments – Wormian bones in the cranium
Rickets	– Osteopenia – Widening and cupping of the metaphyses – Irregularly widened growth plates – Periosteal reactions – Bending deformity of the long bones

Tips and Pitfalls

When in doubt, obtain an additional oblique film • Do not obtain comparative films of the contralateral side, rather obtain MRI studies where indicated • Traumatic effusion in the elbow can also occur without a fracture.

Selected References

Barmada A et al. Premature physeal closure following distal tibia physeal fractures: a new radiographic predictor 2003; 23: 733–739

Donnelly LF et al. Traumatic elbow effusions in pediatric patients: are occult fractures the rule? Am J Roentgenol 1998; 171: 243–245

John SD et al. Expanding the concept of the toddler's fracture. Radiographics 1997; 17: 367–376

O'Driscoll SW et al. Difficult elbow fractures. Pearls and pitfalls. Instr Course Lect 2003; 52: 113–134

Swischuk LE et al. Frequently missed fractures in pediatrics (value of comparative views). Emerg Radiol 2004; 11: 22–28

Definition

- **Epidemiology**

  Violent, nonaccidental physical or psychologic damage to a child • 63% of abused children are younger than 3 years.

- **Etiology, pathophysiology, pathogenesis**

  The younger the child, the more susceptible the skeleton is to injury • Typical locations include the skull, ribs, and long bones.

  - *Subperiosteal ossifications:* These form as result of hemorrhages between the cortex and periosteum (which in a newborn is not firmly adherent to the bone) • Radiologically detectable after 5 days at the earliest and 14 days at the latest • Hemorrhages occur when then infant is grasped too tightly.
  - *Metaphyseal injuries:* Microfractures in the end of the metaphysis with hemorrhages • These occur from excessive compression or traction near the joint.
  - *Epiphyseal injuries:* Typically in the distal humerus, from causes such as hyperextension.
  - *Shaft fractures:* These occur four times more often than metaphyseal injuries • Common sites include the femur and humerus • Transverse fractures occur more often than spiral fractures.
  - Intracerebral hemorrhages produced by vigorous shaking (see Chapter 7).

Imaging Signs

- **Radiographic findings**

  High specificity: Metaphyseal lesions (fracture lines parallel to the end zone of the metaphysis, "corner" fractures [avulsion of a lateral metaphyseal corner fragment], "bucket handle" fractures [oval fracture in the end zone of the metaphysis]) • Posterior rib fractures • Scapula fractures • Fractures of the spinous process • Fractures of the sternum.

  Moderate specificity: Multiple bilateral fractures • Separated epiphyses • Complex skull fractures • Phalangeal fractures • Vertebral fractures and subluxations • Fractures of varying ages.

  Low specificity: Subperiosteal ossification • Fissure fractures of the skull • Shaft fractures of the long bones • Clavicular fractures.

- **Ultrasound findings**

  Separation of nonossified epiphyses is visualized • Subperiosteal hematomas are visualized • Joint effusions • Intracerebral structures are visualized • Associated parenchymal organ or soft tissue injuries can be excluded.

- **CT**

  Intracerebral hemorrhages • Bony injuries to the skull and axial skeleton • Intraabdominal injuries.

- **MRI**

  Used to diagnose the age of hematomas • Visualizes sequelae of cerebral and spinal injuries.

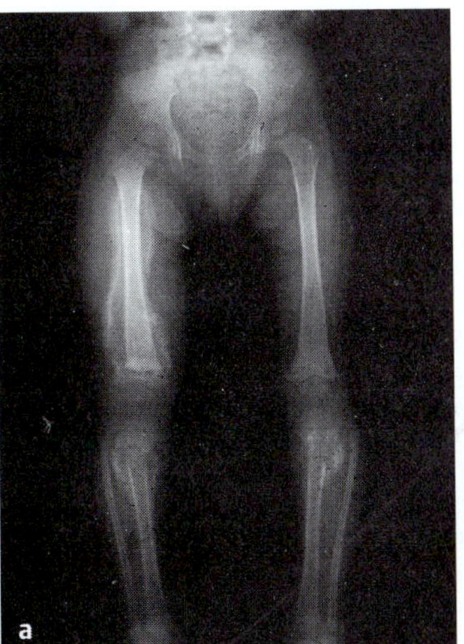

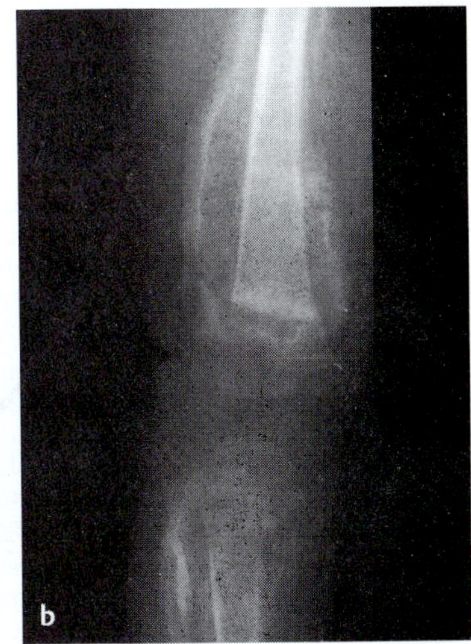

Fig. 6.39 a, b Child abuse. A-P radiograph of the legs. Multiple metaphyseal fractures with extensive subperiosteal ossification (**a**). Magnification (**b**) shows the metaphyseal portion of the right femur and the tibia in greater detail.

- **Bone scan**
  Used for visualizing occult fractures in cases of suspected child abuse. However, scanning cannot reliably demonstrate acute fractures.

Clinical Aspects

- **Typical presentation**
  Multiple hematomas • Wounds • Scars of varying ages • Retinal bleeding produced by vigorous shaking • General signs of neglect and lack of care • Developmental retardation of varying severity including dystrophy • Apathy • Neurologic deficits • Psychic abnormalities • Fractures of varying ages • Atypical head injuries • Intraabdominal injuries.
- **Therapeutic options**
  Surgical treatment of the acute injury • Psychosocial assessment of the home environment • Child should be protected against further abuse and placed in foster care where indicated.
- **Course and prognosis**
  This depends on the nature of the acute and chronic injuries.
- **Complications**
  Highly variable depending on the injury • Intracerebral injuries are much more likely to develop complications than are simple fractures.

Differential Diagnosis

Osteomyelitis	– Periosteal reactions – Varied pattern with osteolytic and sclerotic changes – Chronic Garré osteomyelitis involves purely osteosclerotic changes – Raised inflammation parameters – MRI shows inflammatory joint or soft tissue involvement – Multifocal occurrence in chronic recurrent multifocal osteomyelitis
Osteogenesis imperfecta	– Cortical thinning – Reduced diaphyseal diameter – “Corner sign” is rare – Diaphyseal fractures are common – Family history (autosomal dominant inheritance) – Blue sclerae may occur
Accident	– No fractures of varying ages – Plausible mechanism of injury for the extent of the fracture detected
Congenital indifference to pain	– Attributable to sensory deficits – Fractures and metaphyseal lesions
Physiologic periosteal reaction	– Usually bilateral in the medial femur and medial tibia, < 2 mm – Occurs between the ages of 6 weeks and 6 months – Caused by accelerated growth
Birth trauma	– History – Typical locations, such as the clavicle, humeral head, and skull fractures in forceps delivery (“ping pong ball” fracture).
Acute lymphatic leukemia	– Periosteal reactions – Radiolucent metaphyseal bands – Circumscribed areas of osteolysis and/or osteosclerosis
Rare diseases and metabolic disorders	– Rickets – Scurvy – Vitamin A intoxication – Caffey disease (infantile cortical hyperostosis) – Prostaglandin treatment to delay closure of the ductus arteriosus (cortical hyperostosis)

Tips and Pitfalls

Pelvis radiographs should be obtained when sexual abuse is suspected (these may demonstrate bony changes in the inferior pubic ramus and ischium) • Even typical bony lesions do not exclude a "normal" traumatic etiology • Coagulation disorders and thrombocytopathy should be excluded wherever there is extensive hemorrhaging (including intracerebral hemorrhage) • When a typical radiologic picture is present, the radiologist must mention the possibility of child abuse, especially in the absence of a plausible history of trauma • The psychosocial component of the disorder must not be neglected.

Selected References

Dubowitz H et al. Physical abuse and neglect of children. Lancet 2007; 369: 1891–1899

Kemp AM et al. Which radiological investigations should be performed to identify fractures in suspected child abuse? Clin Radiol 2006; 61: 723–736

Jenny C. Evaluating infants and young children with multiple fractures. Pediatrics 2006; 118: 1299–1303

Kleinman PK. Diagnostic imaging of child abuse. St. Louis: Mosby; 1998: 2–246

Lonergan GJ et al. From the archives of the AFIP. Child abuse: radiologic-pathologic correlation. Radiographics 2003; 23: 811–845

Nimkin K et al. Imaging of child abuse. Radiol Clin North Am 2001; 39: 843–864

Definition

▶ **Epidemiology**

Incidence is 1:1000–2000 • Most often involves the sagittal suture (up to 60% of cases), followed by the coronal suture • Most cases occur sporadically • Boys are affected more often than girls.

▶ **Etiology, pathophysiology, pathogenesis**

Premature fusion of the cranial sutures due to unknown causes • Occurs in disorders such as Crouzon disease, Apert syndrome, and cloverleaf skull (Kleeblattschädel) syndrome • Rarely affects the lambdoid suture alone • Fusion in the primary forms of the disorder begins during pregnancy • The skull base may also be involved • Fusion of the sagittal suture begins at the junction of the middle and posterior thirds; fusion of the coronal suture begins laterally • Normally fusion of the suture progresses uniformly.

- *Scaphocephaly, dolichocephaly (long head):* Fusion of the sagittal suture (60% of cases).
- *Brachycephaly, turricephaly (pointed head):* Bilateral fusion of the coronal suture (20–30%).
- *Plagiocephaly:* Unilateral fusion of the coronal suture (5–10%).
- *Trigonocephaly (triangular skull):* Premature fusion of the frontal and metopic sutures (1–2%).
- *Oxycephaly:* Fusion of all cranial sutures.

Imaging Signs

▶ **Radiographic findings**

Abnormal head shape—the skull grows in the direction of the prematurely fused cranial suture • Sharply demarcated, straight cranial sutures with marginal sclerosis • Later findings include partial or complete bony obliteration of the affected sutures • The resulting increased intracranial pressure produces digital marks and thinning of the skull bones.

- *Scaphocephaly:* Long, narrow cranium • The posterior portion of the coronal suture becomes convex • The anterior fontanelle is very small • The orbits appear large • The head is of normal size or enlarged.
- *Brachycephaly, turricephaly:* Broad and short skull • Small frontal bone • An asymmetric skull results where the coronal suture is not uniformly affected • The head is of normal size or enlarged.
- *Trigonocephaly:* Keel-like, small frontal bone with hyperostosis • Hypotelorism due to hypoplasia of the ethmoid bone • Oval orbits (larger vertical diameter) • Anterior portion of the coronal suture becomes convex at the small anterior fontanelle • The head is of normal size.

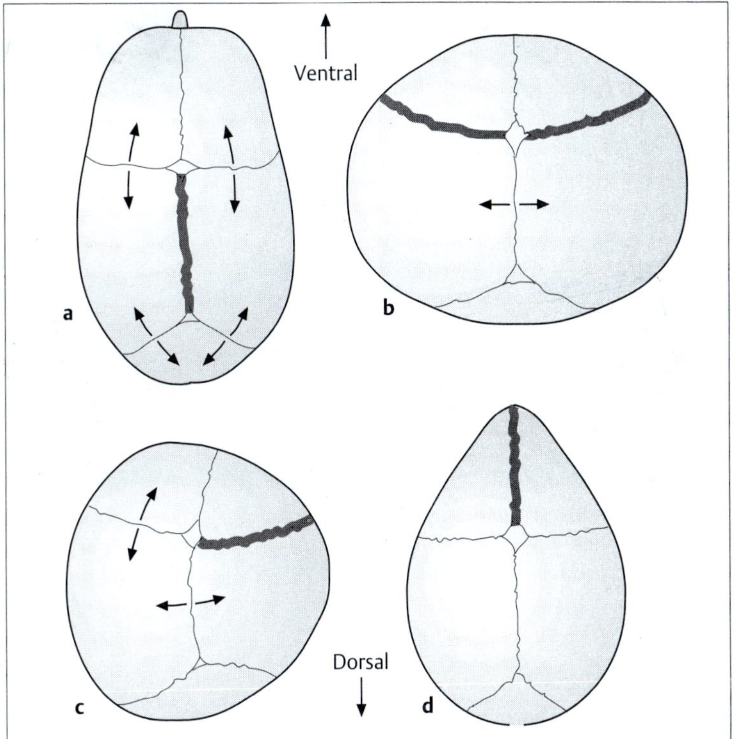

Fig. 7.1 Craniosynostosis. Premature fusion of the cranial sutures with typical skull deformities. The fused suture is marked by the thick gray line and the resultant direction of growth of the skull is indicated by the arrows. **a** Scaphocephaly, **b** brachycephaly, **c** plagiocephaly, **d** trigonocephaly (from Benz-Bohm G. Kinderradiologie. Stuttgart: Thieme; 2005).

- ▸ **Radiographs of the extremities**
  Syndromes are often associated with congenital bony anomalies of the extremities.
- ▸ **CT**
  Used for 3D visualization of the skull in complex deformities • Unobstructed visualization of the sutures.
- ▸ **MRI findings**
  The brain is normal in nonsyndromic forms of craniosynostosis • Abnormal intracerebral findings may be present depending on the underlying syndrome.

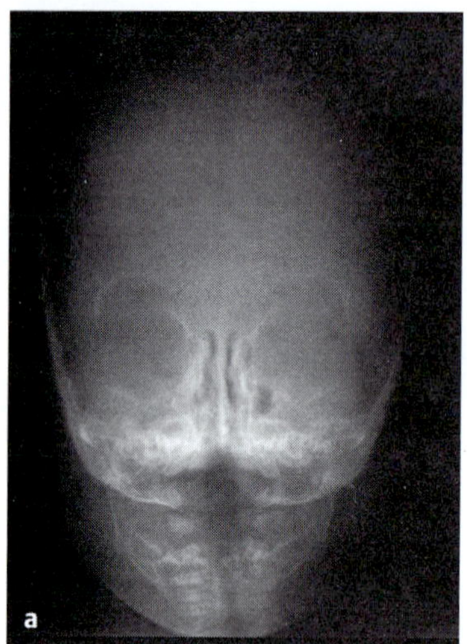

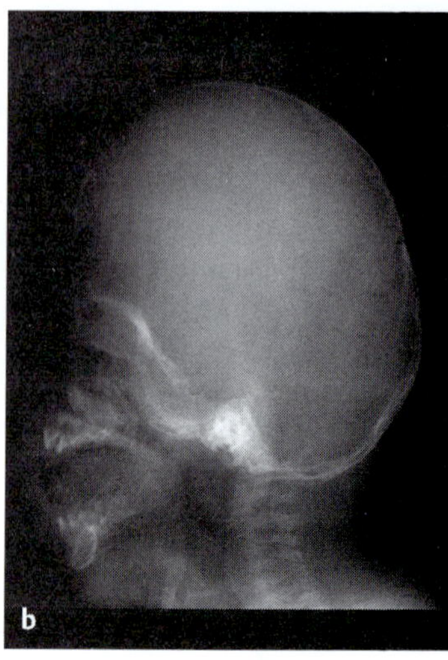

Fig. 7.2 a, b Turricephaly from bilateral premature fusion of the coronal suture. Skull radiographs in two planes. The coronal sutures have fused. Short skull with high cranial vault.

Clinical Aspects

- **Typical presentation**
  Abnormal face and head shape depending on the affected cranial suture • Increased intracranial pressure leads to neurologic symptoms • Loss of vision occurs, especially in oxycephaly and turricephaly • Abnormal bone findings on palpation.
- **Therapeutic options**
  Craniotomy • Craniectomy where indicated • Frontoorbital advancement in turricephaly, plagiocephaly, and trigonocephaly • Parasagittal craniectomy in scaphocephaly.
- **Course and prognosis**
  Where several cranial sutures are affected, growth of the brain will eventually lead to increased intracranial pressure.
- **Complications**
  Microcephaly • Increased intracranial pressure with neurologic complications.

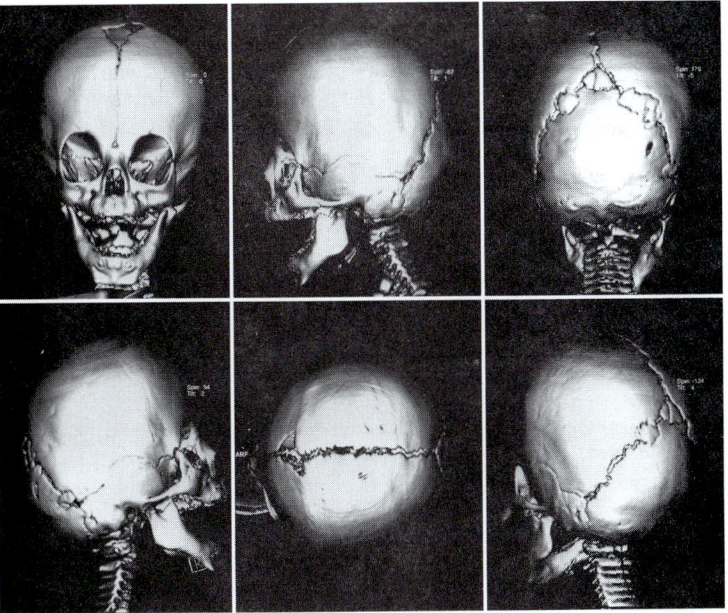

Fig. 7.3 Bilateral fusion of the coronal suture. Preoperative CT of the skull. Surface reconstruction with volume rendering provides unobstructed visualization of the skull anatomy and the pathoanatomy of the cranial sutures. Incidental findings include wormian bones in the lambdoid sutures.

Differential Diagnosis

Postural skull deformations	– Child with motor deficits – Rickets (cranium is very soft) – Osteogenesis imperfecta
Secondary causes	– Microcephaly – Excessively rapid decompression in hydrocephalus (CSF pressure reduced below normal) – Primary hyperthyroidism – Overdose in treatment of hypothyroidism – Hypophosphatasia – Vitamin D resistant rickets – Mucopolysaccharidoses – Osteopetrosis

Tips and Pitfalls

It is possible to misinterpret an apparently patent suture in a child with narrow cranial sutures that travel in straight lines and exhibit marginal sclerosis.

Selected References

Alden TD et al. Mechanisms of premature closure of cranial sutures. Child Nerv Syst 1999; 15: 670–675

Bristol RE et al. The effects of craniosynostosis on the brain with respect to intracranial pressure. Semin Pediatr Neurol 2004; 11: 262–267

Kotrikova B et al. Diagnostic imaging in the management of craniosynostoses. Eur Radiol 2007; 7: 1968–78

Lajeunie E et al. Craniosynostosis: from a clinical description to an understanding of bone formation of the skull. Child Nerv Syst 1999; 15: 676–680

Medina LS et al. Children with suspected craniosynostosis: a cost-effectiveness analysis of diagnostic strategies. Am J Roentgenol 2002; 179: 215–221

Wilkie AO et al. Clinical dividends from the molecular genetic diagnosis of craniosynostosis. Am J Med Genet A 2006; 140: 2631–2639

Definition

- **Epidemiology**
  - *Vermian dysgenesis:* In Dandy-Walker malformation.
  - *Callosal agenesis:* Incidence is 3–7:1000 • Often occurs in association with other CNS malformations (50–80% of cases) • Isolated occurrence is more common in boys than in girls.
  - *Agenesis of the septum pellucidum:* Frequency of isolated agenesis: 2–3:100 000 • More common in association with other syndromes such as septo-optic dysplasia (frequency is 1:50 000).
  - *Dysgenesis of the basal ganglia in holoprosencephaly:* Frequency is 1:16 000–25 000 • More common in boys than girls by a ratio of 1.5:1.
- **Etiology, pathophysiology, pathogenesis**

  Midline anomalies arise as a result of defective organogenesis and affect the cerebellar vermis, corpus callosum, septum pellucidum, and basal ganglia.

  Callosal agenesis: The corpus callosum begins anteriorly and progresses posteriorly (rostrum, genu, corpus, and splenium) • Causes of agenesis include lack of formation of callosal axons. Axons do not grow to the midline due to the absence of adhesion molecules. They extend to the midline but fail to cross it due to absence of a stimulus, growing as thick fibrous bundles (Probst bundles) parallel to the midline • In partial agenesis, usually the posterior portions of the corpus callosum are absent • Can occur as an isolated anomaly or with other malformations.

  Septo-optic dysplasia (de Morsier disease): Etiology is unclear • Usually sporadic • In isolated cases there is autosomal dominant or recessive inheritance or a mutation of the Hesx or Hesx1 gene • Disturbed development of the prosencephalon • Partial or complete agenesis of the septum pellucidum, hypoplasia of the optic nerves and pituitary and hypothalamic dysfunction.

  Holoprosencephaly: 70% of cases involve chromosomal anomalies (trisomy 13, 18q-, 18p-, 3p, 7-) • The embryonal prosencephalon fails to differentiate or differentiates incompletely into the two cerebral hemispheres, thalami, lateral ventricles, and third ventricle • Degrees of severity:
  - *Alobar holoprosencephaly:* Most severe form.
  - *Semilobar holoprosencephaly:* Milder form.
  - *Lobar holoprosencephaly:* Mildest form.

  Intermediate forms that cannot be clearly categorized are common.

Imaging Signs

- **Ultrasound findings**

  Callosal agenesis: Neither the corpus callosum nor the sulcus or cingulate gyrus are visualized • The frontal horns are impressed cranially and medially by Probst bundles, and they are laterally displaced and tapered (bull's horn configuration) • The longitudinal fissure communicates with the third ventricle • The third ventricle is cranially displaced between the two lateral ventricles • The gyri and sulci are arranged radially around the third ventricle • The posterior horns are often dilated and the anterior horns of the lateral ventricles are nar-

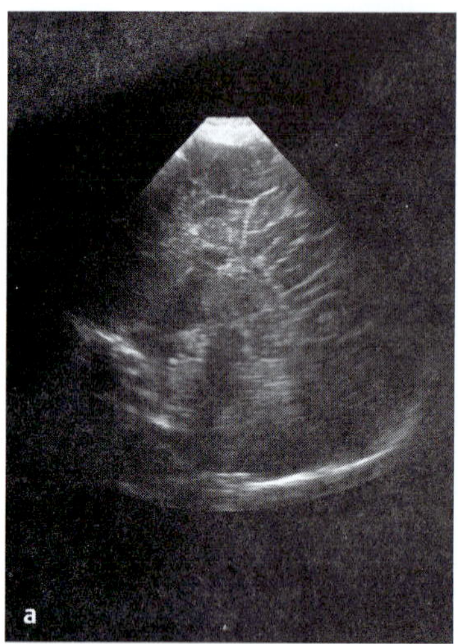

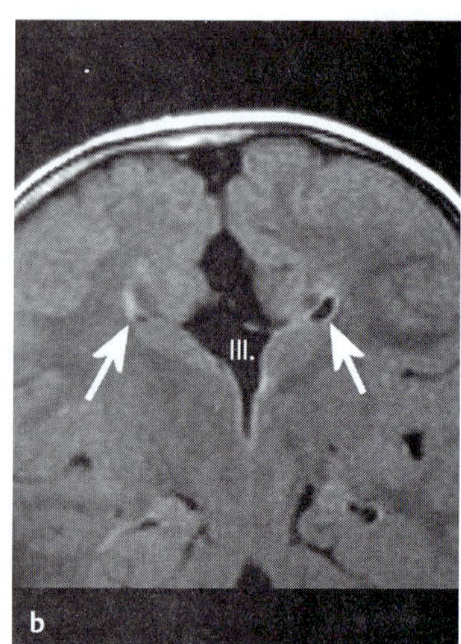

Fig. 7.4 a, b Callosal agenesis. Ultrasound, middle sagittal plane (**a**) and MR image (**b**). Corpus callosum is not visualized on ultrasound. Sulci and gyri are arranged radially around the third ventricle (**a**). The coronal FLAIR image (detail, **b**) demonstrates a lateral ventricle shaped like a bull's horn (arrows) in callosal agenesis.

Fig. 7.5 Septal agenesis in septooptic dysplasia in a 1-year-old boy. Ultrasound. The septum is absent, the anterior horns join to form a monoventricle, and the roof of the anterior horns is flattened.

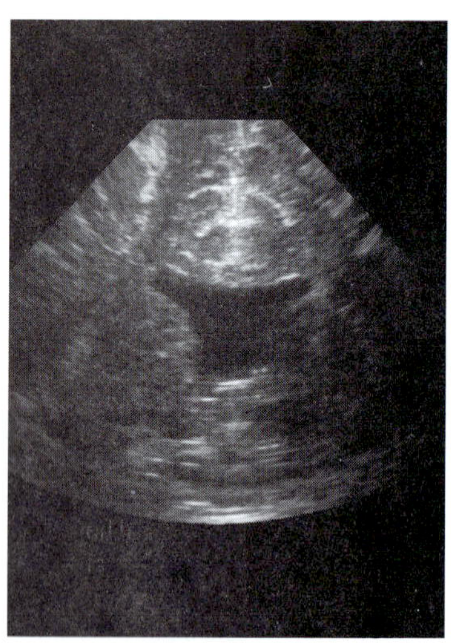

row • The foramina of Monro are elongated • Partial agenesis is often difficult to recognize.
Septo-optic dysplasia: Septum is partially or completely absent • The communicating anterior horns of the lateral ventricles form a monoventricle • The roof of the anterior horns is flattened • The anterior and posterior horns of the lateral ventricles are slightly dilated.
Alobar holoprosencephaly: Large midline horseshoe-shaped monoventricle communicating with a large occipital cyst • The thalamic nuclei and choroid plexus are fused in the midline • The longitudinal fissure, falx cerebri, corpus callosum, third ventricle, and septum pellucidum are absent • There are no occipital lobes • Large parts of the parietal and temporal lobes are missing • The gyri and sulci are arranged radially around the monoventricle • The frontal cerebrum is a single undivided structure • There is one single anterior cerebral artery.
Semilobar holoprosencephaly: A small midline monoventricle is present • Occipital and temporal lobes are present, if only as rudimentary structures • The falx cerebri and longitudinal fissure are rudimentary • The corpus callosum is partially or completely absent • There is no septum pellucidum.
Lobar holoprosencephaly: Only the frontal lobes are fused • Dysplastic falx cerebri • Septum pellucidum is absent • As a result, the anterior horns of the lateral ventricles are fused • The ventricular system is otherwise normal • There is either a normally developed corpus callosum or agenesis of the corpus callosum.

▸ **MRI findings**
Callosal agenesis: Identical findings as on ultrasound (see above) • MRI is superior to ultrasound for demonstrating partial agenesis • Probst bundles are slightly hyperintense to other myelinated fibers on T1-weighted images and slightly hypointense on T2-weighted images • The anterior cerebral arteries exhibit meandering courses on MR angiography.
Septo-optic dysplasia: The optic nerves and chiasm are hypoplastic • Occasionally the pituitary stalk is hypoplastic • Ectopic posterior pituitary • Narrow corpus callosum • Vertical hippocampus.
Holoprosencephaly: Identical to ultrasound (see above).

Clinical Aspects

▸ **Typical presentation**
Callosal agenesis: Epilepsy • Mental defiency • Microcephaly • Metabolic disorders • Syndromic form has a much poorer prognosis.
Septo-optic dysplasia: Affected children are short in stature • Seizures (hypoglycemia) • Apnea • Cyanosis • Hypotension • Prolonged jaundice • Metabolic disorders • Color blindness • Blindness • Nystagmus • Strabismus • Spasticity • Anosmia.
Holoprosencephaly: Hypotelorism or hypertelorism • Cleft lip and palate • Microcephaly • Mental defiency • Metabolic disorders.

▸ **Therapeutic options**
- *Callosal agenesis:* Antiepileptic therapy • Management of possible metabolic disorders.

- *Septooptic dysplasia:* Hormone substitution.
- *Holoprosencephaly:* Hormone substitution • Antiepileptic therapy.

▸ **Course and prognosis**

- *Callosal agenesis:* Nonsyndromic form can remain asymptomatic until age 3 • Syndromic form has a much poorer prognosis.
- *Septooptic dysplasia:* Prognosis depends on the associated CNS anomalies.
- *Holoprosencephaly:* The more severe the anomaly, the worse the prognosis • Severe cases lead to spontaneous abortion.

▸ **Complications**

- *Callosal agenesis:* Occasionally associated with diencephalic cysts that can obstruct the foramina of Monro. This in turn can lead to hydrocephalus requiring a shunt.
- *Septooptic dysplasia:* Metabolic crises • Sudden infant death syndrome.
- *Holoprosencephaly:* Pituitary and hypothalamic dysfunction (diabetes insipidus) may occur • Disturbed regulation of body temperature.

Differential Diagnosis

Callosal hypoplasia	– Corpus callosum is complete but hypoplastic – Occurs in myelination disorders
Agenesis of the corpus callosum with interhemispheric cyst	– Type 1 cyst communicates with the ventricular system – Type 2 cysts (multiple) do not communicate with the ventricular system – Often associated with macrocephaly or hydrocephalus
Schizencephaly	– Congenital malformation of the cortex – Cleft extending from surface of the pia mater to the ependyma of the lateral ventricle – Two forms: “Open lip” and “closed lip” according to the width of the gray matter lining the cleft. – Large bilateral “open lip” schizencephaly can mimic holoprosencephaly

Tips and Pitfalls

In agenesis of the corpus callosum and septum, other malformations should be sought • Partial agenesis of the corpus callosum cannot always be excluded on ultrasound. In such cases, MRI is the most suitable modality for documenting the extent of the anomaly.

Selected References

Antonini Sr et al. Cerebral midline developmental anomalies: endocrine, neuroradiographic and ophthalmological features. J Pediatr Endocrinol Metab 2002; 15: 1525–1530

Barkovich AJ et al. Analysis of the cerebral cortex in holoprosencephaly with attention to the Sylvian fissures. AJNR 2002; 29: 143–150

Campbell CL. Septo-optic dysplasia: a literature review. Optometry 2003; 74: 417–426

Moutard ML et al. Agenesis of corpus callosum: Prenatal diagnosis and prognosis. Child Nerv Syst 2003; 19: 471–476

Definition

- **Epidemiology**
  Incidence is 1:25 000 births • Girls are affected slightly more often than boys.
- **Etiology, pathophysiology, pathogenesis**
  The term Dandy–Walker complex includes similar malformations that do not all exhibit every one of the changes described below.
  Etiology is unclear • Presumably results from failure of development of the rhombencephalon • This leads to persistence of the superior medullary velum, which expands and herniates posteriorly • Cystic expansion of the fourth ventricle, which does not communicate with the subarachnoid space • Posterior cranial fossa is enlarged • The tentorium cerebelli lies at a steep angle with a high attachment • The transverse sinus and confluence of the sinuses are cranially displaced • The straight sinus lies at a steep angle • Hypoplasia and aplasia of the cerebellar vermis • 70% of cases are associated with other CNS anomalies (agenesis of the corpus callosum or callosal dysgenesis, gray matter heterotopias, polymicrogyria or agyria, schizencephaly, occipital encephalocele) • Craniofacial, cardiac, renal, skeletal, and respiratory malformations are occasionally present as well.

Imaging Signs

- **Ultrasound findings**
  Can be diagnosed on ultrasound during pregnancy • Diagnosis should not be made prior to the 18 th week of gestation • Large cystic mass in the posterior cranial fossa • Cyst communicates with the fourth ventricle • Posterior horns of the lateral ventricles diverge • Hypoplastic cerebellar vermis • Often associated with hydrocephalus after the age of 3 months (75% of cases).
- **CT findings**
  For follow-up after shunt procedure • Large posterior cranial fossa with cyst of variable size • Confluence of the sinuses lies cranial to the lambdoid suture • Flattened and remodeled occipital bone • Pons is displaced anteriorly.
- **MRI findings**
  Other CNS anomalies may be present • The posterior fourth ventricle expands into a large cyst • The cyst wall is poorly demarcated • Cyst contents are isointense to CSF • In hypoplasia of the cerebellar vermis, the vermian structures are folded cranially and lie on the cyst • High attachment of the tentorium, which courses cranially at a steep angle • The cerebellar hemispheres are displaced anterolaterally • Occasionally there are slight signal differences between the cyst contents and CSF on the FLAIR image • MR venography demonstrates cranial displacement of the transverse sinus, a steep angle of the straight sinus, and cranial displacement of the confluence of the sinuses.

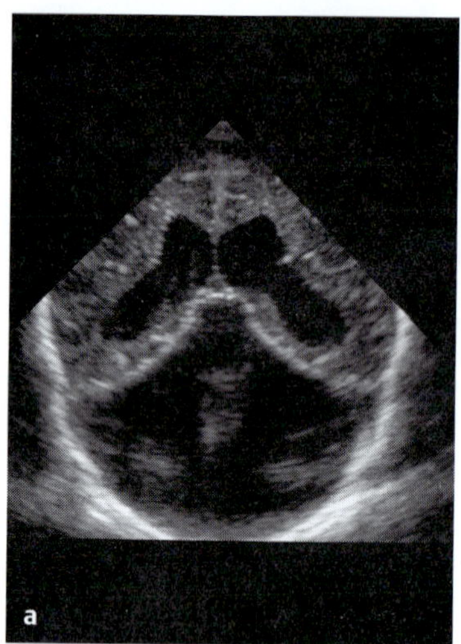

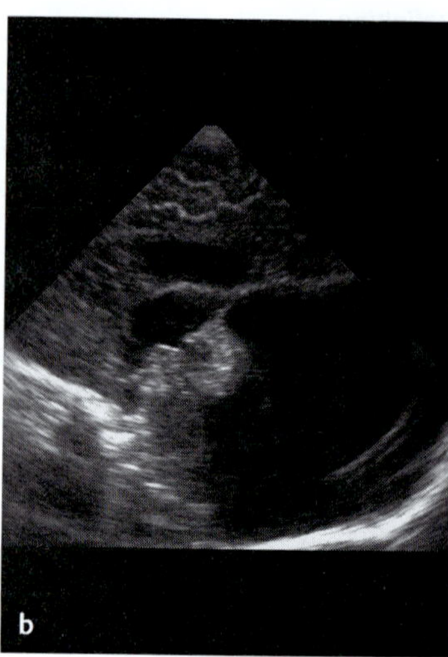

Fig. 7.6 a, b Dandy–Walker malformation in a newborn. Ultrasound. The posterior coronal (**a**) and sagittal images (**b**) demonstrate a large cystic mass that communicates with the fourth ventricle. The cerebellar vermis is hypoplastic. Associated internal hydrocephalus.

Clinical Aspects

- **Typical presentation**
  Macrocephaly • Protrusion of the fontanelle • Headache • Seizures • Retarded motor development • Spasticity • Lack of balance • Respiratory dysfunction.
- **Therapeutic options**
  CSF drainage via a ventriculoperitoneal shunt with or without a cyst shunt • Marsupialization.
- **Course and prognosis**
  Up to 50% of patients exhibit normal intelligence • Prognosis depends on associated supratentorial malformations, hydrocephalus, and complications.
- **Complications**
  Hydrocephalus is present in up to 90% of cases at the time of the diagnosis • Shunt occlusion • Shunt infection.

Differential Diagnosis

Mega-cisterna magna	– Expanded posterior cranial fossa – Normal cerebellar vermis – Normal fourth ventricle – Falx cerebelli and small veins course through the cyst
Arachnoid cyst	– Fourth ventricle is normally developed but compressed and displaced – Falx cerebelli and small veins do not course through the cyst – Cerebellar vermis is cranially displaced
Joubert anomaly	– Cleavage or aplasia of the cerebellar vermis – "Bat's wing" appearance of the fourth ventricle – "Molar tooth" appearance of the mesencephalon
Walker–Warburg syndrome	– Cerebral gyri are absent or greatly reduced – Occipital encephalocele – Corpus callosum is absent – Hypoplasia of the cerebellum

Tips and Pitfalls

Other CNS malformations should be sought as this disorder frequently occurs in association with them • MRI is indicated wherever ultrasound findings suggest a Dandy-Walker malformation.

Selected References

Barkovich AJ et al. Revised classification of posterior fossa cysts and cystlike malformations based on the results of multiplanar MR imaging. Am J Roentgenol 1989; 153: 1289–1300

Nelson MD Jr et al. A different approach to cysts of the posterior fossa. Pediatr Radiol 2004; 34: 720–732

Klein O et al. Dandy-Walker malformation: prenatal diagnosis and prognosis. Childs Nerv Syst 2003; 19: 484–489

Tortori-Donati P et al. Cystic malformations of the posterior cranial fossa originating from a defect of the posterior membranous area. Mega cisterna magna and persisting Blake's pouch: two separate entities. Child Nerv Syst 1996; 12: 303–308

Definition

- **Epidemiology**
  Occurs particularly in premature infants born before 28 weeks' gestation and with birth weight below 1000 g • Frequency is 30–55% • The younger and more immature the infant, the greater the probability of intracranial hemorrhage • Often occurs in the first 3 days of life • No sex predilection.
- **Etiology, pathophysiology, pathogenesis**
  The disorder is caused by the germinal matrix, an immature, highly vascular, and metabolically active zone of neuroepithelial cells • Involution of the germinal matrix begins after 32 weeks' gestation • In this stage of development, the vascular network is very fragile and vulnerable to fluctuations in blood pressure, acidosis, disorders of coagulation, hypoxia, and rapid expansion in volume • Important risk factors are hyperperfusion, hypoperfusion, and hypoxia • Hemorrhages arise from the germinal matrix and spread into the ventricles • Clots can occlude the lateral and median apertures of the fourth ventricle, leading to hydrocephalus • Hemorrhagic infarction secondary to insult occurs in 20% of cases, usually unilaterally, where increasing compression of the superior thalamostriate vein impairs drainage.

Imaging Signs

- **Ultrasound findings**
  Papile classification:
  - *Grade I:* Subependymal bleeding.
  - *Grade II:* Intraventricular hemorrhage without dilation of the ventricle.
  - *Grade III:* Intraventricular hemorrhage with dilation of the ventricle.
  - *Grade IV:* Grades I–III with bleeding into the brain parenchyma may result from venous infarction.

  Grade I: Unilaterally or bilaterally increased echogenicity limited to the germinal matrix on the floor of the lateral ventricle between the head of the caudate nucleus and the thalamus posterior to the ipsilateral foramen of Monro • Usually the clots resolve within a few weeks • Occasionally subependymal cysts develop; these resolve within a few months.

  Grade II: Fresh hyperechoic blood in the ventricle • The blood is occasionally distributed symmetrically in the lateral ventricles, but usually asymmetrically • Clots entering the third ventricle can give it the appearance of a hyperechoic band • Clot deposits on the choroid plexus produce an irregular contour • Aseptic ventriculitis can occur 1 week after the hemorrhage • The ventricular ependyma then appears hyperechoic (findings persist up to 6 weeks) • Clots resolve within a period of weeks to months and their echogenicity decreases.

  Grade III: More severe hemorrhage than in grade II • CSF is only detectable as a hypoechoic halo between the hypoechoic brain and the hyperechoic clots • Blood clots accumulate along the CSF drainage routes • Occlusion of one foramen of Monro leads to asymmetric hydrocephalus • Occlusion of the lateral and median apertures of the fourth ventricle leads to hydrocephalus involving all CSF spaces.

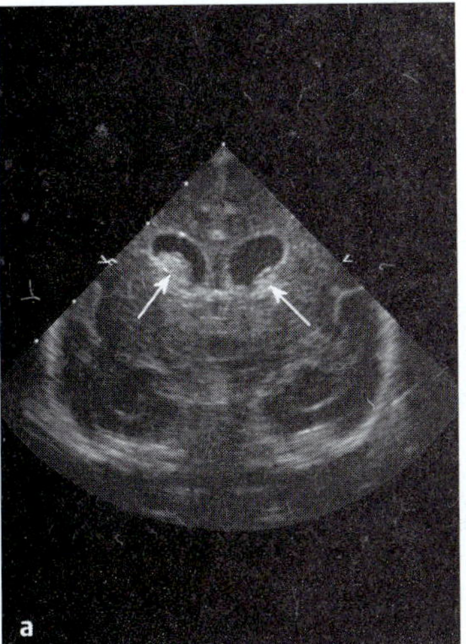

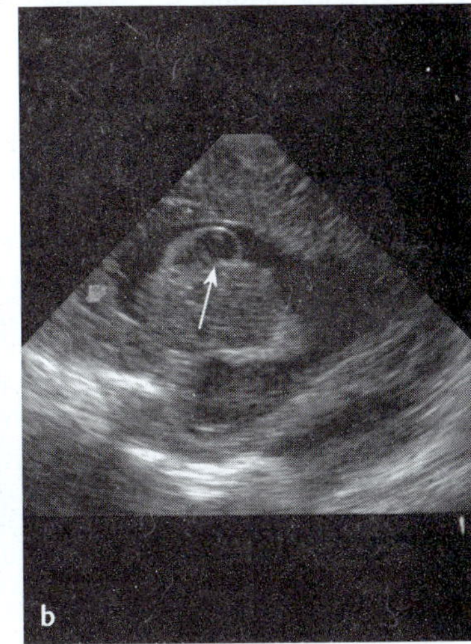

Fig. 7.7 a, b Intraventricular hemorrhage in the premature infant. Ultrasound. The middle coronal image (**a**) demonstrates bilateral hyperechoic subependymal hemorrhage (arrows) arising from the germinal matrix and spreading into the dilated ventricular system (grade III hemorrhage). A follow-up study (parasagittal plane, **b**) performed a few weeks later shows a residual subependymal cyst (arrow) and posthemorrhagic hydrocephalus.

Grade IV: Hemorrhagic infarctions, usually frontoparietal • Wedge-shaped area of increased echogenicity • The apex of the wedge points toward the parenchyma and the base of the wedge toward the ventricular system • Hemorrhagic infarctions can affect large parts of a hemisphere and extend into the subcortical region • Unilateral infarctions can lead to midline shift • Hemorrhagic infarction leaves behind a cystic porencephalic defect corresponding in size to the infarcted area that previously exhibited increased echogenicity.

▸ **CT findings**

Ultrasound is preferable to CT due to the lack of ionizing radiation • Hemorrhages appear hyperdense to brain parenchyma on unenhanced scans.

▸ **MRI findings**

This is only an option where the child is sufficiently stable • Acute hemorrhages are hyperintense on T1-weighted images and hypointense on T2-weighted images.

Clinical Aspects

▸ **Typical presentation**

Clinical symptoms are highly variable • Failure to thrive • Seizures • Hyperreflexia • Slight irritability • Hypotonia • Paresis.

- **Therapeutic options**
  Stabilizing cerebral perfusion • Minimizing risk factors • Ventriculoperitoneal shunt.
- **Course and prognosis**
  Small cysts can occasionally develop from grade I hemorrhages • Grade III hemorrhages lead to hydrocephalus that may require treatment • Following grade IV hemorrhages, porencephalic cysts develop from the infarcted areas and exhibit corresponding neurologic deficits • Grade I and grade II hemorrhages have a very good prognosis • The prognosis worsens with increasing severity (76% of grade IV hemorrhages involve severe neurologic complications).
- **Complications**
  Recurrent hemorrhages • Hydrocephalus • Seizures • Retarded development • Cerebral palsy.

Differential Diagnosis

Choroid plexus grade I hemorrhage	– Normal choroid plexus findings: – Choroid plexus on the floor of the lateral ventricle in the coronal plane – Area of increased echogenicity does not extend posteriorly past the foramen of Monro in the sagittal plane – Choroid plexus narrows toward the foramen of Monro – Clots on the choroid plexus are occasionally separated by fine hypoechoic lines
Periventricular leukomalacia and hemorrhagic infarction	– Usually symmetric – Smaller hyperechoic lesions – Anterior and lateral of the anterior horns – Posterior above the trigone – Periventricular region – Usually associated with minor bleeding – Usually separated from the ventricle by brain tissue

Tips and Pitfalls

Ventriculitis can also occur without bleeding, for example in infections and metabolic disorders • In immature newborns, color Doppler ultrasound with measurement of blood flow in the anterior cerebral artery is indicated to detect risk factors for intracranial hemorrhage (low flow velocity, fluctuating flow pattern).

Selected References

Blankenberg FG et al. Sonography, CT, and MR imaging: a prospective comparison of neonates with suspected intracranial ischemia and hemorrhage. AJNR 2000; 21: 213–318

Fukui K et al. Fetal germinal matrix and intraventriculare haemorrhage diagnosed in MRI. Neuroradiology 2001; 43: 68–72

Futagi Y et al. Neurodevelopmental outcome in children with intraventricular hemorrhage. Pediatr Neurol 2006; 34: 219–224

Vasileiadis GT et al. Uncomplicated intraventricular hemorrhage is followed by reduced cortical volume at near-term age. Pediatrics 2004; 114: 367–372

Definition

- **Epidemiology**
Sequela of a severe hypoxic-ischemic injury to the brain of a premature infant (<28 weeks' gestation) • Occurs in 1.5–6% of live births.
- **Etiology, pathophysiology, pathogenesis**
Causes include reduced oxygen content of the blood and reduced perfusion of the brain • Lesions first occur in the region of the terminal microvasculature • In premature infants, the periventricular white matter is supplied by vessels coursing outward from the ventricles (from the choroid plexus) and inward toward the ventricles (from the cortex to the lateral ventricles); a "watershed" occurs between the two vascular systems • Cerebral vessels in this stage of development do not yet have the capacity for autoregulation.
PVL lesions are found near the anterior horns of the lateral ventricles, in the corona radiata, in the centrum semiovale, above the trigone of the lateral ventricles, and in the parietooccipital region • The internal and external capsules, motor cortex, corticospinal tracts, visual cortex, and speech center are particularly affected • Cysts develop in previously necrotic areas; they may be separated from the ventricular system by septa or may communicate with it • These lesions lead to brain atrophy.
  - *Nonhemorrhagic form (two-thirds of cases):* Bilaterally symmetric around the lateral ventricles.
  - *Hemorrhagic form (one-third of cases):* Unilateral with grade IV hemorrhage.

  Aicardi classification of PVL severity:
  - *Grade 1:* PVL in the region of the posterior horns.
  - *Grade 2:* PVL in the region of the posterior and anterior horns.
  - *Grade 3:* PVL along the lateral wall of the entire lateral ventricle.
  - *Grade 4:* Grade 3 PVL accompanied by cysts in the white matter.

Imaging Signs

- **Ultrasound findings**
Two stages of periventricular leukomalacia can be distinguished on ultrasound.
Stage I (1–2 weeks): Symmetric bands of increased echogenicity (echo pattern corresponds to that of the choroid plexus) cranial and lateral to the lateral ventricles, sharply demarcated from the surrounding parenchyma • Rarely unilateral • A hypoechoic zone 1–2 mm wide separates the lesions from the ventricular system • This zone disappears where additional intraventricular hemorrhaging occurs • The area of increased echogenicity is usually inhomogeneous with patches of greater and lesser echogenicity • One-quarter of these lesions are associated with intraventricular hemorrhage.
Stage II (≥3 weeks): The area of increased echogenicity contains multiple small, diffusely distributed, periventricular cysts • Larger circumscribed cysts suggest a more severe clinical course • Cysts are confluent in the more severe forms • In these cases, large septate cysts arise that communicate with the ventricular system • Cysts also occur in areas of the brain that were not previously hyperecho-

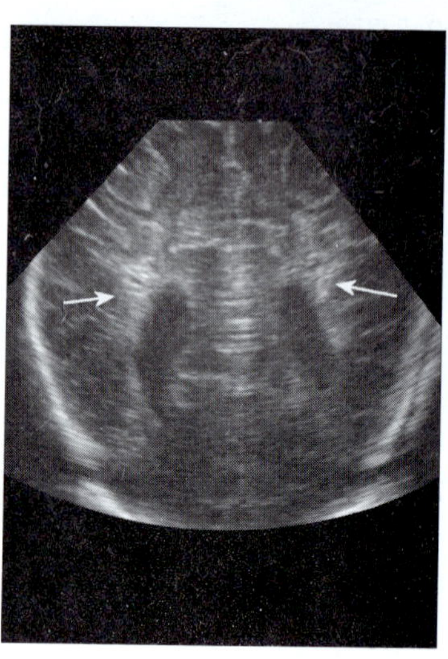

Fig. 7.8 Stage I periventricular leukomalacia in a premature infant born after 28 weeks' gestation. Ultrasound, posterior coronal plane. Typical increased echogenicity in the periventricular region.

ic • A particularly severe form of periventricular leukomalacia is seen in children who also have intraventricular hemorrhage • Small cysts from milder forms can resolve completely • Severe forms lead to brain atrophy with dilation of the inner and outer CSF spaces, primarily the anterior horns of the lateral ventricles and the longitudinal fissure, respectively.

- **CT findings**
  Risks should be weighed against benefits • Areas of decreased density are seen in nonhemorrhagic PVL • Hyperdense periventricular lesions are present in hemorrhagic PVL.
- **MRI findings**
  Only possible in stable children • Nodular and streaky periventricular hyperintensities, especially on FLAIR images • Lateral ventricles exhibit an irregular, wavy contour • Focal or asymmetric dilation of the lateral ventricles • Posterior portion of the corpus callosum is narrowed.

Clinical Aspects

- **Typical presentation**
  Presentation may vary from asymptomatic to cerebral palsy.
- **Therapeutic options**
  No treatment for the underlying causes • Noxious agents should be avoided • Cardiovascular stabilization.

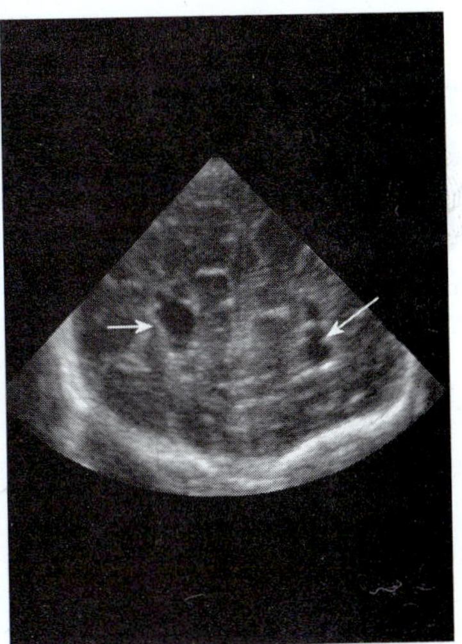

Fig. 7.9 Stage II periventricular leukomalacia in a 4-week old premature infant born after 30 weeks of gestation. Ultrasound, anterior coronal plane. Multiple confluent cystic lesions are present in the frontal periventricular white matter.

- **Course and prognosis**
  Neurologic deficits often develop • Retarded development • Seizures • Prognosis is usually poor for these reasons.
- **Complications**
  Retarded development • Diplegia and paraplegia • Cerebral palsy • Impaired hearing and vision • Epilepsy.

Differential Diagnosis

Multicystic encephalomalacia	– In mature infants with severe perinatal asphyxia – Diffuse generalized brain damage – Multiple cystic cavities of varying size – Cysts may be septated – Typically occur in the cortex and adjacent white matter – Often in the frontal and occipital regions
Vasculitis	– Very rare – Multiple cortical and subcortical lesions – May be associated with hemorrhages – Perfusion defects in the acute stage – Occasionally areas of blood–brain barrier damage are detectable

Tips and Pitfalls

PVL can be difficult to differentiate from hemorrhagic infarction in the presence of severe intraventricular bleeding.

Selected References

Fan GG et al. Potential of diffusion tensor MRI in the assessment of periventricular leukomalacia. Clin Radiol 2006; 61: 358–364

Roelants-van Rijn AM et al. Parenchymal brain injury in preterm infants: comparison of cranial ultrasound, MRI and neurodevelopmental outcome. Neuropediatrics 2001; 32: 80–89

Sie LT et al. Early MR features of hypoxic-ischemic brain injury in neonates with periventricular densities on sonograms. AJNR Am J Neuroradiol 2000; 21: 852–861

Definition

- **Epidemiology**
  Incidence: 1.5–6% of all live births • Risk factors presumably include chorioamnionitis, preeclampsia, diabetes, and maternal drug abuse (specifically cocaine).
- **Etiology, pathophysiology, pathogenesis**
  The cause is asphyxia leading to hypoxia, hypercapnia, and acidosis • Cerebral hypoxia and ischemia, often accompanied by toxic cerebral edema • This leads to a further reduction in brain perfusion • The pattern of damage depends on the extent of the hypoxemia (focal or generalized), its duration (brief or chronic), and the maturity of the brain • In premature infants, lesions occur in the periventricular white matter • In term infants parenchymal damage first occurs in the cerebral cortex and the intravascular boundary zones ("parasagittal watershed areas") of the cerebral hemispheres • In profound hypotension or cardiocirculatory arrest, the injury is initially located in the basal ganglia, thalami, brainstem and perirolandic cortex.
  In immature newborns, intraventricular and periventricular hemorrhages also often occur, and PVL may occur later • In mature infants and older children, hypoxemia can lead to cerebral edema, status marmoratus, and subcortical necrosis.

Imaging Signs

- **Ultrasound findings**
  Premature infants: Sharply demarcated, inhomogeneous periventricular bands of increased echogenicity • Often symmetric • Focal lesions often occur in the centrum semiovale, corona radiata, and peritrigonal at the lateral ventricles • Can be visualized in several imaging planes through the fontanelles • Isoechoic to the choroid plexus • Difficult to differentiate from the ventricle in the presence of hemorrhage (usually low grade) • See the section on "Periventricular Leukomalacia" earlier in this chapter for further details.
  Mature infants: Secondary to asphyxia, a cerebral edema may be present with diffusely increased echogenicity in the brain parenchyma, narrowed inner and outer CSF spaces, and diminished differentiation of brain structures • The acute stage may involve hemorrhagic infarction of the basal ganglia (usually the caudate nucleus and less often the putamen, globus pallidus, or subthalamus) • Infarction appears as symmetrically increased echogenicity • *Status marmoratus (at the earliest, after 2 weeks to 6 months):* Increased echogenicity of the basal ganglia but less than in hemorrhagic infarction • Necrotic areas may later calcify. Within 2–3 weeks of the insult, multiple small cysts appear deep in the sulci at the corticomedullary junction, usually in the parasagittal region • With time, the cysts become confluent and increase in size • Loss of brain substance leads to dilation of the inner and outer CSF spaces • This leads to hydrocephalus ex vacuo • After 2–4 weeks, color Doppler demonstrates increased vascularity in the cerebral cortex and basal ganglia (revascularization).

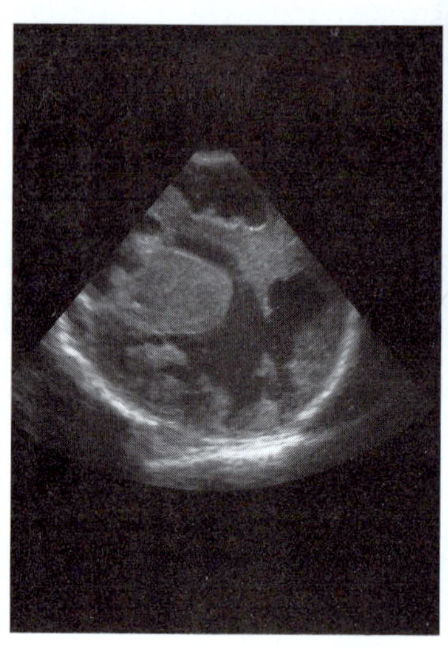

Fig. 7.10 Hypoxic-ischemic brain damage in a 4-week-old mature newborn. Ultrasound, parasagittal plane. Multiple porencephalic defects of varying size in the white matter and hydrocephalus ex vacuo.

▸ **CT findings**

Ultrasound is preferable to CT due to the lack of ionizing radiation.

Premature infants: In the acute stage, more or less hypodense focal or multifocal lesions are present in the periventricular white matter • Intraventricular hemorrhage • In the subacute stage, periventricular cysts are present • In the late stage, the lateral ventricles are dilated.

Mature infants: In hemorrhagic infarction, the basal ganglia are hyperdense • Loss of demarcation between gray and white matter • Later there is loss of volume in the affected areas of the brain • Extensive insults lead to cystic encephalomalacia.

▸ **MRI findings**

Protocol should include T1-weighted, T2-weighted, proton density, diffusion-weighted, and T2*-weighted sequences • This modality is less suitable in premature infants due to the lack of myelination and the unfavorable ambient conditions (loud noise and cold).

- T1-weighted images: Hyperintense signal in the anterolateral thalamus and basal ganglia (brighter than the cortex) • Focal signal increase in the cortex.
- T2-weighted and proton density images: Basal ganglia are hyperintense and poorly demarcated • Hypointense where calcifications and hemorrhage are present • Cortical lesions.
- T2*-weighted images: Used for differentiating hemorrhages.
- Diffusion-weighted images: Hyperintense areas in the cortex • Findings in the basal ganglia are often negative despite the presence of lesions.
- Late findings: Cystic substance defects and hydrocephalus ex vacuo.

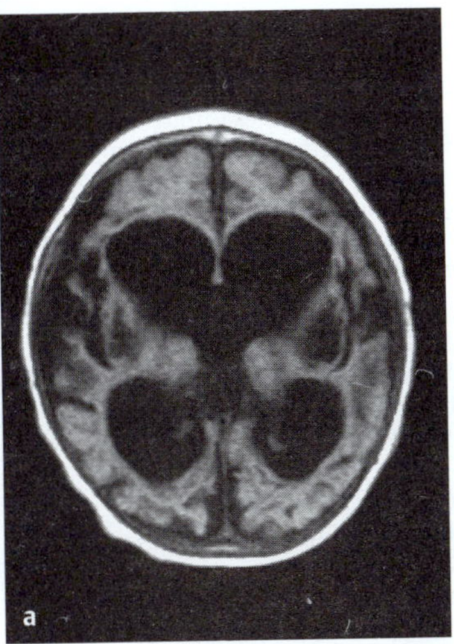

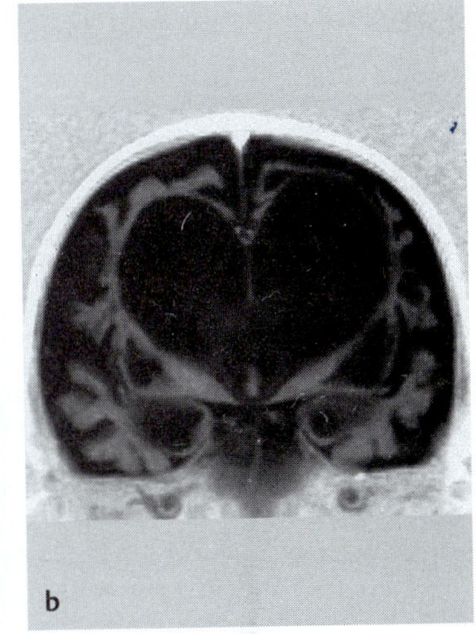

Fig. 7.11 a, b One year after perinatal asphyxia. Low-field-strength MR image. The axial T1-weighted SE image (**a**) and coronal IR TSE image (**b**) show dilation of the inner and outer CSF spaces (hydrocephalus ex vacuo). Cystic defects in the white matter and bilaterally in the basal ganglia.

Clinical Aspects

▸ **Typical presentation**

Sarnat classification:

- *Sarnat grade I:* Agitation • Mydriasis • Tachycardia • Normal EEG.
- *Sarnat grade II:* Apathy • Miosis • Bradycardia • Seizures.
- *Sarnat grade III:* Stupor • Asymmetric pupillary response • Tachycardia or bradycardia • Rarely seizures.

▸ **Therapeutic options**

Restoration of sufficient oxygenation • Correction of hypoglycemia and acidosis • Regulation of blood pressure • Parenteral nutrition may be indicated.

▸ **Course and prognosis**

Clinical course varies from normal development to paraplegia • Prognosis is poor where spontaneous respiration does not occur within the first 20–30 minutes • Prognosis is also poor where neurologic deficits persist longer than 7–10 days • Decreased head growth in the first year is often associated with permanent neurologic deficits.

▸ **Complications**

Retarded development • Microcephaly • Seizures.

Differential Diagnosis

Normal findings	– Increased echogenicity is only visualized in the parasagittal and coronal planes through the anterior fontanelle, not through the posterior fontanelle. – Echogenicity is less than that of the choroid plexus – Echogenicity is homogeneous; ventricles are well demarcated – No cysts after 3 weeks
Hemorrhagic infarction	– Asymmetric – Large areas are affected – Anterior to the lateral ventricles – Extends far into the periphery of the brain – Usually associated with severe intraventricular hemorrhage – Immediately adjacent to the ventricle
Mitochondrial encephalopathy	– Highly variable appearance – Affects gray and white matter – Basal ganglia, brainstem, thalami, and dentate nuclei may be affected, less often the white matter, cortex, and cerebellum – Focal and diffuse atrophy – Edema and swelling in acute lesions – Volume loss in the late stage

Tips and Pitfalls

DWI provides only a brief time window for demonstrating lesions • DWI often does not demonstrate the full extent of the lesion • Ultrasound findings can easily be confused with normal findings or early-stage PVL.

Selected References

Barkovich AJ et al. Perinatal asphyxia: MR findings in the first 10 days. AJNR 1995; 16: 427–438

Barkovich AJ et al. Proton spectroscopy and diffusion imaging on the first day of life after perinatal asphyxia: preliminary report. AJNR 2001; 22: 1658–1670

Sie LT et al. Early MR features of hypoxic-ischemic brain injury in neonates with periventricular densities on sonograms. AJNR 2000, 21: 852–861

Sie LT et al. MR patterns of hypoxic-ischemic brain damage after prenatal, perinatal or postnatal asphyxia. Neuropediatrics 2000; 31: 128–136

Slovis TL et al. Ultrasound in the evaluation of hypoxic-ischemic injury and intracranial hemorrhage in neonates: the state of the art. Pediatr Radiol 1984; 14: 67–75

Definition

- **Epidemiology**
  Most common cause of unilateral proptosis in children • Usually associated with sinusitis • Affected children are often younger than 15 years.
- **Etiology, pathophysiology, pathogenesis**
  Ethmoid and maxillary sinusitis can lead to periostitis of the lamina papyracea or floor of the orbit • Left untreated, the inflammation spreads to the orbit by extension • Inflammation may also spread to the orbit via the valveless orbital veins • If the orbital cellulitis is not promptly detected, a subperiosteal abscess may form in the lamina papyracea and/or floor of the orbit • Inflammation is initially extraconal • Later intraconal spread may occur • Rare causes include opening of the retrobulbar space due to direct trauma and hematogenous spread in the setting of sepsis.

Imaging Signs

- **Radiographs of the paranasal sinuses**
  This is a merely preliminary study • Opacification of the paranasal sinus • Bony erosion of the orbital wall • Soft tissue swelling.
- **Ultrasound**
  Where edema is present, fatty tissue septa are visualized as anechoic bands • A subperiosteal abscess appears as a hypoechoic mass on the medial wall of the orbit. Before liquefaction occurs, these masses may also appear hyperechoic • The medial rectus muscle and globe are displaced • Sound transmission in place of air artifacts suggests mucosal swelling or mucus retention.
- **CT**
  Density of the orbital fat pad is increased • Slight diffuse contrast enhancement • Proptosis • Periorbital soft tissue swelling.
  Findings in subperiosteal abscess:
  - Mass on the medial wall of the orbit (more often than on the cranial wall) isodense to soft tissue.
  - Medial rectus muscle is swollen and displaced.
  - A larger process may also involve the extraocular muscles.
  - Contrast enhancement often demarcates the abscess with its hypodense center.
- **MRI**
  Indicated in optic neuritis • Better differentiates diffuse inflammations from small abscesses.
  - T1-weighted images: Hypointense lesions in the orbital fat pad.
  - T2-weighted images: Diffuse hyperintense signal of the fatty tissue and involved extraocular muscles • Subperiosteal abscess is visualized as a circumscribed hyperintense lesion.
  - Contrast-enhanced T1-weighted images: Diffuse enhancement of the fatty tissue and extraocular muscles • Abscess appears as a central hypointense lesion with marginal enhancement.

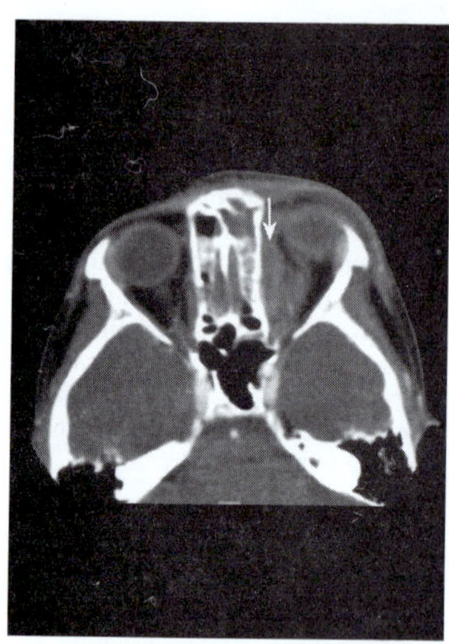

Fig. 7.12 Orbital cellulitis in the left orbit. Contrast-enhanced CT at the level of the ethmoid cells: Inflammatory opacification of the ethmoid cells with subperiosteal abscess (arrow) on the medial wall of the left orbit.

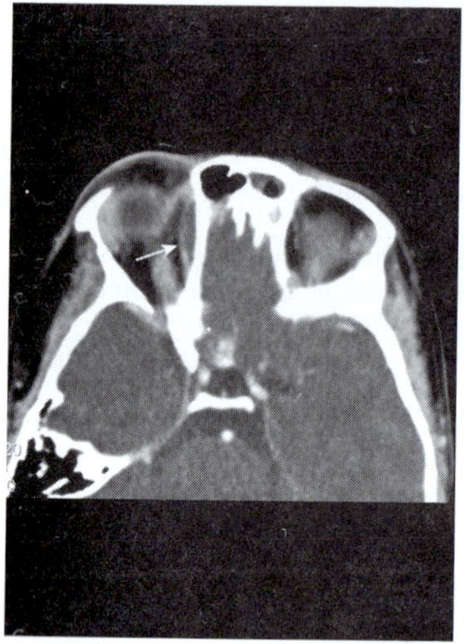

Fig. 7.13 Abscess in the right orbit, a complication of ethmoid sinusitis in an infant. On the contrast-enhanced CT, the subperiosteal abscess is demarcated by the markedly enhancing periosteum (arrow).

Clinical Aspects

- **Typical presentation**
  Proptosis • Upper and lower eyelid edema • Erythema • Ophthalmoplegia • Sensation of congestion in the affected paranasal sinus • Headache.
- **Therapeutic options**
  Antibiotic therapy • Surgical management.
- **Course and prognosis**
  Partial or total loss of visual acuity due to optic neuritis, ischemia due to increased intraorbital pressure, or retinal ischemia due to central retinal artery occlusion • Delayed treatment leads to blindness in 10% of cases.
- **Complications**
  Subperiosteal abscess • Osteomyelitis • Intracranial abscess • Venous thrombosis in the cerebral or sinus veins • Blindness.

Differential Diagnosis

Myositis	– Swelling of the medial rectus, superior rectus, and superior oblique muscles – Tendon insertion is also affected – Often bilateral
Pseudotumor	– Painful exophthalmos without signs of inflammation – Can affect all segments of the eye – Diffuse infiltration of some or all compartments and/or structures – No bony destruction

Tips and Pitfalls

In orbital cellulitis, CT of the orbit should not be performed as a plain scan but with contrast media to visualize subperiosteal abscesses (an indication for surgery) • MRI of the CNS is indicated in symptomatic cases where complications such as optic neuritis, intracranial extension, and especially venous thrombosis of the cerebral and sinus veins are suspected.

Selected References

Givner LB et al. Periorbital versus orbital cellulitis. Pediatr Infect Dis J 2002; 21: 1157–1158

Rahbar R et al. Management of orbital subperiosteal abscess in children. Arch Otolaryngol Head Neck Surg 2001; 127: 281–286

Sobol SE et al. Orbital complications of sinusitis in children. J Otolaryngol 2002; 31: 131–136

Definition

- **Epidemiology**

  Neurofibromatosis type 1: Von Recklinghausen disease • Incidence is 1:2000–3000 • One of the most common hereditary disorders • High rate of spontaneous mutation, but also increased familial incidence • Penetrance is 100% • Expressivity is highly variable • Boys are affected more often than girls.

  Neurofibromatosis type 2: Incidence is 1:35 000 • 50% of cases involve a new mutation • Clinical picture is considerably variable.

  Tuberous sclerosis: Bourneville disease • Incidence is 1:7000–10 000 • New mutations account for 60–70% of cases • Boys are affected more often than girls.

  Von Hippel–Lindau disease: Incidence is 1:35 000–45 000 • There are numerous mutations of the same gene • Spontaneous mutations occur in up to 50% of cases • No sex predilection.

  Sturge–Weber syndrome: Encephalotrigeminal angiomatosis • Incidence: 1:50 000 • Occurs sporadically.

- **Etiology, pathophysiology, pathology**

  Autosomal dominant syndromes with variable penetrance • Associated with tumors or tumor-like malformations of the nervous system, skin, and internal organs.

  Neurofibromatosis type 1: Defect in the NF-1 tumor suppressor gene • This leads to unchecked proliferation of certain cell types • Multiple neurofibromas (plexiform neurofibromas in the intracranial, intraspinal, and intramedullary regions, in the skin, and in internal organs) • Café-au-lait spots • Optic pathway gliomas (15–20% of cases) • Other intracranial astrocytomas and nonneural tumors such as meningioma also occur • Chronic neurofibromas can degenerate into malignant lesions • Slightly increased incidence of medulloblastomas and ependymomas.

  Neurofibromatosis type 2: Defect in the NF-2 tumor suppressor gene • This leads to disruption of cell migration and cell shape or loss of contact inhibition • Bilateral schwannomas of the vestibular nerve (acoustic neurinomas) or other cranial nerves • Multiple schwannomas of the spinal nerve roots (85–90% of cases) • Meningiomas, astrocytomas, and hamartomas of the cerebral cortex • Ependymomas of the conus medullaris.

  Tuberous sclerosis: Gene defect that disrupts cell differentiation and migration during embryogenesis and fetal development • Nodular proliferations of glial tissue occur in individual gyri (tubers) and in the lateral ventricles (subependymal hamartomas, giant cell astrocytomas or gangliogliomas) • Angiofibromas occur in the nasolabial folds and on the forehead, and chin • Ungual fibromas • Benign hamartomas occur in the heart (rhabdomyomas, occurring in 50–65% of cases) and kidney (angiomyolipomas, cysts, 40–80%) • Retinal hamartomas • Hamartomas very rarely degenerate into hamartoblastomas.

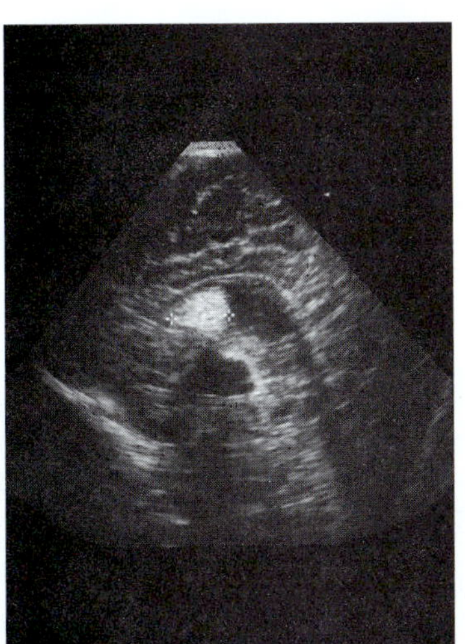

Fig. 7.14 Giant cell astrocytoma. Ultrasound, parasagittal plane. Seven-month-old infant with tuberous sclerosis.

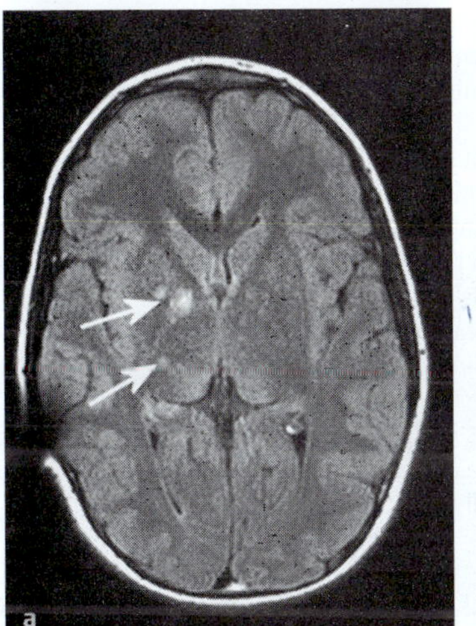

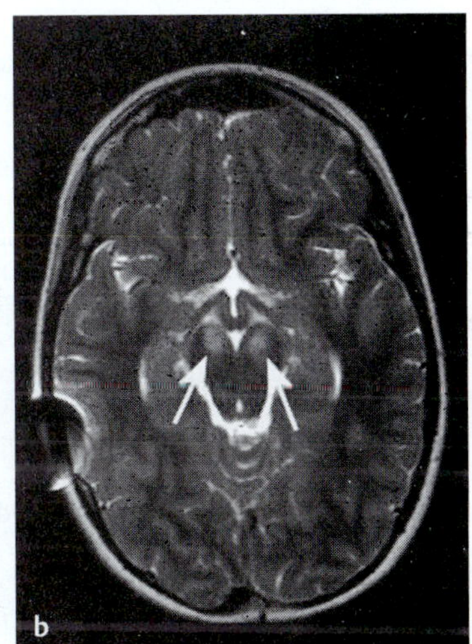

Fig. 7.15 a, b A 9-year-old girl with neurofibromatosis type 1. MR image. Typical hyperintense focal areas (arrows) in the globus pallidus and thalamus on the right (**a**, axial FLAIR) and bilaterally in the cerebral peduncle (**b**, axial T2-weighted TSE).

Von Hippel–Lindau disease: Defect on chromosome 3p25 • Hemangioblastoma in the cerebellum and other regions of the CNS • Unilateral or bilateral hemangioblastomas of the retina • Hemangioblastomas in the spinal cord • Renal cell carcinoma • Pheochromocytoma • Endolymphatic sacciform tumor • Polycystic organs (kidney, pancreas) also occur.
Sturge–Weber syndrome: Etiology is unknown • Angiomatosis of the leptomeninx (often unilateral) • Calcification of the intracortical capillaries • Cortical atrophy • Choroid angiomas • Facial nevus flammeus.

Imaging Signs

- **Radiographic findings**
  Neurofibromatosis type 1: Scoliosis with acute angle • Dural ectasia and lateral meningoceles lead to flattened vertebrae • Posterior elements of the vertebra are hypoplastic • Rib notching • Multiple pseudarthroses.
- **Contrast CT findings**
  Neurofibromatosis type 1: The superior orbital fissure is widened due to optic pathway gliomas, or the foramen ovale due to neurofibromas • Sphenoid wing dysplasia • Lambdoid suture defect • Dural calcifications • Neurofibromas are usually isodense to brain tissue • Variable enhancement • Calcifications are rare.
  Neurofibromatosis type 2: Widening of the internal auditory canal occurs where a mass in the vestibular nerve is present • *Meningioma:* Focal or diffuse hyperdense dural lesion showing marked enhancement • Nontumorous calcifications are often present.
  Tuberous sclerosis: Subependymal nodules occur more often in the lateral ventricles than in the temporal horns • Nodules calcify over time • Supratentorial tubers are more common than infratentorial tubers • Hypodense or isodense subcortical mass • Calcifications occur in the overlying cortex • Tubers themselves also calcify • The ventricular system is dilated.
  Von Hippel–Lindau disease: In 70% of cases cerebellar hemangioblastomas, typical appearance: small isodens tumor nodule in the wall of a hypodens cerebellar cyst • The nodule enhances markedly; the cyst does not.
  Sturge–Weber syndrome: Calcifications in the gyral and subcortical white matter (not in the angiomas themselves) • Calcification progresses from posterior to anterior • Angiomas enhance markedly • Tortuous appearance, often with dilation of the ipsilateral choroid plexus.
- **Contrast MRI findings**
  Neurofibromatosis type 1: In 60–80% of cases, there are focal areas of high signal intensity in the white matter, globus pallidus, thalamus, hippocampus, brainstem, and cerebellum • Slight or absent mass effect • Hyperintense on T2-weighted images • Variable on T1-weighted images • Rarely enhancing (in 11% of cases, with proliferation).
  Optic pathway gliomas: Affected structures can include the optic nerve, optic chiasm, or hypothalamus • Occurs less often along the optic tract • Structures exhibit fusiform thickening • Tortuous optic nerve with dilated nerve sheath •

Lesion is isointense on T1-weighted images, hyperintense on T2-weighted images • Moderate to pronounced enhancement on T1-weighted images.
Plexiform neurofibroma: Affected structures include the skull base, orbits, and scalp. Paraspinal and intraspinal lesions may also occur, leading to widening of the spinal canal and neural foramina • Hypointense to isointense on T1-weighted and T2-weighted images • Intramedullary lesions exhibit inhomogeneous contrast enhancement on contrast T1-weighted images; other lesions show variable contrast enhancement.
Neurofibromatosis type 2: Schwannomas: Well demarcated lesions in the vestibular nerve (unilateral or bilateral mass in the inner auditory canal, occasionally with cysts) and in the spinal nerve roots • Intraspinal and/or extraspinal growth may occur in these lesions • Hypointense to isointense on T1-weighted images • Isointense to hyperintense on T2-weighted images • Pronounced but inhomogeneous contrast enhancement on T1-weighted images.
Ependymomas, astrocytomas: Often in the cervicothoracic region • Thickening of the spinal cord • Hypointense to isointense on T1-weighted images • Hyperintense on T2-weighted images • Contrast enhancement on T1-weighted images.
Meningioma: Circumscribed, occasionally diffuse dural lesion • Isointense to cerebral cortex on T1-weighted and T2-weighted images • Pronounced contrast enhancement on T1-weighted images.
Tuberous sclerosis: Cortical and subcortical tubers: Thickened gyrus and cortex, occasionally with a central notch • In order of decreasing frequency, lesions occur in the frontal, parietal, occipital, and temporal regions • Signal intensity varies with myelination • Hypointense to hyperintense on T1-weighted images • Hyperintense on T2-weighted images • Rarely contrast enhancing.
Subependymal nodules: Isointense to hyperintense on T1-weighted images • Hyperintense on T2-weighted images • 30–80% of cases show contrast enhancement • Enhancing subependymal nodules in the foramen of Monro are often giant cell astrocytomas.
White matter lesions: T2-weighted images show streaky or ill-defined lesions along the migration lines from the ventricle to the cortex.
Von Hippel–Lindau disease: Cerebellar hemangioblastomas: T1-weighted images show isointense nodule and hypointense cyst • Hyperintense on T2-weighted images • The nodule enhances markedly on T1-weighted images • Flow artifacts may be present within the mural nodule • Lesions in the spinal canal are often associated with syrinx • Several small nodules may be present.
Sturge–Weber syndrome: Accelerated myelination in the early stage • Leptomeningeal angiomas show marked contrast enhancement • The choroid plexus is frequently enlarged • In the late stage: gliosis in the white matter (hyperintense signal on T2-weighted images) • Hardly any enhancement in the leptomeninx • Increasing calcifications • Cerebral hemiatrophy.
MR venography: Superficial cerebral veins are absent • Flow in the transverse sinus and jugular veins is reduced • Medullary veins are prominent.

Clinical Aspects

- **Typical presentation**

Neurofibromatosis type 1: Presence of two or more of the following signs is diagnostic: More than six café-au-lait spots occur during the first year of life, more than two neurofibromas during puberty or one plexiform neurofibroma • Axillary and/or inguinal pigment spots • Optic pathway glioma • Typical bone changes • Immediate relative has neurofibromatosis • Learning disability • Mental deficiency.

Neurofibromatosis type 2: The following situations are diagnostic: Bilateral acoustic schwannomas, or immediate relative with neurofibromatosis type 2 and unilateral acoustic schwannoma, or two of the following changes: meningioma, schwannoma, glioma, neurofibroma, juvenile lens opacity (posterior subcapsular or cortical cataract). Acoustic schwannomas produce symptoms such as tinnitus, hearing loss and vertigo, headache, balance impairment, and unsteady gait.

Tuberous sclerosis: Mental deficiency (50–80% of cases) • Seizures (80–90%) • Presence of two primary criteria or one primary criterion and one secondary criterion is diagnostic.

Primary criteria: Facial angiofibroma or plaque on the forehead • Subungual fibroma • More than two pigmented spots • Multiple retinal hamartomas • Cortical tubers • Subependymal nodules • Subependymal giant cell astrocytomas • Cardiac rhabdomyoma • Lymphangioleiomyomatosis • Renal angiomyolipoma.

Secondary criteria: Pitting in dental enamel • Hamartomatous rectal polyps • Bone cysts • Cerebral radial migration lines in the white matter • Gingival fibromas • Nonrenal hamartomas • Retinal achromatic spot • Confetti skin lesions • Multiple renal cysts.

Von Hippel–Lindau syndrome: Heterogeneous picture • Visual symptoms • Headache • Gait disturbances • Diagnosis based on CNS or retinal hemangioblastoma and one of the associated tumors or a positive family history.

Sturge–Weber syndrome: Seizures (75% of cases) • Flat nevus flammeus in the area supplied by the trigeminal nerve • Glaucoma • Buphthalmos • Strokelike episodes.

- **Therapeutic options**

Neurofibromatosis type 1: Observation • Radiation therapy and chemotherapy may be indicated for optic pathway glioma • Partial resection of neurofibromas may be indicated where they block the airway or compress the gastrointestinal tract • Stabilization of the spine in scoliosis.

Neurofibromatosis type 2: Acoustic schwannoma should be resected wherever possible.

Tuberous sclerosis: Antiepileptic treatment • Dermabrasion or laser treatment of angiofibromas • Surgical management of epilepsy involving resection of the epileptogenic tubers may be indicated • Resection of subependymal giant cell astrocytomas is indicated in obstructive hydrocephalus.

Von Hippel–Lindau syndrome: Annual physical and neurologic examinations • Ophthalmologic examination • Resection of cerebellar and spinal hemangioblastomas • Stereotactic radiation treatment • Laser treatment of retinal angiomas.

Sturge–Weber syndrome: Antiepileptic treatment • Neurosurgery is indicated for epilepsy resistant to treatment.

- **Course and prognosis**

Neurofibromatosis type 1: Focal hyperintense areas increase from 2 to 10 years and decrease again after age 20 • Cutaneous manifestations increase with age • Optic pathway glioma increases the risk of developing other CNS tumors • Prognosis is relatively good • However, life expectancy is reduced.

Neurofibromatosis type 2: Multiple schwannomas often occur early (earlier than sporadic lesions) • They can involve any cranial or peripheral nerve • Prognosis is slightly worse than for type 1.

Tuberous sclerosis: Mild cases have a good prognosis • Prognosis is worse with lung and kidney involvement.

Von Hippel–Lindau disease: Often only becomes symptomatic between the ages of 10 and 40 years • Renal cell carcinoma is the most common cause of death.

Sturge–Weber syndrome: Seizures begin during the first year of life • This often leads to retarded development • A third of all patients develop progressive hemiparesis • Hemianopia occasionally occurs • Progressive atrophy of the affected hemisphere.

- **Complications**

Neurofibromatosis type 1: Malignant degeneration of the plexiform neurofibromas • Blindness in optic pathway gliomas • Paraplegia in spinal tumors • Scoliosis.

Neurofibromatosis type 2: Vertigo • Deafness • Cataract • Facial palsy.

Tuberous sclerosis: Obstructive hydrocephalus • Epileptic seizures • Mental deficiency • Autism • Kidney failure • Bronchopneumonia in pulmonary lymphangioleiomyomatosis • Cardiac arrhythmia and heart failure in rhabdomyoma.

Von Hippel–Lindau disease: Retinal bleeding • Retinal detachment • Blindness • Progressive myelopathy • Intracerebellar and intraspinal hemorrhages • Tumor-associated complications (renal cell carcinoma, pheochromocytoma) • Deafness.

Sturge–Weber syndrome: Glaucoma and buphthalmos • Seizures • Neurologic deficits • Tonic-clonic and myoclonic spasms.

Differential Diagnosis

Gliomatosis cerebri (neurofibromatosis type 1 with multiple hyperintense areas)	– Affects two or more lobes – Diffuse proliferation of white matter (basal ganglia, thalamus, corpus callosum, brainstem, spinal cord, cerebellum) that increases the volume of the affected lobes but preserves cerebral architecture – Isointense to hypointense on T1-weighted images – Hyperintense on T2-weighted images – Slight enhancement
Multiple schwannomas without neurofibromatosis type 2	– No cutaneous changes – No meningiomas
X-linked subependymal heterotopia	– Isointense to gray matter – No enhancement – No calcifications
Pilocytic astrocytoma	– Younger patients – Solid component hypointense to isointense to CSF and cystic component slightly hyperintense to CSF on T1-weighted images – Hypointense solid component and hyperintense cyst on T2-weighted images – Highly inhomogeneous enhancement – Cyst wall enhances as well
Wyburn–Mason syndrome	– Congenital nonhereditary arteriovenous malformations of the CNS, retina, and maxillofacial region – Involving the ipsilateral hemisphere of the affected eye – No mass effect – Large lesions exhibit flow artifacts

Tips and Pitfalls

MR spectroscopy is helpful in differentiating white matter lesions from gliomas • Most differential diagnoses require examination of the spinal axis • A thin slice examination of the orbits is recommended in Sturge–Weber syndrome.

Selected References

He FJ et al. Von Hippel-Lindau disease: strategies in early detection (renal-, adrenal-, pancreatic masses). Eur Radiol 1999; 9: 598–610

Maria BL et al. Central nervous system structure and function in Sturge-Weber syndrome: evidence of neurologic and radiologic progression. J Child Neurol 1998; 13: 606–618

Maria BL et al. Tuberous sclerosis complex: pathogenesis, diagnosis, strategies, therapies, and future research directions. J Child Neurol 2004; 19: 632–642

Quigg M et al. Clinical findings of the phakomatoses: neurofibromatosis. Neurology 2006; 66: 23–24

Ruggeri M. The different forms of neurofibromatosis. Childs Nerv Syst 1999; 15: 295–308

Definition

- **Epidemiology**
  Brain tumors are the second most common tumor disorder in children and adolescents after the leukemias • Incidence is 4:100 000 • 50% of these tumors are located in the posterior cranial fossa.
  - *Medulloblastoma:* Most common tumor of the posterior cranial fossa (40% of cases) • Usually occurs before age 10 years • More common in boys than girls (1.5:1).
  - *Pilocytic astrocytoma:* Most common brain tumor and second most common tumor of the posterior cranial fossa in children • Usually occurs before age 20 years • Peak age is 5–9 years • No sex predilection.
  - *Ependymoma:* Third most common tumor of the posterior cranial fossa in children • Accounts for 10% of all brain tumors • Peak age is 5–6 years • A third of the affected children are under age 3 years • No sex predilection.
  - *Epidermoid cyst:* Third most common mass of the cerebellopontine angle and internal auditory canal • Rare intracranial mass.
- **Etiology, pathophysiology, pathogenesis**
  Medulloblastoma: Belongs to the primitive neuroectodermal tumors (PNET) • Arises from the vermis cerebelli • Tumor growth is usually round and displaces adjacent structures • Progressive growth gradually obliterates the fourth ventricle • This leads to hydrocephalus • Tumor spreads by direct extension (into the cerebellar peduncles and/or to the floor of the fourth ventricle, brainstem, spinal cord, and supratentorial region) or by metastasis via the CSF (to the supratentorial region, into the leptomeninx, and into the spinal canal) • Extracranial metastases can also occur in rare cases • WHO grade IV.
  Pilocytic astrocytoma: Arises from precursor cells of the astrocytes in the cerebellar hemispheres • Slow-growing, circumscribed, often cystic tumor • Metastasizes and degenerates only very rarely • Spontaneous regression can occur • Often occurs in the cerebellum • Less often involves the optic nerve, optic chiasm, hypothalamus, thalamus, basal ganglia, and cerebral hemispheres • Rarely involves the brainstem • Progressively compresses the fourth ventricle, leading to hydrocephalus.
  Ependymoma: Arises from the ependyma • Presumably results from genetic defects • There are four subtypes: Cellular, papillary, clear cell, and tanycytic • Two-thirds of all lesions are infratentorial (on the floor of the fourth ventricle), one-third are supratentorial • Tumor is usually lobulated and circumscribed • It can contain cysts • Occasionally necrosis and hemorrhage are present • Calcifications occur in 50% of lesions • The tumor can expand through the lateral apertures of the fourth ventricle as far as the cerebellopontine angle and into the basal cisterns; it can expand posteriorly through the median aperture into the cisterna magna • Spinal ependymomas are very rare in children • In up to 20% of cases, the tumor metastasizes via the CSF.
  Epidermoid cyst: Arises during embryogenesis from ectoderm enclosed within the neural tube • Usually outside the midline • Most often at the cerebellopontine angle • Less often in the fourth ventricle • Cyst wall consists of squamous epithelium, the contents of crystalline cholesterol, and cellular debris • Grows very slowly • Encases neurovascular structures.

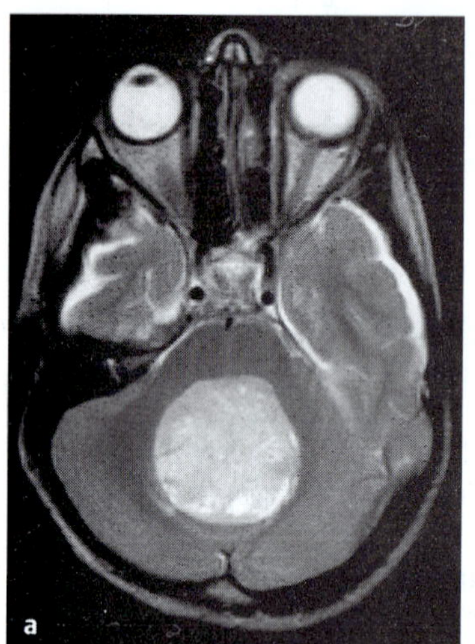

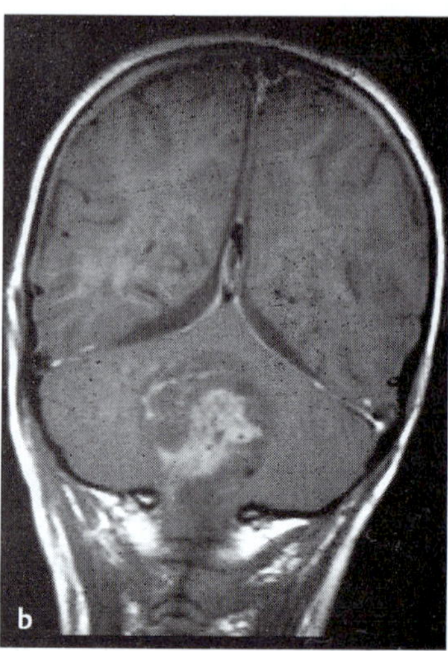

Fig. 7.16 a, b Medulloblastoma in a 9-year-old boy. MR images. On the T2-weighted image (**a**), tumor is isointense to gray matter with isolated hyperintense cysts. The post-contrast T1-weighted image (**b**) shows inhomogeneous enhancement of the tumor tissue.

Imaging Signs

- **Ultrasound findings**

  Most intracranial tumors occur after age 2 years • By then the fontanellae are no longer patent and only the temporal bone is available as an acoustic window.

  Medulloblastoma: Increased echogenicity • Occasionally cysts and calcifications • Obstructive hydrocephalus.

  Pilocytic astrocytoma: Hyperechoic solid component • Usually large anechoic cystic component • Hydrocephalus.

- **Contrast CT findings**

  Medulloblastoma: Solid, isodense to hyperdense mass in the roof of the fourth ventricle • Small cysts or necroses are present in 40–50% of all lesions • Calcifications are rare • Hemorrhages are very rare • Over 90% of cases involve hydrocephalus • Tumor tissue enhances homogeneously.

  Pilocytic astrocytoma: Mass with cystic component isodense to CSF and solid component hypodense or isodense to brain parenchyma • Often there is a halo of decreased density in the surrounding brain parenchyma (edema) • Calcifications and hemorrhages are rare • Hydrocephalus is usually present • The solid component enhances homogeneously, necrosis inhomogeneously • The cystic component enhances in only half of all tumors • Contrast agent occasionally fills the cysts.

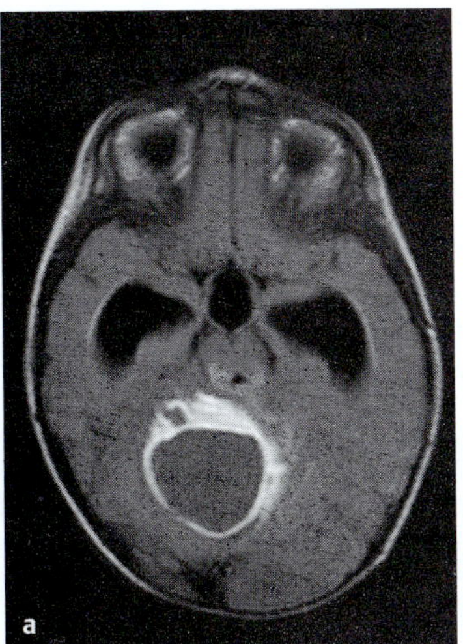

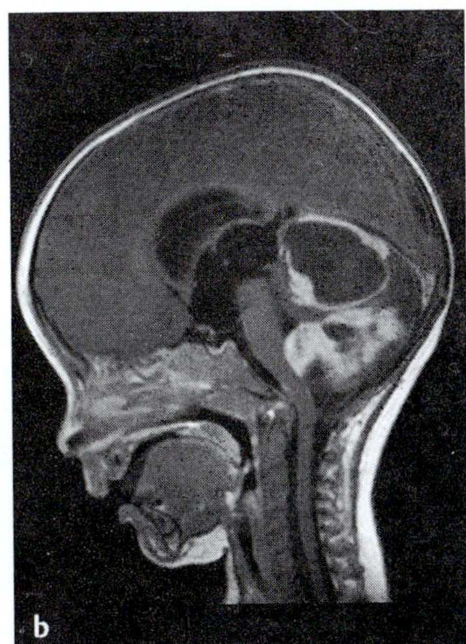

Fig. 7.17 a, b Pilocytic astrocytoma in a 2-year-old boy. MR axial FLAIR (**a**) and sagittal T1-weighted post-contrast (**b**) images. Large inhomogeneous tumor with solid and cystic components and secondary internal hydrocephalus (used with the kind permission of Dr. G. Hahn, Department of Pediatric Radiology, Institute of Diagnostic Radiology and Polyclinic, Carl Gustav Carus University Medical Center, Dresden).

Ependymoma: Mass on the floor of the fourth ventricle, usually isodense to brain tissue • May spread into the cerebellopontine angle and cisterna magna • Calcifications are common • Hemorrhages and cysts occasionally occur • Contrast enhancement is variable and inhomogeneous.

Epidermoid cyst: Hypodense mass (isodense to CSF) • Calcifications are present in up to 25% of cases • Rare variant: Dense epidermoid • Usually does not enhance after contrast administration.

▸ **MRI findings**

Medulloblastoma: Preoperative staging • Postoperative follow-up • Hypointense to gray matter on T1-weighted images • Isointense on T2-weighted images • Hyperintense on proton density and FLAIR images • Reduced diffusion on DWI • Inhomogeneous enhancement on T1-weighted images • Leptomeningeal enhancement occurs where the tumor spreads via the meninges.

Pilocytic astrocytoma: T1-weighted images: Solid component is hypointense or isointense to gray matter • Cyst contents are isointense or slightly hyperintense to CSF.

T2-weighted images: Solid component is hypointense to gray matter • Cyst contents are isointense or slightly hyperintense to CSF.

FLAIR: Solid component is hyperintense • Cyst contents are hyperintense to CSF.

Contrast-enhanced T1-weighted images: Markedly inhomogeneous enhancement of the solid component • Cyst walls only occasionally enhance.

Ependymoma: T1-weighted images: Hypointense to isointense • Calcifications and hemorrhages appear as slightly hyperintense areas • Cyst contents are hyperintense to CSF.
T2-weighted images: Isointense to hyperintense • Cystic areas appear hyperintense • Calcifications and hemorrhages appear as hypointense areas.
FLAIR: Tumor is more clearly demarcated • Cyst contents are markedly hyperintense.
T1-weighted images with contrast: Slight to moderate inhomogeneous enhancement.
Epidermoid cyst: T1-weighted images: Slightly hypointense to CSF • Can resemble a complex arachnoid cyst • Occasionally septated • A dense epidermoid is hyperintense.
T2-weighted images: Isointense or hyperintense to CSF.
FLAIR: Hyperintense.
Contrast-enhanced T1-weighted images: Slight or absent marginal enhancement.

Clinical Aspects

- **Typical presentation**
Medulloblastoma: Symptoms of cerebellar involvement (ataxia of the trunk and extremities, intention tremor, nystagmus) • Signs of increased intracranial pressure (vomiting, headache, sixth cranial nerve palsy) • Symptoms of local tumor spread (cranial nerve palsy, dysregulation in vital centers; deficits in long pathways).
Pilocytic astrocytoma: Symptoms of increased intracranial pressure and cerebellar involvement.
Ependymoma: Symptoms of increased intracranial pressure • Symptoms of cerebellar involvement • Occasional neck pain • Torticollis • Vision loss.
Epidermoid cyst: Remains clinically asymptomatic for many years • First symptoms usually appear around age 40 • Symptoms depend on the location • Headache • Cranial neuropathies (fifth, seventh, and eighth cranial nerves).
- **Therapeutic options**
Medulloblastoma: Radical surgery is best wherever possible • Chemotherapy • Irradiation of the entire CNS (in children over age 3).
Pilocytic astrocytoma: Resection • Adjuvant combined radiation and chemotherapy is indicated to treat residual tumor.
Ependymoma: Complete tumor resection • Postoperative radiation therapy • Efficacy of chemotherapy has not been established.
Epidermoid cyst: Resection.
- **Course and prognosis**
Medulloblastoma: Prognosis depends on the age of the child, the size of the residual tumor postoperatively, and evidence of distant metastases (M classification).
Pilocytic astrocytoma: Where total resection of the tumor is feasible, the 10-year survival rate is nearly 100%.
Ependymoma: In up to 20% of cases, metastases are present at the time of the diagnosis • Resectability is a decisive factor in the prognosis • Where total resection

is possible, the survival rate is 51–80% • Where only subtotal resection is possible, it decreases to 0–26% • Prognosis in infants younger than 1 year is very poor.

Epidermoid cyst: Prognosis is good where the cyst is completely resected.

▶ **Complications**

Medulloblastoma: Hydrocephalus • Neurologic deficits • Pain • Treatment-related complications such as endocrinopathy, retarded growth, leukomalacia and encephalomalacia, microangiopathy, hearing loss including deafness, and secondary CNS malignancies.

Pilocytic astrocytoma: Identical to medulloblastoma.

Ependymoma: Identical to medulloblastoma.

Epidermoid cyst: Residual cyst wall left in situ after resection often leads to recurrence.

Differential Diagnosis

Choroid plexus papilloma	– More common in the lateral ventricles (70% of cases) – Lobulated appearance – Highly homogeneous enhancement – Lesser mass effect – Choroidal artery dilated
Hemangioblastoma	– Older patients – Nodule adjacent to the pia mater – Marked homogeneous enhancement of the nodule – Tumor lacks soft tissue component
Brainstem gliomas	– See section on "Brainstem Gliomas"
Atypical teratoid or rhabdoid tumor	– Younger children – Usually indistinguishable from medulloblastoma – Very heterogeneous appearance – Tumor appears as a cystic and solid hemorrhagic mass – Variable enhancement

Tips and Pitfalls

Examination of the spinal axis is indicated in medulloblastoma to exclude drop metastases • Pilocytic astrocytomas compress the fourth ventricle, medulloblastomas fill it • Ependymomas are far less common than medulloblastomas and pilocytic astrocytomas.

Selected References

Cheng YC et al. Neuroradiological findings in atypical teratoid/rhabdoid tumor of the central nervous system. Acta Radiol 2005; 46: 89–96

Koeller KK et al. From the archives of the AFIP: pilocytic astrocytoma: radiologic-pathologic correlation. Radiographics 2004; 23: 1693–1708

Marmuth-Metz M et al. Neuroradiological differential diagnosis in medulloblastomas and ependymomas: results of the HITk91-study. Klin Padiatr 2002; 214: 162–166

Strother D. Atypical teratoid rhabdoid tumors of childhood: diagnosis, treatment and challenges. Expert Rev Anticancer Ther 2005; 5: 7621–7631

Definition

- **Epidemiology**

  These tumors account for 15% of all pediatric brain tumors • They account for 20–30% of all tumors of the posterior cranial fossa • Often occur between ages 3 and 10 years • May be associated with neurofibromatosis type 1 • No sex predilection.

- **Etiology, pathophysiology, pathogenesis**

  The definition of a high-grade glioma is usually histologic • Brainstem gliomas represent an exception because the risk of morbidity of the operation is high and the prognostic value of histologic findings is slight.

  Typical diffuse intrinsic pons gliomas: Cause: Genetic mutation • Diffuse infiltration of the anterior pons • This causes the pons to appear distended • Tumor spreads along the spinal nerve tracts.

  Typical midbrain gliomas: Slowly or not at all progressive • May lead to obstruction of the cerebral aqueduct.

  Posterior exophytic cerebellomedullary gliomas: Identical to typical midbrain gliomas.

  Atypical brainstem gliomas: These do not fall into any of the categories mentioned and include tumors such as exophytic pons tumors and gliomas showing primary enhancement • Metastases are rare; spread is usually through the CSF.

Imaging Signs

- **CT findings**

  Midbrain gliomas, exophytic cerebellomedullary gliomas: Usually well demarcated • Slightly hyperdense where calcifications are present • Enhancement is variable and decreases with increasing calcification • Hydrocephalus may be present.

  Diffuse intrinsic pons glioma: Hypodense to isodense • Fewer calcifications • Usually does not enhance.

- **Contrast MRI findings**

  Midbrain gliomas and exophytic cerebellomedullary gliomas: Isointense to slightly hyperintense on T1-weighted images • Hyperintense on T2-weighted and FLAIR images • Slight or absent enhancement on T1-weighted images • Lead to early obstruction of the cerebral aqueduct • Displace the tectum cranially • Remain circumscribed • Can infiltrate the cerebral peduncles.

  Diffuse intrinsic pons glioma: Hypointense on T1-weighted images • Hyperintense on T2-weighted and FLAIR images • Absent or slight enhancement on contrast-enhanced T1-weighted images • Pons is distended • Only occasionally obstructs the cerebral aqueduct • Can encase the basilar artery and vertebral arteries.

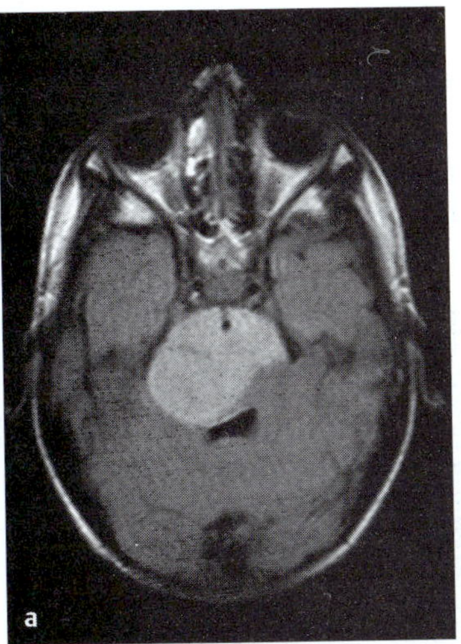

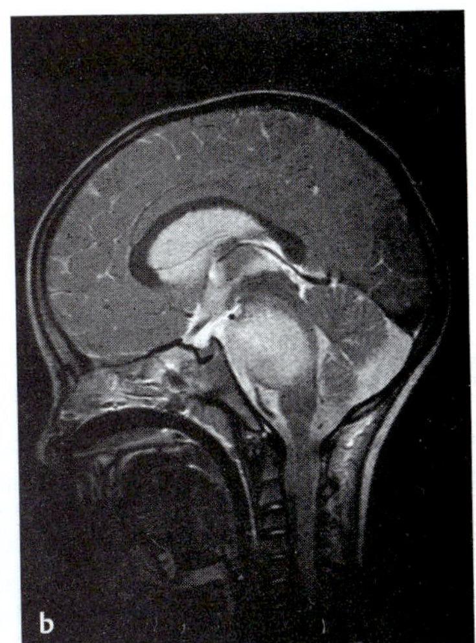

Fig. 7.18 a, b Diffuse intrinsic pons glioma in a 4-year-old boy. MR axial FLAIR (**a**) and sagittal T2-weighted TSE (**b**) images. Hyperintense tumor leading to diffuse enlargement of the pons. The tumor is compressing the fourth ventricle and has encased the basilar artery (used with the kind permission of Dr. G. Hahn, Department of Pediatric Radiology, Institute of Diagnostic Radiology and Polyclinic, Carl Gustav Carus University Medical Center, Dresden).

Clinical Aspects

- **Typical presentation**
  Nausea and vomiting • Headache • Cranial nerve deficits with bulbar symptoms • Ataxia • Dysarthria • Nystagmus • Sleep apnea • Pyramidal tract signs.
- **Therapeutic options**
  Pons gliomas are treated with radiation therapy and chemotherapy (children under age 3 years) • Surgery may be indicated for midbrain gliomas.
- **Course and prognosis**
  Prognosis for pons gliomas is poor • Mean survival time is about 1 year • Midbrain gliomas and exophytic cerebellomedullary gliomas have a better prognosis • Prognosis worsens for lesions showing primary contrast enhancement • Lesions associated with neurofibromatosis type 1 have a better prognosis.
- **Complications**
  Increasing brainstem symptoms • Cranial nerve deficits • Dissemination • Hydrocephalus.

Differential Diagnosis

Brainstem encephalitis	– Acute clinical course, fever – Ill-defined areas with cytotoxic edema – With or without hemorrhage – Associated meningitis may be present
Acute disseminated encephalomyelitis	– Supratentorial and spinal patches of demyelination, hyperintense on T2-weighted images – Bilateral asymmetric occurrence – Involvement of gray and white matter – Focal or ring enhancement
Neurofibromatosis type 1	– Multiple focal lesions without mass effect, hyperintense on T2-weighted images and variable on T1-weighted images – Dentate nuclei more often affected – Optic pathway gliomas – Focal hyperintense lesions increasing between 2 and 10 years and decreasing after 20 years
Osmotic myelinolysis	– Due to excessively rapid compensation of hyponatremia – Findings can be highly variable, rendering differentiation difficult – Acute: isointense to slightly hypointense on T1-weighted images, hyperintense on T2-weighted images – Subacute: hyperintense (after 1–4 weeks) on T1-weighted images, slightly hyperintense on T2-weighted images – Spares the pyramidal tracts
Hamartoma	– In conjunction with tuberous sclerosis – Subcortical lesions are hyperintense on T1-weighted images and hypointense on T2-weighted images – Signal behavior changes with age – Calcifications occur in up to 50% of cases

Tips and Pitfalls

In isolated stenosis, the cerebral aqueduct has a funnel-shaped appearance on the sagittal image • CT findings are rarely decisive in cranial nerve deficits.

Selected References

Barkovich AJ. Pediatric Neuroimaging. Philadelphia: Lippincott Williams & Wilkins; 2005: 514–551

Broniscer A et al. Intratumoral hemorrhage among children with newly diagnosed, diffuse brainstem glioma. Cancer 2006; 106: 1364–1371

Donaldson SS et al. Advances towards an understanding of brainstem glioma. J Clin Oncol 2006; 24: 1266–1272

Hargrave D et al. Diffuse brainstem glioma in children: critical review of clinical trail. Lancet Oncol 2006; 7: 241–248

Schumacher M et al. Magnetic resonance imaging compared with biopsy in the diagnosis of brainstem diseases of childhood: a multicenter review. J Neurosurg 2007; 106 (Suppl 2): 111–119

Definition

- **Epidemiology**
  The frequency of tethered cord can only be estimated as not all affected children get symptoms • It is often associated with meningomyelocele (25–50% of all occult cases of spinal dysraphism) or a dermal sinus • No sex predilection.
- **Etiology, pathophysiology, pathogenesis**
  The neural tube closes in the third to fourth week of gestation • When this occurs, the neural ectoderm separates from the cutaneous ectoderm • The distal portion of the spinal cord then involutes • Where this involution fails to occur, a thickened filum terminale remains in situ and fuses with the mesenchymal fat (tethered cord) • Longitudinal growth places tension on the filum terminale • Possible sequelae: Syringomyelia, myelomalacia.

Imaging Signs

- **Ultrasound findings**
  Used in children younger than 1 year • Most suitable in infants up to 4 weeks old • The panoramic ultrasound shows the level of the conus medullaris • M-mode shows mobility of the filum terminale with breathing • The spinal cord is hypoechoic with a central linear hyperechoic structure • Physiologic level of the conus medullaris is between T12 and L3, on average at L1–L2 • In tethered cord, the filum terminale is too far distal, thickened, and fixed • Intraspinal lipoma • The fibers of the cauda equina course in an atypical pattern.
- **Spine radiographs**
  Radiographic findings depend on the severity of the dysraphism • Scoliosis • Segmental anomalies • Vertebral fusion anomalies.
- **CT**
  For evaluating the severity of bony anomalies.
- **Contrast MRI findings**
  Low conus medullaris (farther distal than L2) • Thickened filum terminale (> 2 mm at the level of L5) • Intraspinal lipoma • The conus medullaris is better demarcated on T2-weighted images • Fast T2-weighted sequences obtained with the spine flexed demonstrate the mobility of the conus medullaris • STIR images allow evaluation of the spine and surrounding soft tissue • T1-weighted images with contrast media are used in complications such as an infected dermal sinus.

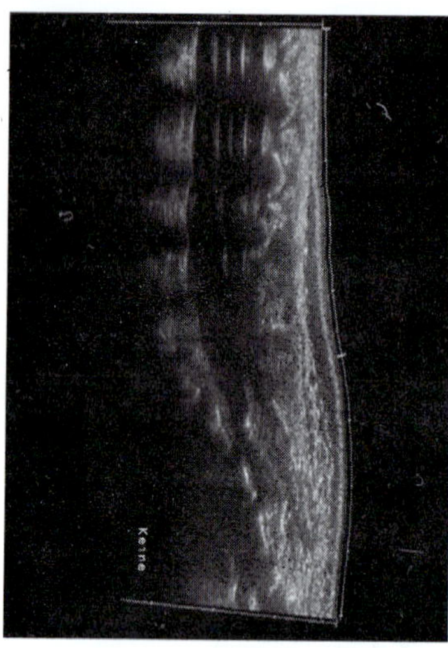

Fig. 7.19 Lipomyelocele and tethered cord. Panoramic ultrasound. The conus medullaris is fixed at the level of vertebra S3, and a hyperechoic intraspinal lipoma is visualized in the sacral spinal canal.

Clinical Aspects

- **Typical presentation**
  Affected children are frequently symptomatic during a growth spurt • Back and leg pain • Scoliosis • Progressive gait disturbance • Talipes equinus deformity • Loss of reflexes • Difficulties with bladder and bowel control.
- **Therapeutic options**
  Surgical mobilization of the filum terminale and resection of the lipoma.
- **Course and prognosis**
  This depends on the severity of the adhesion of the filum terminale and the associated anomalies.
- **Complications**
  Recurrent tethering • Surgical and postoperative complications.

Differential Diagnosis

Sacrococcygeal teratoma	– Tumor can contain hair, teeth, cartilage, and fat – Arises from the coccyx – Exhibits external growth more often than internal growth – Mixed signal intensity, chemical shift artefacts
Cauda equina regression syndrome	– Hypoplasia or absence of the distal lumbar spine and sacrum – Cauda equina is not tapered – Often associated with other anomalies – More common in children of diabetic mothers

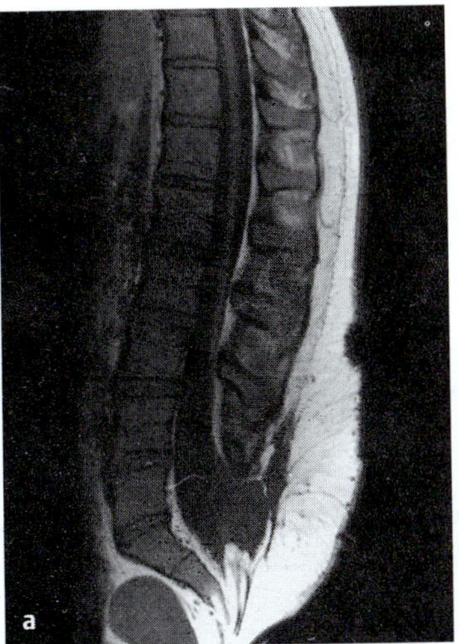
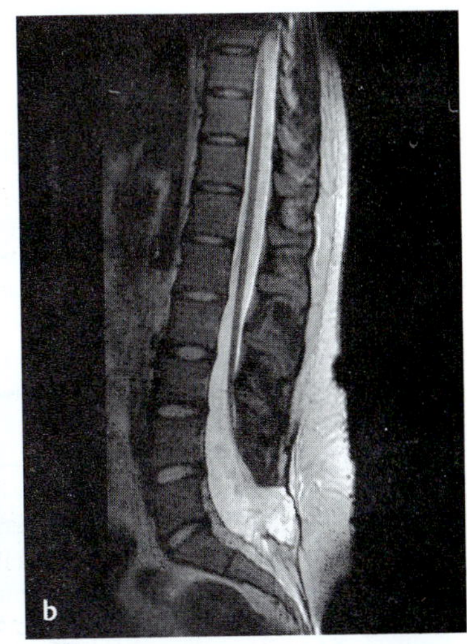

Fig. 7.20 a, b Meningomyelocele in a 15-year-old girl. MR images of the spinal canal. Sagittal T1-weighted SE image (**a**) and T2-weighted TSE image (**b**). Dural sac is expanded posterior to vertebrae L5, S1, and S2. The conus medullaris extends to the superior margin of vertebra L5, where it attaches posteriorly. The cauda equina can be traced all the way into the posteriorly expanded dural sac.

Tips and Pitfalls

Normal level of the conus medullaris does not exclude a tethered cord • Most intraspinal lipomas are incidental findings.

Selected References

DiPietro MA. The conus medullaris: normal US findings throughout childhood. Radiology 1993; 188: 149–153

Haro H et al. Long-term outcomes of surgical treatment for tethered cord syndrome. J Spinal Disord Tech 2004; 17: 16–20

Lam WW et al. Ultrasound measurement of lumbosacral spine in children. Pediatr Neurol 2004; 30: 115–121

Rinaldi F et al. Tethered cord syndrome. J Neurosurg Sci 2005; 49: 131–135

Xenos C et al. Spinal lipomas in children. Pediatr Neurosurg 2000; 32: 295–307

Yamada S et al. Pathophysiology of tethered cord syndrome and other complex factors. Neurol Res 2004; 26: 722–726

Definition

- **Epidemiology**

  Closed craniocerebral trauma is the most common type of trauma in children • Multiple trauma also involves craniocerebral trauma in up to 60% of cases • Epidural hematoma occurs in 1% of cases of craniocerebral trauma.

- **Etiology, pathophysiology, pathogenesis**

  Cause: Trauma to the vault of the cranium • Brain injuries are either open or closed • Craniocerebral trauma is classified according to the severity of neurologic findings as slight (Glasgow Coma Scale [GCS] > 12), moderate (GCS 9–12), or severe (GCS ≤ 8) • Components of craniocerebral trauma include skull fractures; epidural, subdural, and intracerebral hemorrhages; and diffuse brain damage.

  Extracranial hemorrhage: Cephalic hematoma and subgaleal hematoma • Blindness occurs in 2% of cases.

  Epidural hematoma: Associated with fractures that cross the cranial sutures • Almost always at the site of the incident force • Often in the temporoparietal region • Hemorrhage between the cranium and dura mater • In 80–90% of cases bleeding occurs from the middle meningeal artery, and in 10–20% from the sinus • Rare in child abuse.

  Subdural hematoma: Occurs as a result of direct trauma and indirect injury (from shear or rotation forces) • Bleeding between the dura mater and arachnoid • Due to traumatic tearing of the bridging veins, especially in the superior sagittal sinus • Classified as acute, subacute, or chronic • In child abuse, this often occurs bilaterally along the convexity of the brain, extends into the longitudinal fissure, and can also occur in the posterior cranial fossa.

  Subarachnoid hemorrhage: Tearing of fine leptomeningeal vessels or bridging veins • Adjacent to contusions or subdural hematomas • More often occurs in the sulci of the convexity than in the basal cisterns.

  Cerebral contusion: The injury occurs at the time of the trauma • Brain parenchyma is impacted against the cranium • Most common parenchymal lesion in craniocerebral trauma • Occurs in almost half of cases of moderate or severe craniocerebral trauma • Usually bilateral and multiple • Often associated with galeal or subgaleal hematoma, subarachnoid bleeding, subdural hematoma, or intraventricular bleeding • Often occurs in the anterior basal temporal and frontal lobes or in the cortex adjacent to the Sylvian fissure.

  Shear injuries (axonal injuries): Due to strong shear forces • Hemorrhagic or nonhemorrhagic • These may occur at the corticomedullary junction, close to the ventricles, in the corpus callosum, and in the brainstem.

Imaging Signs

- **Radiographic findings**

  Detection of fractures • Detection of simple linear skull fractures usually has no impact on treatment • CT is indicated in emergency situations or where neurologic symptoms are present • Findings in child abuse include multiple fractures, growing fractures, and impression fractures.

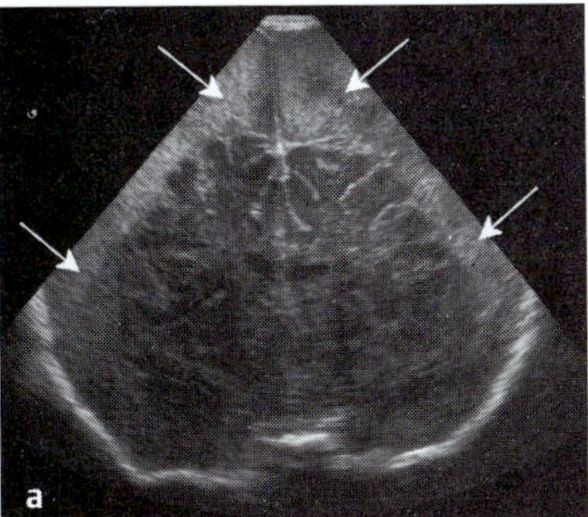

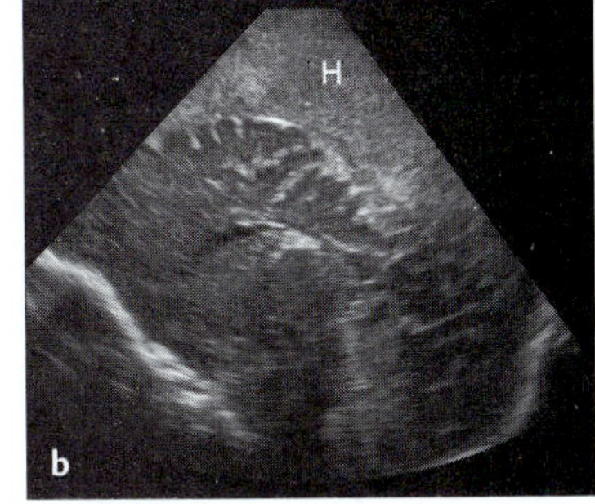

Fig. 7.21 a, b Subdural hematomas in an infant injured because of violent shaking. Ultrasound, paracoronal (**a**) and sagittal (**b**) imaging planes. Bilateral subdural hematomas (arrows).

- **Ultrasound**

  Epidural hematoma: Inhomogeneous hyperechoic mass between the hypoechoic brain and the hyperechoic cranium • Biconvex shape • Findings may include midline shift • The medial portions of the temporal lobe can herniate through the tentorial hiatus; herniation into the foramen magnum can also occur • Often associated with cerebral edema.

  Subdural hematoma: Crescentic hyperechoic accumulation of fluid with its concavity facing the surface of the brain • Injury from violent shaking (child abuse) often produces bilateral hemorrhages and hemorrhages of varying ages • Blood accumulates between the dura mater and arachnoid • Findings may include midline shift and ventricular compression.

  Subarachnoid hemorrhage: Ultrasound visualization is difficult at best and sometimes impossible • The Sylvian fissure is widened and may be irregularly demarcated • Gyri and sulci are hyperechoic • The affected hemisphere exhibits diffusely increased echogenicity.

- **CT findings**

  Cranial CT is indicated where skull base fracture, intracranial hemorrhage, or brain edema is suspected • A Glasgow Coma Scale score ≤ 8 is an absolute indication.

  Epidural hematoma: Biconvex extraaxial mass that appears hyperdense in two-thirds of cases, and mixed hypodense to hyperdense in one-third • Brain tissue beneath the lesion is displaced • A vortex within the hematoma is indicative of acute bleeding • Associated lesions such as contusion are present in up to 50% of cases.

  Subdural hematoma: Crescentic lesion, usually hyperdense, but appearing as mixed hypodense to hyperdense lesion in a third of cases • Concave toward the brain parenchyma • Lesion can cross suture lines but not dural attachments • Often spreads into the longitudinal fissure and along the tentorium • Often associated with other lesions such as subarachnoid hemorrhage.

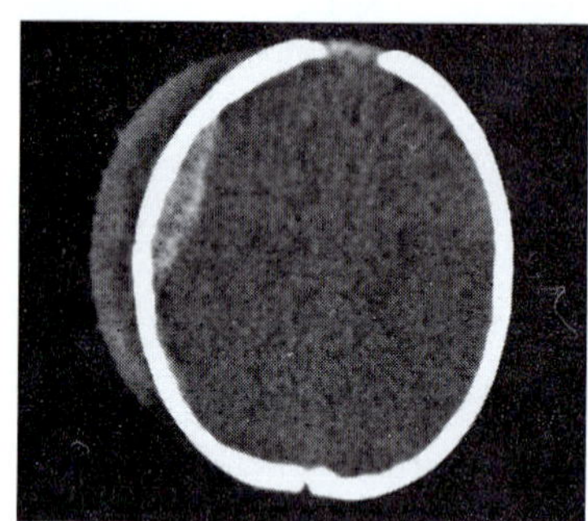

Fig. 7.22 Epidural hematoma in a 9-month-old girl. Cranial CT. Typical epidural hematoma in the right parietal region.

Subarachnoid hemorrhage: Hyperdense area in the subarachnoid space, occasionally limited to the interpeduncular cisterns • Hemorrhage in the ventricles usually subsequent to contusions and deep hematomas (indicated by blood and CSF levels).

Contusion: Initial CT findings may be normal • Hypodense cortex with focal hyperdense lesions • Contrast enhancement occurs in the subacute stage.

► **MRI findings**

Very sensitive in detecting parenchymal injuries and hemorrhages of varying ages • Demonstrates axonal injuries in the thalamus, hypothalamus, or corticomedullary junction in child abuse.

Epidural hematoma:

- T1-weighted images: Isointense in the acute stage • Hyperintense in the subacute stage • Linear signal void between the hematoma and brain (displaced dura mater).
- T2-weighted images: Findings in the acute stage are variable (hypointense to hyperintense) • Hyperintense in the subacute stage • Linear signal void between the hematoma and brain.
- Contrast-enhanced T1-weighted images: Bleeding from the sinus may be demonstrated • Sinus thrombosis.

Subdural hematoma: Signal intensity varies with the age of the hematoma.

- T1-weighted images: Hypointense to slightly hyperintense in the acute stage.
- T2-weighted images: Hypointense in the acute stage.

Subarachnoid hemorrhage: Isointense on T1-weighted and T2-weighted images • Hyperintense on FLAIR images • Focal bleeding in the choroid plexus • Blood and CSF levels in the ventricles.

Contusion: Multifocal lesions of mixed signal intensity • Acute hemorrhage is isointense on T1-weighted images and hyperintense on T2-weighted images • Cortical edema is hyperintense on T2-weighted images • Hemosiderin (residual blood product) is hypointense on T2*-weighted images.

Clinical Aspects

- **Typical presentation**

  Unconsciousness • Vomiting • Retrograde amnesia • Headache • Vertigo • Transitory cortical blindness may occur • Episodes of screaming • Hemorrhage may produce focal neurologic symptoms • Skull base fracture may lead to bleeding and/or CSF leakage from the nose and/or ears and to periorbital hematoma • Palpable fracture line • Palpably unstable skull in burst injuries.

  Epidural hematoma: Headache • Nausea • Vomiting • Seizures • Neurologic deficits.

  Subdural hematoma: Varies from asymptomatic to unconsciousness.

  Subarachnoid hemorrhage: Headache • Nausea • Vomiting • Decreased vigilance.

  Contusion: Occasional unconsciousness • Confusion • Focal neurologic deficits • Personality changes.

- **Therapeutic options**

  Slight and moderate craniocerebral trauma: Hospitalization and observation for 48 hours • Where vomiting occurs, gastric tube and fasting are indicated • Cardiovascular parameters, pupils, and vigilance (Glasgow Coma Scale) should be regularly monitored.

  Severe craniocerebral trauma: Cardiovascular stabilization • Early intubation and ventilation; this is absolutely indicated with a Glasgow Coma Scale score < 8 • Adequate blood volume management • Cranial impressions exceeding the thickness of the cranium should be decompressed • Epidural and subdural hematomas should be evacuated where mass effect and neurologic symptoms are present • Prophylaxis against and treatment of increased intracranial pressure are indicated.

- **Course and prognosis**

  Mild and moderate craniocerebral trauma usually have a very good prognosis • Severe craniocerebral trauma is often associated with residual neurologic deficits and is life-threatening in a third of patients • Primary areflexia and generalized brain edema are unfavorable prognostic signs.

  Epidural hematoma: Brief unconsciousness occurs initially • An asymptomatic interval may follow • Left untreated, this progresses to coma.

  Subdural hematoma: Half of cases exhibit an initial asymptomatic interval • Patient is initially conscious • This is followed by loss of consciousness hours after the trauma • Hemorrhage can gradually increase in size • Increasing displacement and compression of brain parenchyma.

  Subarachnoid hemorrhage: Prognosis is worse where associated contusions are present.

  Contusion: Initial contusions often increase in size.

- **Complications**

  Permanent paralysis or spasticity from focal brain damage • Permanent psychomotor dysfunction • Progressive increase in intracranial pressure that is refractory to treatment • This leads to reduced perfusion of the brain and impingement of the brainstem • Diffuse axonal damage with severe psychomotoric sequelae.

Differential Diagnosis

Empyema	– Biconvex extraaxial mass – Slightly hyperdense or isodense to CSF – Usually bilateral – Between cranium and dura mater – Pronounced marginal enhancement
Nontraumatic subarachnoid bleeding	– Due to rupture of an aneurysm or arteriovenous malformation – Usually no history of previous trauma
Meningitis	– Ultrasound shows widening of the sulci, increased echogenicity in the subarachnoid space, and thickened meninges – Usually no abnormal findings on CT – Meningeal exudate is isointense on T1-weighted images and hyperintense on T2-weighted and FLAIR images – Leptomeningeal enhancement
Meningioma	– No acute onset of symptoms – Sharply demarcated mass attached to the dura mater – Hyperdense in most cases – Cranial hyperostosis in the tumor region – Calcifications – Marked homogeneous enhancement

Tips and Pitfalls

High parietal hemorrhages can be missed on ultrasound. Therefore, CT is indicated wherever neurologic symptoms are present • Where bleeding is suspected and cranial ultrasound is feasible, examination through the temporal acoustic window is invariably indicated as well • Where subdural hematomas of varying ages are present, child abuse must be considered and examination of the ocular fundus is indicated to detect possible retinal bleeding • When reading CT images, reduce the size of the window to better detect small acute hemorrhages.

Selected References

Halley MK et al. Loss of consciousness: when to perform computed tomography? Pediatr Crit Care Med 2004; 5: 230–233

Holsti M et al. Pediatric closed head injuries treated in an observation unit. Pediatr Emerg Care 2005; 21: 639–644

Simon B et al. Pediatric minor head trauma: indications for computed tomographic scanning revisited. J Trauma 2001; 51: 231–237

Tung GA et al. Comparison of accidental and nonaccidental traumatic head injury in children on noncontrast computed tomography. Pediatrics 2006; 118: 626–633

A

abdomen, free fluid 165
abdominal trauma 162–165, *163, 164, 165*
abscess
Brodie 225, 227, *227*, 247
pericecal 135, *136*
pulmonary 21, 24, 27, 33
retropharyngeal 98–100, *99*
subperiosteal 319, *320*
accidental injuries 294
acetabular index 269
acoustic neurinomas (vestibular schwannomas) 322, 324, 325, 326
acute disseminated encephalomyelitis 336
acute lymphatic leukemia (ALL) 263–265, *264*, 294
adolescents
acute hematogenous osteomyelitis 225
transitional fractures 288–289, 290
adrenal hemorrhage 195–197, *196, 197*, 200
adrenal hyperplasia, congenital 196
air portogram 105, *106*, 107
Alagille syndrome 149
anal atresia 122–125, *123*
anal stenosis 129
Andre von Rosen line 269
aneurysmal bone cyst 233–236, *234, 235*, 256
anomalous pulmonary venous connection 76, 86–89, *88*
partial (PAPVC) 86, *87*, 89
total (TAPVC) 86, *87*
antrum 134
aorta
coarctation 62–65, *63*
pseudo-coarctation 65
aortic arch
discontinuous 65
double 57, 59–61, *60*, 68
right, with aberrant left subclavian artery 60, 68
aortopulmonary collateral arteries, major (MAPCAs) 71, 73
Apert syndrome 296
appendicitis 134, 135–137, *136*, 144
apple peel deformity 119
arachnoid cyst 307
arteria lusoria 57–58, *58*
arteriovenous malformation (AVM) 280–283
aspiration
foreign body 44–46, *45, 46*
pneumonia 118
recurrent 43
asthma 43, 45
astrocytoma *323*, 325
pilocytic *see* pilocytic astrocytoma
atrial septal defect (ASD) 80–82, *81*
differential diagnosis 70, 79, 84, 89
avascular necrosis of femoral head 273
axonal injuries, intracranial 340

B

basal ganglia, dysgenesis of 301
battered child syndrome *see* child abuse
Beckwith–Wiedeman syndrome 159, 190
bell clapper deformity 215
benign fibrous histiocytoma 232
biliary atresia 148–150, *149*, 159
biloma 154
birth trauma 90, 195, 294
bizarre parosteal osteochondromatous proliferation 243
bladder
masses 179
neurogenic 182
rhabdomyosarcoma 201, *202*, 203, 204
Blalock–Taussig shunts 71, 72, 76
Blount disease 220
Bochdalek hernia 28
bone abscess *see* Brodie abscess
bone cysts 261

Page numbers in *italics* refer to illustrations.

aneurysmal 233–236, *234*, *235*, 256
juvenile 235
bone metastases 228, 256
bone pseudotumor, hemophilia 236
Bourneville disease
see tuberous sclerosis
brachycephaly 296, *297*
brain injuries 340, 342
brainstem
encephalitis 336
gliomas 333, 334–336, *335*
brain tumors 329–336
Brodie abscess 225, 227, *227*, 247
bronchial atresia 17
bronchiectasis 21, 41, *42*
bronchiolitis
obliterans 45
respiratory syncytial virus (RSV) 31–32, *32*
bronchogenic cyst 25–27, *26*
cervical 93
differential diagnosis 21, 52
bronchopulmonary dysplasia (BPD) 11, 12–14, *13*
bronchopulmonary foregut malformation *see* pulmonary sequestration
bucket handle fractures 292
bull's eye sign
appendicitis 135, *136*
Crohn disease 138
intussusception 131, *132*, 134

C

Caffey disease 294
calcifications
brain tumors 330, 331, 332
hepatoblastoma 159, *160*
neuroblastoma 51, 53, 198, *199*
teratoma 47, *49*, 209
tuberous sclerosis 324
Wilms tumor 190
callosal agenesis 301–303, *302*, 304
with interhemispheric cyst 304
callosal hypoplasia 304
Capener triangle sign 271
carcinoid tumor 45
cardiac multivalvular defects 70
Caroli disease 151
cauda equina regression syndrome 338
CCAM *see* congenital cystic adenomatoid malformation
cecum, right upper abdomen 110
cerebellar hemangioblastoma 324, 325
cerebellar vermis
dysgenesis 301
hypoplasia 305
cerebral contusion 340, 342, 343
cervical cysts 92–94, 287
differential diagnosis 91, 100
lateral 92, *93*
median 92
cervical lymphadenitis 95–97, *96*
cervical meningocele 287
child abuse 292–295, *293*
craniocerebral trauma 340, 341, *341*, 344
differential diagnosis 291, 294
chimney figure *3*, *55*
Chlamydia trachomatis 213
chlamydial pneumonia 32, 33
cholecystolithiasis 156–158, *157*
choledochal cyst 149, 151–155, *152*, *153*
chondroma, juxtacortical periosteal 243
chondrosarcoma
adjacent to exostosis 243
differential diagnosis 256
secondary 238, 242, 244
chordoma 207
choroid plexus
grade I hemorrhage 310
papilloma 333
ciliary dyskinesia syndrome, primary 43
clear cell sarcoma, kidney 190, 193
cloverleaf skull 296
coarctation of aorta 62–65, *63*
Codman triangle 249, *250*
coffee bean sign 112
comb sign, Crohn disease 139, *141*
concentric ring sign *see* bull's eye sign

congenital adrenal hyperplasia 196
congenital cystic adenomatoid malformation (CCAM) 19–21, *20*
  differential diagnosis 11, 18, 27, 30
congenital diaphragmatic hernia
  see diaphragmatic hernia, congenital
congenital indifference to pain 294
congenital lobar emphysema 17–18, *18*, 21, 30
congenital megacolon
  see Hirschsprung disease
congenital mesoblastic nephroma 190, 194
congenital skeletal deformity 220
constipation, habitual 129
corkscrew sign 112
corner fractures 292
cor pulmonale 41
corpus callosum
  agenesis *see* callosal agenesis
  hypoplasia 304
cortical island 247
cor triatriatum 89
coxa magna 276
craniocerebral trauma 340–344, *341*, *342*
craniosynostosis 296–300, *297*, *298*, *299*
creeping fat 138, 139
Crohn disease 137, 138–142, *139*, *140*, *141*
Crouzon disease 296
cystic adenomatoid malformation, congenital *see* congenital cystic adenomatoid malformation
cystic fibrosis 41–43, *42*
cystic teratoma *see* dermoid cyst
cystitis, chronic 204
cytomegalovirus (CMV) 31

D

Dandy–Walker malformation 305–307, *306*
de Morsier disease 301
dermoid cyst (mature cystic teratoma)
  differential diagnosis 27, 93, 287
  ovary 209, *211*
desmoid, periosteal 232
developmental dysplasia of hip (DDH) 266–270, *268*
diaphragmatic hernia, congenital 18, 21, 28–30, *29*
diuresis ultrasound 170
dolichocephaly 296
double aortic arch 59–61, *60*, 68
double bubble sign 108
double gallbladder sign 151, *153*
double outlet right ventricle (DORV) 76
Down syndrome (trisomy 21) 57, 71, 101, 115, 128, 271
duodenal atresia 110, 121
duodenal duplication, cystic 154
duodenal ectasia, annular pancreas 154
duodenal stenosis 110, 126
duodenum, air filled 157
duplex kidney 177–180, *178*, *179*

E

Ebstein anomaly 69–70, *70*
Eisenmenger reaction
  atrial septal defect 80, 81
  ventricular septal defect 77, *78*, 79
emphysema
  congenital lobar 17–18, *18*, 21, 30
  pulmonary interstitial (PIE) 9–11, *10*
empyema
  intracranial 344
  thoracic 33
encephalitis, brainstem 336
encephalocele 287
encephalomalacia, multicystic 313
encephalomyelitis, acute disseminated 336
encephalotrigeminal angiomatosis
  see Sturge–Weber syndrome
enchondroma 235, 238
enchondromatosis 237–240, *238*, *239*
endobronchial tumor 45
enteric cyst 27

enteric duplication with ectopic
  gastric mucosa 144
eosinophilic granuloma
  251, 257, *258*, 265
ependymoma
  neurofibromatosis 2 325
  posterior cranial fossa 329, 331, 332–333
  spinal 208
epidermoid cyst 329, 331, 332, 333
epididymitis 213–214, *214*
epididymo-orchitis 213, 217
epidural hematoma 340, 341, 342, *342*, 343
epiglottitis 100
epiphyseal fractures/injuries
  288, 289, 292
Escherichia coli 184, 213, 225
esophageal atresia 115–118, *116*, *117*
Ewing sarcoma 249–252, *250*
  differential diagnosis
    228, 229, 256, 260, 265
exostosis
  chondrosarcoma adjacent to 243
  osteocartilagenous
    see osteochondroma
extracranial hemorrhage 340

F

Fanconi syndrome 220
femoral epiphysis, slipped capital
  see slipped capital femoral epiphysis
femoral focal deficiency,
  proximal 270
femoral head, avascular necrosis 273
fibroma, nonossifying 230–232, *231*
fibromatosis colli 90–91, *91*
fibrosarcoma 238
fibrous cortical defect 230–232, *231*
fibrous dysplasia 232, 236, 261
  polyostotic 240
fistulas
  anal atresia *123*, 124
  Crohn disease 140, *140*, *141*
  tracheoesophageal 115, *116*, 117, 118
foramen ovale, patent 80
foreign body aspiration 44–46, *45*, *46*
fractures 288–291, *289*, *290*
  child abuse 292, *293*
  impacted/buckle 288, 289, *289*
  incomplete 288
  pathologic 233, 234, 251, 263
  rickets 218, *219*
  see also specific types
fungal pulmonary infections 39
furosemide test 170

G

galactosemia 149
gallbladder
  "double" 151, *153*
  hydrops 154
  polyp 157
  porcelain 157
  sludge 157, *157*
gallstones 156–158, *157*
gastroenteritis 134
gastroesophageal reflux 110
Ghon focus 36
giant cell tumor of bone 235
gliomas
  atypical brainstem 334
  brainstem 333, 334–336, *335*
  midbrain 334, 335
  optic pathway 322, 324–325
  posterior exophytic cerebello-
    medullary 334, 335
  typical diffuse intrinsic pons
    334, 335, *335*
gliomatosis
  cerebri 328
  peritoneal 209, 211
glomerulonephritis 186
goiter
  diffuse nodular 101
  Hashimoto thyroiditis 101–102, *102*
  retrosternal 50
Graves disease 101
greenstick fractures *219*, 288, 289, *290*
Group B streptococcal pneumonia 8, 31

H

Haemophilus influenzae pneumonia 32, 33
hamartomas
  intracranial 336
  tuberous sclerosis 322, 326
Hand–Schüller–Christian disease 257
Hashimoto thyroiditis 101–102, *102*
head shape, abnormal 296–300, *297, 298, 299*
head trauma 340–344, *341, 342*
hemangioblastoma 333
  cerebellar 324, 325
hemangioendothelioma 161
hemangioma 207, 280–283, *281, 282*
hematoma
  craniocerebral 340
  intra-abdominal 154, 162
  scrotal 197, 214
hemihypertrophy 190, *191*
hemophilia, pseudotumor in 236
hepatic cyst 154
hepatitis, neonatal 149
hepatoblastoma 159–161, *160*
hepatocellular carcinoma, fibrolamellar 161
hernia, scrotal 214, 217
hilar lymph nodes, enlarged
  cystic fibrosis 41, *42*
  Hodgkin lymphoma 54, *55*
  tuberculosis 36, 38
Hilgenreiner line 269
hip
  developmental dysplasia (DDH) 266–270, *268*
  transient synovitis (irritable) 222–224, *223*, 274, 278
Hirschsprung disease 128–130, *129*
  complications 105, 129
  differential diagnosis 104, 114, 121, 125
histiocytoma, benign fibrous 232
histiocytosis
  Langerhans cell *see* Langerhans cell histiocytosis
  thymus 2
Hodgkin disease
  mediastinal 52
  thoracic 39, 54–56, *55*
holoprosencephaly 301, 303, 304
Hutch diverticulum 166, 179
hydrocele 147
hydrocephalus
  Dandy–Walker malformation 305, 306
  posthemorrhagic 308, *309*
  tumor-associated 329, 330, *331*, 333
  in vacuo 315, *316, 317*
hypertrophic pyloric stenosis (HPS) 126–127, *127*
hypoplastic left heart syndrome 8
hypoxic-ischemic brain damage 315–318, *316, 317*

I

ileal atresia 104, 114
infants
  acute hematogenous osteomyelitis 225
  neuroblastoma 198
  RSV bronchiolitis 32
  see also neonates
inflammatory pseudotumor 204
inguinal hernia 145–147, *146*
intestinal nonrotation/malrotation 108–111, *109, 110*, 119
  differential diagnosis 114, 121
intraventricular hemorrhage 308–310, *309*
intussusception 131–134, *132*, 137
invertography/Wangensteen view 122–124, *123*, 125

J

Joubert anomaly 307
juvenile bone cyst 235
juvenile osteonecrosis 278
juxtacortical periosteal chondroma 243

K

Kartagener syndrome 43
Kasabach–Merritt syndrome 283
kidneys
  clear cell sarcoma 190, 193
  compensatory hypertrophy 186
  duplex 177–180, *178*, *179*
  medullary sponge 175
  microabscesses 184
  multicystic dysplastic 173, 174–176, *175*, *176*
  parenchymal bridge 179
  rhabdoid tumor 190, 193
  traumatic injury 162, *165*
  tumors 179
Kleeblattschädel syndrome 296
Klein tangent 271
Klinefelter syndrome 47

L

Ladd peritoneal bands 108, 109
Landouzy septicemia 36
Langerhans cell histiocytosis 228, 257–262, *258*
large bowel volvulus 112–114
Larrey hernia 28
laryngocele 93
Legg–Calvé–Perthes disease 222, 275–279, *276*, *277*
  differential diagnosis 224, 274
Letterer–Siwe disease 257
leukemia, acute lymphatic (ALL) 263–265, *264*, 294
leukemic bands 263
lipomyelocele *338*
liver trauma 162, *163*
lung disease, idiopathic fibrosing 261
Lutembacher syndrome 80
lymphangioma 284–287, *285*, *286*
  neck 93, 100
  sacrococcygeal region 207
lymphatic malformation 283
lymphoma
  differential diagnosis 91, 97, 228, 261, 265
  gastrointestinal 137, 142
  mediastinal 39–40, 50, 52, 54–56, *55*
  thymus 2, 56

M

Maffucci syndrome 238
MAG3 nuclear medicine imaging 167, 170, *172*, 178, 181
major aortopulmonary collateral arteries (MAPCAs) 71, 73
McCune–Albright syndrome 240
Meckel diverticulum 137, 143–144, *144*
meconium aspiration syndrome 15–16, *16*
meconium ileus 103, 107, 114, 121, 125
meconium peritonitis 120
meconium plug syndrome 103–104, *104*, 121, 125, 129
mediastinal lymph nodes, enlarged
  Hodgkin lymphoma 54, *55*
  tuberculosis 36, 38, 39
mediastinum
  lymphoma 39–40, 50, 52, 54–56, *55*
  teratoma 47–50, *48–49*, 56
  tumors 60, 68
medullary sponge kidney 175
medulloblastoma 329, 330, *330*, 331, 332, 333
megacalicosis 175
mega-cisterna magna 307
megacolon, congenital *see* Hirschsprung disease
megaureter, primary 168, 182
meningioma 324, 325, 344
meningitis 344
meningocele, cervical 287
meningomyelocele 207, 337, *339*
mesenchymal hamartoma 161
mesenteric cyst 144, 154, 287
mesenteric duplication 287
mesenteric lymphadenitis 137
metabolic disorders 294
metaphyseal dysplasia 240
metaphyseal injuries, *293* 292
metaphyseal radiolucent bands 263, 265

Meyer dysplasia 278
Meyer–Weigert rule 177
MIBG (metaiodobenzylguanidine) imaging 51
microcolon 129
midbrain gliomas 334, 335
midgut volvulus 112
midline anomalies 301–304, *302*
mitochondrial encephalopathy 318
Moraxella catarrhalis 33
Morgagni hernia 28
multicystic dysplastic kidneys 173, 174–176, *175*, *176*
multilocular cystic nephroma 190, 194
mycobacterial disease, atypical 97
Mycobacterium tuberculosis 36
Mycoplasma pneumoniae infection 32, 33
myelinolysis, osmotic 336
myositis 321
myositis ossificans 256

N

necrotizing enterocolitis (NEC) 105–107, *106*
neonates
  adrenal hemorrhage 195
  congenital cystic adenomatoid malformation 19
  congenital diaphragmatic hernia 28, 29
  esophageal atresia 115–118, *116*, *117*
  fibromatosis colli 90–91, *91*
  hepatitis 149
  hypoxic-ischemic brain damage 315–318, *316*
  meconium aspiration syndrome 15–16, *16*
  pneumonia 16
  respiratory syncytial virus (RSV) bronchiolitis 31
  sacrococcygeal teratoma 205–208, *206*
  testicular torsion 215
  transient tachypnoea 8, 16
  see also premature infants
nephroblastoma *see* Wilms tumor
nephroblastomatosis *193*, 194
nephrocalcinosis 188–189, *189*
nephroma
  congenital mesoblastic 190, 194
  multilocular cystic 190, 194
neuroblastoma 198–200, *199*
  differential diagnosis 91, 193, 196
  metastases 161, 251, 265
  pelvic 204
  thoracic 51–53, *52*, *53*
neurocutaneous syndromes 322–328
neuroenteric cyst 27
neurofibromas, plexiform 322, 325
neurofibromatosis type 1 322, 326, 327
  differential diagnosis 220, 328, 336
  imaging signs *323*, 324–325
neurofibromatosis type 2 322, 324, 325, 326, 327
neuromuscular disorders 270
neuronal hypoplasia 107
newborn infants *see* neonates
nidus 245, *246*, *247*, 248
non-Hodgkin lymphoma 40, 56
nonossifying fibroma 230–232, *231*
Noonan syndrome 71, 284

O

Ollier disease 237
orbital cellulitis 319–321, *320*
orbital pseudotumor 321
orchitis 213
osmotic myelinolysis 336
ossifications, subperiosteal 292
osteoblastoma 236, 247
osteochondroma 240, 241–244, *243*
  multiple 241, 242, *242*
  solitary 241, 242
osteochondromatous proliferation, bizarre parosteal 243
osteoclastoma 235
osteogenesis imperfecta 220, 291, 294
osteoid osteoma 245–248, *246*, *247*, *248*
osteoma 247
osteomalacia 218
osteomyelitis 225–229, *226*, *227*

acute hematogenous 225
chronic 225, 227, 228, 256
chronic recurrent multifocal (CRMO) 225
differential diagnosis 251, 252, 260, 265, 294
plasma cell 225
sclerosing, nonsuppurative Garré 225, 227
osteonecrosis, juvenile 278
osteosarcoma (osteogenic sarcoma) 253–256
differential diagnosis 228, 229, 251, 261
enchondromatosis-associated 238
parosteal 243, 253, *255*
periosteal 253
telangiectatic 235, 253, *254*
ovarian cyst 212
torsion 137
ovarian cystadenoma 212
ovarian hernia 145, *146*
ovarian teratoma 209–212, *210*, *211*
ovarian torsion 212
ovarian tumors 204
oxycephaly 296

P

pain, congenital indifference to 294
pancreas
annular 110, 154
pseudocyst 154
trauma 162, *163*
parapneumonic effusion 33
parathyroid cyst 93
partial anomalous pulmonary venous connection (PAPVC) 86, *87*, 89
patent ductus arteriosus (PDA) 83–85, *84*, *85*
differential diagnosis 79, 82
patent foramen ovale 80
pentalogy of Fallot 71
perianal fistulas 140, *141*
pericardial effusion 70
pericecal abscess 135, *136*
periosteal chondroma, juxtacortical 243
periosteal desmoid 232
periosteal reaction 249, 253, 294
periostitis, long bones 263
peritoneal gliomatosis 209, 211
periventricular hemorrhagic infarction 310, 318
periventricular leukomalacia (PVL) 310, 311–314, *312*, *313*
Perkins–Ombrédanne line 269
phakomatoses 322–328
pharynx, perforation 118
pilocytic astrocytoma 329, 332, 333
differential diagnosis 328, 333
imaging signs 330, 331, *331*
plagiocephaly 296, *297*
plasmacytoma 261
pleural effusion, complicated 33
pneumatocele 18, 21, 107
pneumatosis intestinalis 105, *106*, 107
pneumonia
with abscess formation 24
aspiration 118
atypical 261
cavitary necrosis complicating 21, 27, 33
chronic recurrent 24
differential diagnosis 31–32, 39, 52
Group B streptococcal 8
lobar and segmental 33–35, *34*
neonatal 16
peripheral 33
round 27
viral 39
polycystic kidney disease, autosomal recessive 175, 189
polymyelitis 270
pons gliomas 334, 335, *335*
porencephalic cysts 310, *316*
portogram, air 105, *106*, 107
posterior cranial fossa tumors 329–333, *330*, *331*
postpericardiotomy syndrome 79
post-splenectomy infection syndrome 164
premature infants
bronchopulmonary dysplasia 12
hypoxic-ischemic brain damage 315, 316

inguinal hernia 145
intraventricular hemorrhage 308–310, *309*
necrotizing enterocolitis 105–107, *106*
periventricular leukomalacia 311–314, *312*, *313*
pulmonary interstitial emphysema 9
respiratory distress syndrome 6–8, *7*
see also neonates
primitive neuroectodermal tumors (PNET) 329
processus vaginalis, patent 145
prostate, rhabdomyosarcoma 201, *202*
pseudo-coarctation 65
pseudokidney sign 131
pseudomembranous colitis 142
pulmonary abscess 21, 24, 27, 33
pulmonary arteriovenous fistula 24
pulmonary artery
aberrant origin of left 60
stenosis of left 71
pulmonary artery sling 66–68, *67*
pulmonary atresia 73, 76
pulmonary contusion 24
pulmonary cysts 17, 21
pulmonary hemorrhage, bilateral 8
pulmonary hypertension
atrial septal defect 80, 81
ventricular septal defect 77, *78*, 79
pulmonary hypoplasia 20, 28, 29, *29*
pulmonary interstitial emphysema (PIE) 9–11, *10*
pulmonary sequestration 21, 22–24, *23*, 52
pulmonary tumors, primary 27
pulmonary valve, bicuspid 71
pulmonary venous connection, anomalous *see* anomalous pulmonary venous connection
pulmonary venous obstruction 88
pyelonephritis
acute 184–187, *185*, *186*
xanthogranulomatous 193, 194
pyloric stenosis, hypertrophic (HPS) 126–127, *127*
pylorospasm 127

R

rachitic rosary 218, *219*
radiation therapy 141
Ranke's complex 36
rectum, cystic duplication anomaly 207
renal infarction 186
renal osteopathy 218
renal tubular acidosis 220
renal tumors 179, 190, 193–194
respiratory distress syndrome (RDS) 6–8, *7*
congenital diaphragmatic hernia and 29
patent ductus arteriosus and 83, 84
respiratory syncytial virus (RSV) bronchiolitis 31–32, *32*
retroperitoneal teratoma 200
retropharyngeal abscess 98–100, *99*
retropharyngeal inflammation, diffuse 100
rhabdoid tumor
intracranial 333
kidney 190, 193
rhabdomyosarcoma
cervical 91
embryonal, infiltrating bone 251
pelvic 201–204, *202*, 208, 212
rheumatoid arthritis, juvenile 224, 279
rib notching 62, *63*
rickets 218–221, *219*, 291
Rokitansky protuberance 209
Roviralta syndrome 126

S

sacrococcygeal teratoma 204, 205–208, *206*, 338
sail sign *3*
salmonellosis 141
Salter–Harris fractures 288, 289, 291
SAPHO syndrome 225

sarcoidosis 40, 261
scaphocephaly 296, *297*
schizencephaly 304
schwannomas
  multiple, without
    neurofibromatosis 2 328
  neurofibromatosis 2 322, 325, 326
scimitar syndrome 89
scrotal hematoma 197, 214
septic arthritis 225–229, *226, 227*
  differential diagnosis
    224, 270, 279
septo-optic dysplasia
  301, *302,* 303, 304
septum pellucidum, agenesis of 301
sexual abuse 295
shear injuries, cerebral 340
Shenton's line 269
Shone complex 62
shoulder sign 126, *127*
skeletal deformity, congenital 220
skin appendage, simple 208
skull deformation 296–300
  postural 299
  secondary causes 299
skull fractures 340
slipped capital femoral epiphysis
  271–274, *272*
  differential diagnosis 224, 279
  traumatic 274
small bowel atresia 119–121, *120*
small bowel volvulus
  112–114, *113, 114,* 121
snowman figure 86
soft tissue sarcoma 283, 287
spinal cord, tethered
  337–339, *338, 339*
spinnaker sign *3*
spleen, traumatic injury 162, *164*
spondylodiskitis, thoracic 52
Staphylococcus aureus 31, 33, 225
status marmoratus 315
sternomastoid tumor of infancy
  90–91, *91*
Streptococcus pneumoniae 33
stress fractures 247
Sturge–Weber syndrome
  322, 324, 325, 326, 327
subarachnoid hemorrhage
  nontraumatic 344
  traumatic 340, 341, 342, 343
subclavian artery
  aberrant left 57, 60, 68
  aberrant right 57–58, *58*
subdural hematoma 340, 341, *341,*
  342, 343, 344
subependymal heterotopia,
  X-linked 328
subgaleal hematoma 340
subperiosteal abscess 319, *320*
subperiosteal ossifications 292
subpulmonary stenosis 74, 76
suppurative arthritis *see* septic arthritis
supracondylar fractures 288
supracondylar process 243
Swyer-James syndrome 45

T

Takayasu arteritis 65
Tamm-Horsfall protein 189
T-cell leukemia, thymus 56
tea test 126
telangiectatic osteosarcoma 235
teratoid tumors
  atypical intracranial 333
  mediastinal 2
teratoma
  benign 205
  immature 209, *210*
  malignant 205, 207, 211
  mature cystic *see* dermoid cyst
  mediastinal 47–50, *48–49,* 56
  monodermal 209
  ovarian 209–212, *210, 211*
  retroperitoneal 200
  sacrococcygeal 204, 205–208,
    206, 338
testicular appendages, torsion of 217
testicular torsion 213, 215–217, *216*
testicular trauma 217
testicular tumors 217
testis
  hydrocele of 147
  inguinal undescended 147
tethered cord 337–339, *338, 339*

tetralogy of Fallot 71–73, *72*, 76
thymoma 1, 50, 56
thymus 1–5, *2*, *3*, *4–5*, 50
  cysts 2, 27, 93, 287
  histiocytosis 2
  hyperplasia 1
  lymphoma 2, 56
thyroiditis
  acute 101
  Hashimoto 101–102, *102*
thyroid tissue, cyst arising in ectopic 27
toddler fractures 288, 289–290
tonsillitis, complicated 98, *99*
total anomalous pulmonary venous connection (TAPVC) 86, *87*
tracheobronchial compression, extrinsic 45
tracheoesophageal fistula 115, *116*, 117, 118
transient synovitis of hip 222–224, *223*, 274, 278
transient tachypnoea of newborn 8, 16
transitional fractures of late adolescence 288–289, 290
transposition of great arteries (TGA) 74–76, *75*
trauma
  abdominal 162–165, *163*, *164*, *165*
  adrenal hemorrhage 195
  birth 90, 195, 294
  craniocerebral 340–344, *341*, *342*
  slipped capital femoral epiphysis 274
  testicular 217
triangular cord sign 148
tricuspid atresia 73
tricuspid insufficiency 70
trigonocephaly 296, *297*
triple bubble sign 119
triple sign, coarctation of aorta 62
trisomy 21 *see* Down syndrome
tuberculosis 36–40, *37*, *38*
  differential diagnosis 97
  gastrointestinal tract 141
  miliary 36, *38*, 39
  organ stage 38
  postprimary 36, 38, 39
  primary 36, *37*, 38, 39
tuberous sclerosis 322, *323*, 324, 325, 326, 327
Turner syndrome 62, 101, 284
turricephaly 296, *298*

U

ulcerative colitis 141
urachal cyst 144
ureterocele 177, *178*, 179, 180
  prolapsed 182
ureteropelvic junction obstruction 170–173, *171*, *172*
  differential diagnosis 182
  multicystic dysplastic kidneys with 175, *176*
ureters
  bifid 177
  double 177, *179*
  isolated stenosis 173
urethral valves 181–183, *182*
urinoma 162

V

VACTERL association 115, 122
varicocele 147
vascular malformation 287
vasculitis, cerebral 313
venous malformation 283
ventricular septal defect (VSD) 77 79, *78*
  differential diagnosis 73, 82
  transposition of great arteries 74
vesicoureteral reflux 166–169, *167*, *168*, *169*, 174
vestibular schwannomas 322, 324, 325, 326
voiding cystourethrography (VCUG)
  bladder fistulas *123*, 124
  urethral valves 181, *182*, 183
  vesicoureteral reflux 167, 169, *169*
volvulus 107, 112–114, *113*, *114*
Von Hippel–Lindau disease 322, 324, 325, 326, 327
Von Recklinghausen disease *see* neurofibromatosis type 1

W

Walker–Warburg syndrome 307
Wangensteen view/invertography 122–124, *123*, 125
Waterhouse–Friderichsen syndrome 195
wave sign *3*
wet lung disease 8
whirlpool sign 112, *113*, *114*
Wilms tumor (nephroblastoma) 190–194, *191*, *192*
  differential diagnosis 159, 186, 200
  multicystic 196
Wolman disease 196
Wyburn–Mason syndrome 328

X

xanthogranulomatous pyelonephritis 193, 194

Y

yersiniosis 141
Y line 269